PRACTICAL ETHICS IN CLINICAL NEUROLOGY

A Case-Based Learning Approach

EDITOR

Michael A. Williams, MD, FAAN

Medical Director, The Sandra and Malcolm Berman Brain & Spine Institute
Director, Adult Hydrocephalus Center
Co-Director, Center for Gait and Mobility
Sinai Hospital of Baltimore
Baltimore, Maryland

CO-EDITORS

Dawn McGuire, MDiv, MD, FAAN

Adjunct Professor of Neurology
Morehouse School of Medicine, Neuroscience Institute
Atlanta, Georgia
Physician Specialist, Department of Medicine
Laguna Honda Hospital
San Francisco, California

Matthew Rizzo, MD, FAAN

Professor of Neurology, Mechanical and Industrial Engineering and
Public Policy
Founding Director, University of Iowa Aging Mind and Brain Initiative
Vice Chair, Translational and Clinical Research
Director, Division of Neuroergonomics
University of Iowa Hospitals and Clinics
Iowa City, Iowa

Wolters Kluwer | Lippincott Williams & Wilkins
Health

Philadelphia · Baltimore · New York · London
Buenos Aires · Hong Kong · Sydney · Tokyo

Acquisitions Editor: Julie Goolsby
Product Manager: Tom Gibbons
Vendor Manager: Alicia Jackson
Senior Manufacturing Manager: Benjamin Rivera
Marketing Manager: Alexander Burns
Design Coordinator: Steven Druding
Production Service: Integra Software Services Pvt. Ltd.

LIPPINCOTT WILLIAMS & WILKINS, a WOLTERS KLUWER business
Two Commerce Square
2001 Market Street
Philadelphia, PA 19103 USA
LWW.com

Printed in China

Library of Congress Cataloging-in-Publication Data

Practical ethics in clinical neurology : a case-based learning approach / editor, Michael A. Williams; coeditors, Dawn McGuire, Matthew Rizzo.
     p. ; cm.
  Includes bibliographical references and index.
  ISBN 978-1-4511-1405-8 (alk. paper)—ISBN 1-4511-1405-2 (alk. paper)
  I. Williams, Michael A. (Michael Allan), 1959- II. McGuire, Dawn, 1954- III. Rizzo, Matthew.
  [DNLM: 1. Neurology—ethics. 2. Ethics, Clinical. WL 21]

  174.2'968—dc23

                                                                        2012031791

Care has been taken to confirm the accuracy of the information presented and to describe generally accepted practices. However, the authors, editors, and publisher are not responsible for errors or omissions or for any consequences from application of the information in this book and make no warranty, expressed or implied, with respect to the currency, completeness, or accuracy of the contents of the publication. Application of the information in a particular situation remains the professional responsibility of the practitioner.

The authors, editors, and publisher have exerted every effort to ensure that drug selection and dosage set forth in this text are in accordance with current recommendations and practice at the time of publication. However, in view of ongoing research, changes in government regulations, and the constant flow of information relating to drug therapy and drug reactions, the reader is urged to check the package insert for each drug for any change in indications and dosage and for added warnings and precautions. This is particularly important when the recommended agent is a new or infrequently employed drug.

Some drugs and medical devices presented in the publication have Food and Drug Administration (FDA) clearance for limited use in restricted research settings. It is the responsibility of the health care provider to ascertain the FDA status of each drug or device planned for use in their clinical practice.

To purchase additional copies of this book, call our customer service department at (800) 638-3030 or fax orders to (301) 223-2320. International customers should call (301) 223-2300.

Visit Lippincott Williams & Wilkins on the Internet: at LWW.com. Lippincott Williams & Wilkins customer service representatives are available from 8:30 am to 6 pm, EST.

10 9 8 7 6 5 4 3 2 1

RRS1209

DATE DUE

roach

CONTRIBUTORS

Jennifer L. Berkeley, MD, PhD
Neurointensivist
The Sandra and Malcolm Berman
Brain & Spine Institute
Department of Neurology
Sinai Hospital of Baltimore
Baltimore, Maryland

William Brannon Jr., MD, FAAN, FACP
Distinguished Professor Emeritus
of Neurology
University of South Carolina School
of Medicine
Consultant in Neurology
WJB Dorn Veterans Administration
Hospital
Columbia, South Carolina

William P. Cheshire, Jr., MD, MA, FAAN
Professor of Neurology
Mayo Clinic
Jacksonville, Florida

Thomas I. Cochrane, MD, MBA
Assistant Professor of Neurology
Harvard Medical School
Associate Neurologist
Brigham and Women's Hospital
Boston, Massachusetts

Jill Conway, MD, MA
Neurology Clerkship Director
University of North Carolina School of
Medicine-Charlotte Campus
Director, Multiple Sclerosis Center
Carolinas HealthCare System
Charlotte, North Carolina

Patricia A. Evans, MD, FAAN, FAAP
Associate Professor of Neurology and
Pediatrics
University of Texas Southwestern
School of Medicine
Director, Neurodevelopmental
Disabilities Residency Program
Children's Medical Center of Dallas
Dallas, Texas

Jacqueline J. Glover, PhD
Professor of Pediatrics
Center for Bioethics and Humanities
University of Colorado Anschutz
Medical Campus
Aurora, Colorado

Amalia M. Issa, PhD, MPH
Professor and Chair of Health Policy
and Public Health
Director, Program in Personalized
Medicine and Targeted Therapeutics
University of the Sciences in Philadelphia
Philadelphia, Pennsylvania

Peter Lars Jacobson, MD, FAAN
Professor of Neurology
Director, UNC Neurology Palliative Care
Program
University of North Carolina School of
Medicine
Chapel Hill, North Carolina

Don W. King, MD, JD, FAAN
Professor Emeritus of Neurology
Medical College of Georgia
Augusta, Georgia

Eran P. Klein, MD, PhD
Assistant Professor of Neurology
Oregon Health and Sciences University
Staff Physician, Neurology Service
Portland VA Medical Center
Portland, Oregon

Jerome E. Kurent, MD, MPH, FAAN
Professor of Medicine and Neurosciences
Medical University of South Carolina
Attending Neurologist
Ralph H. Johnson Veterans Affairs
Medical Center
Charleston, South Carolina

Dan Larriviere, MD, JD, FAAN
Acting Chair of Neurology
Residency Program Director
Ochsner Medical Center
New Orleans, Louisiana

Dawn McGuire, MDiv, MD, FAAN
Adjunct Professer of Neurology
Morehouse School of Medicine,
Neuroscience Institute
Atlanta, Georgia
Physician Specialist, Department
of Medicine
Laguna Honda Hospital
San Francisco, California

Michael P. McQuillen, MD, MA, FAAN
Ethics, Law and Humanities Committee,
American Academy of Neurology
Member, 1994–2005
ELHC Neurology Resident Elective
Clinical Ethics Subcommittee
Chair, 1999–2005
Palo Alto, California

Ann E. Mills, Msc(Econ), MBA
Assistant Professor and Co-director
Program in Ethics and Policy in
Healthcare Systems
Center for Biomedical Ethics and
Humanities
University of Virginia
Charlottesville, Virginia

**Lois Margaret Nora, MD, JD,
MBA, FAAN**
Professor of Internal Medicine (Neurology)
President and Dean Emerita
Northeastern Ohio Medical University
Rootstown, Ohio

Thomas R. Pellegrino, MD, FACP
Associate Dean for Medical Education
Professor of Neurology
Eastern Virginia Medical School
Norfolk, Virginia

Tyler Reimschisel, MD
Assistant Professor of Pediatrics and
Neurology
Vanderbilt University School of Medicine
Nashville, Tennessee

Steven P. Ringel, MD, FAAN
Professsor and Vice Chair of Neurology
University of Colorado Anschutz
Medical Campus
Vice President, Clinical Effectiveness
and Patient Safety
University of Colorado Hospital
Aurora, Colorado

Matthew Rizzo, MD, FAAN
Professor of Neurology, Mechanical and
Industrial Engineering and Public Policy
Founding Director, University of Iowa
Aging Mind and Brain Initiative
Vice Chair, Translational and Clinical
Research
Director, Division of Neuroergonomics
University of Iowa Hospitals and Clinics
Iowa City, Iowa

Katherine G. Shearer, MD
Resident Physician in Pediatrics
University of Iowa Hospitals and Clinics
Iowa City, Iowa

**Michael Shevell, MDCM, FRCPC,
FANA, FAAN**
Chair of Pediatrics
McGill University
Pediatrician-in-Chief
Montreal Children's Hospital
Montreal, Quebec, Canada

Russell D. Snyder, MD, FAAN
Professor of Neurology and Pediatrics
University of New Mexico School of
Medicine
Albuquerque, New Mexico

Robert M. Taylor, MD, FAAN
Associate Professor of Neurology and
Internal Medicine
The Ohio State University College
of Medicine
Director, Division of Palliative Medicine
Wexner Medical Center at The Ohio
State University
Columbus, Ohio

Patricia H. Werhane, PhD
Wicklander Professor of Business Ethics
DePaul University
Chicago, Illinois

Michael A. Williams, MD, FAAN
Medical Director
The Sandra and Malcolm Berman
Brain & Spine Institute
Director, Adult Hydrocephalus Center
Co-Director, Center for Gait and Mobility
Sinai Hospital of Baltimore
Baltimore, Maryland

Allison W. Willis, MD
Assistant Professor of Neurology
Movement Disorders Division
Washington University School of Medicine
St. Louis, Missouri

Mark Yarborough, PhD
Dean's Professor of Bioethics
Bioethics Program
University of California Davis Health
System
Sacramento, California

PREFACE

Almost no one reads an ethics textbook from cover to cover, or a whole ethics chapter from beginning to end. Yet, almost every neurologist encounters ethical issues every day.

The content of our medical school ethics lectures long forgotten, we tend to learn ethics when we have to—when we encounter difficult cases—but our learning is informal and piecemeal, without the guidance or framework to learn *how* to resolve not only today's challenging case, but future cases as well.

Most practitioners want an ethics textbook to tell them how to resolve today's difficult case. *Practical Ethics in Clinical Neurology* (*PECN*) was created to meet that need for learners, for teachers, and for practicing neurologists. *PECN* meets the needs of students, residents, fellows, and practicing neurologists who want an accessible case-based text for learning, and it meets the needs of directors of medical student clerkships and residency programs in neurology who want an accessible case-based text for teaching.

I understand these needs. My background is like that of most neurologists— I have extensive formal training in neurology but have no formal training in ethics. I wish a book like this had been available when I was in residency and fellowship, *and* I wish it had been available when I started teaching ethics.

I went into the field of neurology because I fell in love with it in medical school in the early 1980s at Indiana University. The patients were (and are) fascinating to me. The way that neurologists think about patients was intuitive to me—take a history by listening carefully and asking the right questions, examine patients to "localize the lesion," synthesize the imaging and laboratory information to reach a working diagnosis, and explain the diagnosis and prognosis to patients and their families in words that they can understand so that patient care can be a collaborative venture. I went into the field of neurology because it felt right and because I could not imagine myself being happier in any other specialty.

By contrast, I first learned ethics out of necessity. After a neurology residency at Indiana University, I trained as a neuroICU fellow at Johns Hopkins Hospital, and to care for patients in the neuroICU, I had to learn ethics. With no formal training program available, I learned as the need arose with challenging cases, discussing them with my mentors and learning how to identify the ethical issues and negotiate them with patients themselves (if they were conscious) and families (if they were not). By the end of my fellowship, I felt comfortable with most of the "routine" ethical issues that we encountered, *but I never intended a career in ethics.*

AN ACCIDENTAL ETHICIST

My career in ethics is accidental. One year after I joined the neurology faculty at Johns Hopkins, the hospital's ethics committee had an opening for a representative from our department. Our department chair, Richard T. Johnson, said, "Mike, we need someone from neurology on the ethics committee. You're it." At the time, neither he nor I knew what he had just set in motion.

Just as with neurology, I fell in love with ethics and, for that, I am indebted to the incredible expertise and wisdom of my friends and mentors on the ethics committee who taught me how to think systematically and creatively like an ethicist. Our role as a committee was to provide ethics case consultation. As a result, we saw the mundane and the challenging. In the process, I learned the principles of ethics and how to analyze and apply them, and I learned how to elicit and appreciate the views and values of everyone involved in an ethics consultation. I also learned how to access and read the ethics literature for self-directed learning.

From these experiences stems my belief that the purpose of teaching ethics is not to tell learners *what* to think or to do but, rather, to show them *how* to think so that they can reach the most ethically permissible choices and courses of action.

I brought my emerging and expanding knowledge of ethics to the neuroICU, teaching on rounds with the intent of helping residents, students, and fellows learn how to think about ethical issues for their patients and incorporate this habit into daily practice. It worked. I am proud that many of them, especially the neuroICU fellows, developed independent skills in ethical analysis and problem solving. I sought to develop novel ways, in addition to bedside teaching, to teach ethics, including the use of simulations with standardized patients. As a teacher, I learned from my students that, by using case-based learning, ethics can be taught and learned by everyone and that ethics need not be the purview of a few experts.

In 1996, I joined the Berman Institute of Bioethics at Johns Hopkins University, and in 1999, I began serving as Co-Chair of the Ethics Committee at Johns Hopkins with my close friend and mentor Cynda Rushton, a pediatric nurse ethicist and internationally recognized expert in pediatric palliative care. Expanding the role of the committee beyond ethics case consultation to include organizational ethics, we took on the task of identifying institution-wide ethics issues to the hospital administration and advocating for better policies and practices that would support ethical problem solving at the bedside.

My career took another turn when, in 2003, then incoming AAN President Sandra Olson appointed me Chair of the AAN Ethics, Law and Humanities Committee (ELHC). Once again, I found myself surrounded by colleagues with incredible expertise and wisdom in ethics, and together over the next 6 years, we expanded the scope and availability of ethics within the AAN, creating the AAN Ethics Section, establishing ethics as a topic of abstracts for the AAN annual meeting, increasing the number of ethics education courses offered at the annual meeting, and working with Aaron Miller, the editor of *Continuum*, to include case-based learning in the Ethical Perspectives section of each issue of *Continuum* since 2006.

THE ORIGINS OF THIS BOOK

PECN is the brainchild of the ELHC, as it is the successor to *Ethical Dimensions of Neurologic Practice: A Case-Based Curriculum for Neurology Residents,*[1] an ELHC pilot project that was created in 2000 and distributed to all residency program directors, but it was never formally published. With the emerging need for more formal ethics training in neurology residency programs, as recommended by the ACGME[2] and the American Board of Psychiatry and Neurology,[3] the ELHC agreed that we should update the curriculum, design it to be a companion to James Bernat's book, *Ethical Issues in Neurology, 3rd ed.,*[4] and publish it as an AAN-branded product.

ASSUMPTIONS

In designing the book, we made several assumptions based on the results of a needs assessment completed by directors of neurology residency programs regarding the uses and users of the book:

a. The book will be used either for self-directed learning or for group learning by case review and discussion taught by a group leader, such as a neurology attending or ethicist.
b. Most learners are novices in ethics and have limited experience in the analysis and direct application of ethical theory in clinical situations.
c. Most learners have had an introductory exposure to ethics and ethical theory in lectures or self-directed learning in medical school or residency.
d. Case-based or problem-based learning (casuistry) is an effective and accessible teaching and learning method for learners with limited experience, especially if the teaching cases are similar to cases commonly encountered in clinical practice.[5]
e. Gaining experience and comfort in the analysis of ethical theory and applying it to individual cases is assisted by the consistent use of a single framework (Clinical Pragmatism Model) for all cases in the book, just as clinical diagnosis in neurology is assisted by learning and applying a consistent framework for the neurologic history and examination.
f. Learners have access to James Bernat's book, *Ethical Issues in Neurology, 3rd ed.,*[4] for which *PECN* is a companion text, and to internet-based resources such as www.PubMed.gov and the website of the American Academy of Neurology (www.aan.com/).

THE CLINICAL PRAGMATISM MODEL

In nearly all chapters in *PECN,* the study questions are based on John Fletcher's Clinical Pragmatism Case Method of Moral Problem-Solving (see the easily accessible grey-edged pages at the end of chapter 1 of this text).[6]

The purpose of consistently applying the Clinical Pragmatism Model is to aid in learning a practical and systematic approach to ethical problems. Additionally, learners will be able to see how different authors apply the same framework to different types of cases. However, the use of only Fletcher's Clinical Pragmatism Model has its limitations, as no single method is ideal for all cases. We recognize that many other frameworks for ethical analysis exist, and our hope is that as learners become comfortable and accomplished with the framework of the Clinical Pragmatism Model, they will investigate and learn to apply other frameworks.

LEARNING OBJECTIVES FOR *PRACTICAL ETHICS IN CLINICAL NEUROLOGY*

Upon reading, discussing, and synthesizing the content of this book, learners will be able to meet these primary learning objectives:

■ Use the clinical-pragmatism framework to analyze the ethical issues in a clinical situation.
■ Provide an opinion informed by ethical and legal principles regarding ethically permissible actions in a given clinical case.
■ Negotiate and implement an action plan with patients, families, or other healthcare professionals based on the analysis.

CHAPTER TOPICS AND CASE CONTENT

The topics and content of the 69 cases in 29 chapters in *PECN* individually and collectively reflect commonly encountered issues in neurology, and we have included separate chapters for pediatric and adult neurology where significant distinctions are present. The chapters are written as stand-alone learning modules that are intended for novices in the field of ethics. Thus, learners can read a chapter from beginning to end for a complete and coherent discussion of the chapter topic. Readers will note some recurring points of discussion among chapters, which reflects the fact that common ethical principles must be considered in a variety of cases. Associated with *PECN* is an extensive online appendix that contains ethics guidance publications from the AAN that are useful in consideration of the cases.

CHAPTER FORMAT

All chapters in *PECN* are similarly formatted to include:

■ Learning Objectives
■ Learning Resources
  • Key chapters in Bernat's 3rd edition of *Ethical Issues in Neurology*
  • Key AAN documents relevant to the chapter topic
■ One or more clinical vignettes
■ Questions to guide self-study or group discussions

- Commentary related to the discussion questions, with reference to specific applicable sections of Bernat's *Ethical Issues in Neurology*.
  - Pages and chapter numbers for the Bernat references are highlighted in the margin callouts.
- Key Points
- Key Words
- References
- Suggestions for Further Reading (optional)

A WORD ABOUT THE LEARNING RESOURCES

The Learning Resources box at the beginning of each chapter lists the key relevant chapters in the third edition of Bernat's *Ethical Issues in Neurology.* As noted above, specific references in *PECN* to content in the Bernat book will be highlighted by callouts in the margins in addition to being listed among the references at the end of each chapter.

PECN makes use of a web-based appendix to give readers ready access to key AAN documents. For ease of identification, each document has been assigned a letter (A–S). The Learning Resources box for each chapter lists, by letter, the key AAN documents relevant to the chapter topic. These documents are available in the Appendix Folder at the password-protected website for *PECN* that is provided by Lippincott Williams & Wilkins and is accessible with the purchase of the text. The documents are also available via open access at the AAN website, and the website url (www.aan.com/view/PECN) is provided in each Learning Resources box. Because it is cited in nearly every chapter, the AAN Code of Professional Conduct (*PECN* document A) is reprinted in the appendix of this text. Lastly, the Learning Resources box contains QR codes for the individual documents, providing readers who have smartphones direct access to these resources.

PHRONESIS

My nearly 25-year sojourn has taught me that ethics is about pragmatism—using principles for problem solving and doing what is right—also known as *phronesis,* Greek for "practical wisdom or prudence, the application of good judgment to human conduct . . ."[7] In fact, once I learned the principles and a basic framework for application early in my career, I realized that *thinking like an ethicist was just like thinking like a neurologist*—take a history by listening carefully and asking the right questions of the patients, families, and healthcare professionals involved; elicit their values and goals; identify conflicts; examine the context and principles to define and analyze the moral problem; explain it to patients, families, and healthcare professionals in words that they can understand; and help them to work collaboratively to find an ethically permissible resolution to their situation. As with neurology, some cases are straightforward, and others are exceptionally complex and require much thought and consultation with colleagues.

*Even the most rational approach to ethics is defenseless
if there isn't the will to do what is right.*

—ALEXANDER SOLZHENITSYN

The goal of *PECN* is to prepare its readers to do what is right by providing them with the knowledge, skills, and confidence to recognize, evaluate, and take action to resolve ethical problems in daily practice. In presenting this text, it is our hope that we have achieved our goal.

REFERENCES

1. American Academy of Neurology. Ethics, Law and Humanities Committee. Ethical Dimensions of Neurologic Practice: A Case-based Curriculum for Neurology Residents. March 2000. Available at www.aan.com/globals/axon/assets/2711.pdf. Accessed April 17, 2012.
2. Accreditation Council for Graduate Medical Education. Program Requirements for Graduate Medical Education in Neurology. Effective July 1, 2010. Available at www.acgme.org/acWebsite/downloads/RRC_progReq/180_neurology_07012010.pdf. Accessed April 17, 2012.
3. Scheiber SC, Kramer TAM, Adamowski SE, American Board of Psychiatry and Neurology. *Core Competencies for Neurologists. What Clinicians Need to Know.* Waltham, MA: Butterworth-Heinemann, 2003.
4. Bernat JL. *Ethical Issues in Neurology, 3rd ed.* Philadelphia: Lippincott Williams & Wilkins, 2008.
5. Barrows HS. Authentic problem-based learning. In: Distlehorst LH, Dunnington GL, Folse JR, eds. *Teaching and Learning in Medical and Surgical Education.* Mahwah, NJ: Lawrence Erlbaum Associates, Inc., 2000, Ch. 23.
6. Fletcher JC, Spencer EM, Lombard PA (eds). *Fletcher's Introduction to Clinical Ethics, 3rd ed.* Hagerstown, MD: University Publishing Group, 2005.
7. Laboratorio di Epistemologia Informatica. Università degli Studi di Bari. A Dictionary of Philosophical Terms and Names. Definition of the word *phronesis*. Available at www.swif.uniba.it/lei/foldop/foldoc.cgi?phronesis. Accessed April 18, 2012.

ACKNOWLEDGMENTS

Of the making of books there is no end.
—ECCLESIASTES 12:12

At times, the creation of this book seemed as if it had no end. It progressed in fits and starts and was a much harder undertaking than we imagined. Working initially with Tyler Reimschisel in 2006, we conducted a needs assessment and created the framework for the book, including the chapter topics. We recruited multiple authors who agreed to the chapter framework and began to submit chapters to us in 2007. Between 2007 and 2008, both Tyler and I experienced career moves to new institutions that placed us in positions of more responsibility, and our work on the text fell dormant. In 2010, after discussion with the members of the ELHC, we resurrected the book, and with the agreement of everyone involved, brought in two new co-editors, Dawn McGuire and Matt Rizzo, and resumed our efforts to complete the text. The editing process was complex for the authors, as the editors aimed not to have redundant cases and thus had to ask some of the authors to omit or change cases. I am grateful to all of the authors for their patience with me in bringing the book slowly to completion, and wish to acknowledge their substantial contributions. I also wish to thank Dawn McGuire and Matt Rizzo for their significant effort in reviewing and revising many chapters and for their patience with the completion of the book.

AAN policy does not allow AAN committee members to earn royalties on AAN products. Thus, because *Practical Ethics in Clinical Neurology* is an AAN-branded text, the work of Tyler, Dawn, Matt, and myself (all members of the ELHC during the creation of the text) is completely unremunerated. Our completion of this project is a sign of our commitment to ethics education. All royalties from the book will go to the AAN, and it is our hope that the AAN will use the royalties to support education and policy development in ethics and the law that will benefit AAN members.

I could not have finished this book without the help of Tzipora Sofare, MA, an extraordinary medical editor and a friend. Her love of both the precision and nuance of language and her attention to detail, structure, grammar, content, and book design is the reason you find such a polished book in your hands.

Many friends and mentors have inspired and guided my career and played a direct or indirect role in the creation of this book, including Cynda Rushton, James Bernat, Murray Sagsveen, Dan Larriviere, James Russell, John Shatzer, Dan Hanley, Cecil Borel, and many others on the Johns Hopkins Hospital Ethics Committee, the Johns Hopkins Berman Institute of Bioethics, and the AAN Ethics, Law and Humanities Committee.

I am the product of my upbringing and want to thank my mother, Mary N. Williams, and my late father, Robert M. Williams, DPM, for instilling in me a love of learning, the ability to communicate clearly, the patience to listen, a knowledge of right and wrong, the belief that just because someone says, "you're not capable of it," doesn't make it so, and the inspiration and freedom to follow my interests and my talents where they lead me.

Lastly, I want to express my love and gratitude to my life partner of 28 years, Clifton G. Scott, whose support through my career has been unwavering and unconditional.

Michael A. Williams, MD, FAAN
Medical Director
The Sandra and Malcolm Berman Brain & Spine Institute
Department of Neurology
Sinai Hospital of Baltimore
September 2012

CONTENTS WITH CASE SYNOPSES

5. Responding to Medical Errors   57

Michael A. Williams, MD, FAAN

- CASE 1

A patient with epilepsy is mistakenly given 10 times the dose of IV lorazepam than she should have received. The neurologist does not want to disclose the error to the patient and her husband.

- CASE 2

A neurologist has a near-miss medical error upon learning from a patient referred for a lumbar puncture that she had a baclofen pump in place that was not disclosed in the records received from the referring physician.

- CASE 3

A patient's neurologic condition significantly worsens after a third-year neurosurgery resident allows a first-year neurology resident, while they are on call and unsupervised, to insert an intraventricular catheter in the ICU. Because they had looked at the wrong CT scan, the IVC was inserted on the wrong side. The neurosurgeon wants to hide the error, and the neurologist wants to disclose it to the ICU attending physician.

6. Gifts from Industry   72

Jacqueline J. Glover, PhD • Steven P. Ringel, MD, FAAN • Mark Yarborough, PhD

- CASE 1

The manufacturer's sales representative for a new antiepileptic medication (a) provides lunch at a weekly epilepsy conference, (b) invites the neurologist to speak at an all-expense-paid, industry-sponsored meeting, and (c) later asks the medical director of the EMU why the medication is not on the hospital formulary and why the neurologist's partners are not prescribing the medication.

- CASE 2

A neurologist has both a business relationship and a social relationship with the sales representative for a manufacturer of epilepsy-monitoring equipment. During a business meeting to discuss the purchase of equipment, the sales representative offers to take the neurologist to the NCAA Final Four.

7. Gifts from Patients   85

Tyler Reimschisel, MD

- CASE 1

A 6-year-old gives his neurologist a hand-drawn picture.

- CASE 2

The mother of the child in Case 1, who is a prominent local artist, gives the neurologist a large painting that she created.

- CASE 3

An elderly patient gives her epileptologist homemade cookies and then explains that she is planning to add the physician as a beneficiary in her will.

- CASE 4

A patient who often gives his neurologist bottles of wine to show his appreciation also frequently reschedules visits and becomes more demanding.

8. Termination of the Physician–Patient Relationship   96

Jill Conway, MD, MA

- CASE 1

A patient repeatedly fails to appear for scheduled appointments.

- CASE 2

A practice decides to no longer see patients who have public health insurance and gives patients 3 months' warning to that effect. One of the patients says she cannot find another physician.

- CASE 3

A divorced 60-year-old man appears to be scheduling frequent appointments more for social contact than for medical need and has been asking personal questions of the neurologist and staff.

- CASE 4

A 40-year-old patient who is consistently angry, rude, and belligerent with physician and staff is escorted from the office by a security guard.

SECTION IV   COGNITIVE IMPAIRMENT

SECTION V   ISSUES IN DEATH AND DYING

SECTION VI   OTHER TOPICS

APPROACHES TO ETHICAL PROBLEM SOLVING

Tyler Reimschisel, MD • Michael A. Williams, MD, FAAN

On a daily basis, neurologists encounter a variety of ethical questions at the bedside, in their research, and in the classroom. *Medical ethics* is the discipline that systematically studies the rationale and justification for appropriate professional behavior in these situations. The purpose of this chapter is to provide a practical introduction to the field of ethics for neurologists, and it will address the components of most ethical problems, decisions, or conflicts. Particular attention will be given to the factors that influence patients and healthcare professionals when they are making ethical decisions, the impact that external forces (e.g., hospital administration, the law, health insurance companies, and other health-related entities) have on the decision-making process, and the philosophical foundations for ethical problem solving in medicine.

SKEPTICAL RESPONSES TO THE DISCIPLINE OF CLINICAL ETHICS

Although clinicians encounter ethical questions frequently, many view the study of ethics as irrelevant to their practice or think that the ethics that is taught in medical school has no connection to the "real life" application of ethics in clinical practice. They might maintain that ethical decision making is rarely required; yet, many are unable to recognize important ethical aspects of patient care. Some neurologists believe that ethical decisions are no more than complicated medical or legal decisions and contend that adequate medical information will result in a resolution of all ethical problems. Some believe that mastery of the medical and scientific aspects of neurology guarantees competency in the field of ethics.

To the contrary, ethical problem solving requires competency in a unique set of skills and knowledge that is distinct from competency within neurology or any other field of medicine. Some neurologists acknowledge that ethics requires additional expertise but prefer to defer all ethical questions to ethicists—a wholly unrealistic solution, as nearly every aspect of clinical practice requires consideration of ethical issues. Therefore, neurologists must be equipped to independently recognize and resolve a variety of ethical questions and conflicts. Consultations with an ethicist or ethics consultation service can then be reserved for the more difficult cases.

1

THE NATURE AND RANGE OF MORAL DISAGREEMENTS

Neurologists frequently make ethical decisions during their clinical practice, and some of those decisions can be made without significant contemplation. However, when a difficult ethical decision arises, the neurologist becomes acutely aware of the challenges involved in bringing the question or conflict to a satisfactory resolution. Ethical decisions are especially difficult when stakeholders disagree about what is morally appropriate in a particular situation. Moral disagreements between conscientious physicians, other healthcare professionals, patients, and patients' families occur for a variety of reasons, including attempting to make decisions based on different understandings or interpretations of the medical facts, having different goals of care, determining the ethically permissible uses and limitations of novel medical technologies, placing varying amounts of importance on competing ethical principles, and using different moral frameworks and approaches to address medical situations. Further, in many circumstances, multiple decisions are ethically permissible, which means that the goal is not to find "the single right choice"; rather, it is to guide patients and other participants through the process so that the patients arrive at the decision that best fits their personal values and goals.

The complexity of the practice of modern medicine presents a myriad of ethical decisions for practicing neurologists. These decisions can be placed on a continuum that is based on the degree to which there is consensus regarding acceptable options within the medical community. Fortunately, a great deal of consensus exists regarding a large number of ethical issues, such as maintaining patient confidentiality, the requirement for informed consent for nonemergent medical treatment, and the need for physicians to be honest, trustworthy, and competent professionals. Other medical situations, e.g., end-of-life care and some forms of assisted reproductive technology, are more controversial and are often the subject of institutional and societal debate before consensus is achieved. Indeed, for some medical issues, such as physician-assisted suicide or elective termination of a pregnancy, no consensus exists within the healthcare community or society at large.

One category of issues, called "ethical dilemmas," is unique. An ethical dilemma is a problem in which fundamental ethical principles or values are in tension or conflict, and no decision can be made without violating one of them. Although by their very nature, true ethical dilemmas are emotionally charged, they also are rare and are the type of ethical problem for which ethics consultation can be most helpful. This is not to suggest, however, that difficult ethical problems or situations are rare for practicing physicians. In fact, for neurologists, they can be quite common. Therefore, having a practical framework with which to analyze these situations can be extremely helpful.

THE CONTEXT OF THE PHYSICIAN-PATIENT RELATIONSHIP

Most clinical ethics problems are identified and addressed within the context of the physician–patient relationship, which provides a basis for discussing, deliberating, and resolving ethical decisions. As described in the Hippocratic Oath and reiterated in many codes of ethics,[1,2] physicians have profound fiduciary duties and obligations to patients and patient interests that emanate from the physician–patient relationship, including holding the patients' interests paramount, effacing physician self-interest in favor of patients' interests, maintaining confidences and privacy, telling the truth, and not abandoning patients, to name but a few.

In most cases, though, the physician is but one member of a team of healthcare professionals with obligations to the patient and to each other, including consulting physicians, nurses, nurse practitioners, physician assistants, social workers, physicians in training, medical students, and others. All of these team members can and should play an active role in the identification and resolution of ethical problems. Indeed, one of the most common indications for an ethics consultation is to resolve conflicting viewpoints among members of the healthcare team.

Physicians must appreciate the factors that influence the view of a patient who is confronted with an ethical question or problem. To begin, physicians must ensure that patients have an accurate understanding of their medical condition and treatment options; i.e., they must do their best to ensure that patients' decisions are informed. Patients expect their physicians to be competent to provide their medical care — or, if they are not, to refer them to another physician with appropriate expertise. Physicians must also identify and address patients' emotional and psychological needs. When faced with an ethical question or problem, patients will be influenced by their personal interests, values, goals, and life experiences; by their family and friends; and by various religious, cultural, and ethnic factors. Physicians who seek to understand the influence of these factors on their patients are better equipped to help their patients make difficult decisions.

Physicians should also appreciate the factors that influence their own perceptions and thinking in the ethical problem-solving process. They should understand that their professional obligations may supersede their personal interests, particularly placing the patients' interests above their own. As long as they do not let their beliefs unduly influence their patients' decisions, they need not violate their own belief systems to provide medical care. Nonetheless, physicians' personal values, principles, culture, and religion will influence their practice, and they must be aware of their biases (defined as a *mental tendency* or *inclination*).

COMMUNICATION IN THE PROCESS OF ETHICAL PROBLEM SOLVING

Effective communication between physicians, patients, patients' families, and other healthcare professionals is invaluable to the problem-solving process; thus, it is regrettable that ineffective communication between any of these stakeholders is a common cause for an ethics consultation. In fact, most ethics cases do not involve a true ethical question or problem,[3] and conflicts caused by ineffective communication are preventable. The ethics consultation provides a forum for conflict resolution through mediation and facilitates effective communication among the concerned parties.[3-5] Effective communication includes explaining the medical situation in language that the patient and family can understand, ascertaining their understanding, listening carefully to appreciate their values and goals, taking time to answer their questions, and discussing the medical plan with all involved healthcare professionals.[4]

Bernat, 119–24, Ch. 5

THE SHARED DECISION MAKING MODEL

Physicians should use the Shared Decision Making model to approach ethical questions or problems with their patients and their patients' families. In this model, the physician provides the medical information necessary for an informed decision and then elicits the patient's values and goals to help guide the patient or patient's family to a decision that is most consistent with the goals. The physician may recommend a resolution for the ethical question and problem, provided that the recommendation reflects both the physician's understanding of the medical issues *and* the patient's values and frame of reference. This approach is preferable to *nondirective counseling* in which the physician merely provides medical information without making a recommendation, leaving the patient or family to decide independently. Because patients and families rarely have the same depth and breadth of understanding of the medical and scientific issues that physicians have, the nondirective counseling approach may lead them to base decisions on incomplete information, which is antithetical to the tenets of informed consent. Further, the nondirective approach can leave patients and families feeling overwhelmed, alone, or even abandoned.

EXTERNAL FORCES ON THE PROCESS OF ETHICAL PROBLEM SOLVING

The impact of the law on the practice of medicine should be secondary in most circumstances. Although the law certainly influences the physician–patient relationship, it primarily dictates the minimally acceptable conduct for a physician and does not define the behavior of an exemplary physician. As Bernat points out, "…the law says what a physician *must* do, whereas medical ethics says what the physician *should* do."[6] Occasionally, the law

Bernat, 81, Ch. 4

clearly prohibits specific conduct; for example, physician-assisted suicide is prohibited in most states. One limitation of the law is that frequently no case law or statutes are relevant for a given ethical question.

Other external factors that contribute to ethical problems include hospital administration decisions and policies, health insurance and other third-party payers, pharmaceutical and medical device industries, political entities, special-interest groups, and the media. Depending on the ethical situation, these external forces may be absent or could dramatically affect the process. For example, a hospital or practice policy to refuse outpatient care to individuals with out-of-state Medicaid, or an insurance company's denial of coverage for the cost of diagnostic testing, may constrain whether physicians may treat certain patients or how physicians may diagnose and treat patients (assuming that patients cannot afford to pay the costs out of pocket).

PHILOSOPHICAL APPROACHES TO THE PROCESS OF ETHICAL PROBLEM SOLVING

Of the many robust philosophical approaches to the ethical dimensions of the practice of medicine, 3 are worth highlighting: *virtue ethics*, the *principles of biomedical ethics*, and the *ethics of care*. Though the tenets of these approaches overlap considerably, each has its own emphasis, such as the personal ethics of *physicians* (virtue ethics), the values and principles of the *profession of medicine* (principles of biomedical ethics), and the needs of the *patient within the physician–patient relationship* (ethics of care).

Virtue Ethics and Professionalism

Virtue ethics is a philosophical perspective that emphasizes the importance of the virtues of individual physicians. This philosophical approach contends that the physician–patient relationship is unique, creating special ethical obligations for physicians. Virtue ethicists reject the notion that patients are merely "clients" who "make a contract" with their doctors to obtain medical goods and services, much the way that services are obtained from an auto mechanic. Virtue ethics maintains that rather than being *contractual*, the relationship is *covenantal,* obligating physicians to a higher standard of conduct and commitment to their patients.[7,8] The personal character of each physician is fundamental to the ethical practice of medicine. The virtuous physician is altruistic, trustworthy, compassionate, reliable, humble, objective, and courageous.[9] Many aspects of professionalism underscore the importance of a physician's personal moral character, including respect, compassion, integrity, responsiveness to the needs of patients and society that supersedes personal interest, and sensitivity to patients' culture, age, gender, and disabilities.[10]

The Principles of Biomedical Ethics

Virtue ethics lacks a mechanism for resolving conflicts when conscientious, virtuous physicians have honest disagreements regarding ethical questions or problems. In these situations, the values and principles of the profession take on increased importance. Beauchamp and Childress developed a set of 4 principles that characterize the fundamental features of bioethics and the practice of medicine: beneficence, nonmaleficence, respect for autonomy, and justice.[11] These principles, also known as *principalism,* have become the most popular guidelines for bioethical discourse and problem solving in the United States.

Beneficence is the active pursuit of the good of the patient. *Nonmaleficence* is the avoidance or minimization of harm to the patient. A practical application of these 2 principles is the analysis of the benefits and burdens of undertaking a medical intervention in comparison to the benefits and burdens of other interventions or of "doing nothing." For example, in treating a patient with epilepsy, the benefits (seizure control) and risks (side effects) of a medication or medications should be compared to the benefits (avoidance of side effects) and risks (recurrent seizures, loss of driving privileges) of not starting medication.

Respect for autonomy is also known as "self-determination."[12] Patients with decision-making capacity have the right to make their own medical decisions without coercion. Adults may consent to or refuse any medical care, including life-saving treatment. The informed-consent process is the practical application of the principle of respect for autonomy. For example, once the rationale for starting an anti-epileptic medication has been explained, the patient can make an informed decision to accept or refuse the physician's recommendation. As a demonstration of respect for patient autonomy, the physician should respect the patient's right to decide, even if the physician disagrees with the patient's informed choice.

Bernat, 13–14, Ch. 1

Justice addresses the fair distribution of healthcare resources among patients or within society[13] and encompasses the concepts of *distributive justice* (allocation of scarce resources, access to healthcare) and *justness,* or just treatment (fairness in individualized treatment and establishment of just and fair protocols, guidelines, and policies such that 2 patients whose clinical circumstances are similar should be treated similarly).

Bernat, 9–11, Ch. 1

The principles of nonmaleficence, beneficence, and respect for autonomy are applicable to ethical analysis and the process of ethical problem solving for individual patients, whereas the principle of justice primarily informs ethical analysis and problem solving for healthcare entities that provide care to populations of patients, including hospitals, medical centers, and governments. Ultimately, *respect for persons* is the fundamental basis for all of these principles. We respect patients solely because they are human beings, not contingent on any quality or merit that they may individually possess. Respect for persons means treating all persons as unique individuals of worth; respecting their dignity, feelings, thoughts, and experiences; and treating them with consideration, courtesy, and civility. The concept of respect for persons as the cornerstone for medical ethics is contained in The Belmont Report.[14]

The Ethics of Care

The *ethics of care* is a philosophical perspective that focuses on the unique ethical dimensions of close relationships, such as the professional relationship between patient and physician or between patient and nurse. This philosophy is based largely on the work of feminist philosopher Carol Gilligan[15] and is more commonly cited in the nursing literature than in the medical literature. Unlike principalism, the ethics of care emphasizes relationships over rules and principles. According to this philosophy, the physician–patient relationship creates in the physician a sense of partiality and attachment to the patient, which is the basis for compassion and empathy for patients and their families. These feelings—not absolute truths or principles—create the ethical basis for the obligation of physicians and other healthcare professionals to meet the needs of their patients.

THE CLINICAL PRAGMATISM MODEL

As illustrated above, various philosophical models can be used for ethical analysis. Each has utility because each provides an important lens for viewing and evaluating ethics cases. How can learners make the leap from philosophical models to the application of ethics in patient care? John Fletcher developed the Clinical Pragmatism Model with inspiration from John Dewey's philosophy of pragmatism.[16] Called "clinical pragmatism" because it provides a useful tool to guide the process of problem solving in clinical practice, it incorporates the Shared Decision Making model discussed above. Although a basic understanding of ethics is required to use this model, it does not require extensive knowledge of ethical theory or philosophy.

Fletcher's Clinical Pragmatism Model is used for nearly every case in this book. Briefly, the model includes 4 main sequential steps that are akin to the approach used to solve clinical problems:

1. Assessment of the case (analogous to the history, physical examination, and laboratory evaluation)
2. Moral diagnosis (analogous to the differential diagnosis)
3. Goal setting, decision making, and implementation (analogous to the therapeutic trial)
4. Evaluation of results (analogous to clinical follow-up)[17]

The *assessment* of the case (the first step) includes a robust analysis of several aspects of the clinical circumstances of the case and the persons involved:

- Understanding the patient's medical condition
- Determining the relevant contextual features for the case (demographics, family, culture, religion, socioeconomic factors)
- Assessing the patient's decision-making capacity
- Determining the patient's preferences (from the patient or the patient's surrogate decision maker)

- Assessing the needs of the patient as a person (interpersonal dynamics, resources)
- Identifying competing interests (family interests, competing needs for scarce resources, integrity of the physician and healthcare organization)
- Identifying issues of power or conflict (between patient and family members, between patient/family members and members of the healthcare team, or among members of the healthcare team)
- Allowing all parties to be heard
- Determining institutional factors (cost constraints, fear of medical malpractice, involvement of legal affairs) that may contribute to the moral complexity of the case

The next step (*moral diagnosis*) is to examine the moral problems in the case. For each ethical problem, one can (a) consider how each participant in the case perceives the problem or frames the issue; (b) identify institutional policies, guidelines, or standards that may address the problem; and (c) determine a range of ethically permissible options for resolving the problem.

In the third step (*goal setting, decision making, and implementation*), goals of care for the patient are established, various interventions are considered in light of the goals of care, and the merits of each option for resolving the ethical problems are determined. If goals cannot be established or a plan of treatment cannot be negotiated, then an ethics consultation should be considered. Finally a plan of action should be implemented.

Evaluation of the plan of action and the ethical problem-solving process is the final step. In this step, efficacy of the plan of action is determined. In addition, if the clinical situation has changed, the plan may need to be reconsidered. When appropriate, the process itself should be evaluated, including understanding the factors that led to the ethical problem, determining if opportunities for resolving the conflict were missed, and deciding if institutional policies should be modified or educational interventions should be implemented.

SUMMARY

Because ethical issues are embedded in nearly all clinical situations encountered by neurologists in their practices, research, and administrative activities, neurologists should have a working knowledge of philosophical approaches to ethics and of methods for systematically assessing and resolving ethical concerns. The Clinical Pragmatism Model provides a useful framework for many cases, and in most, neurologists can work with patients and their families to resolve ethical problems without difficulty. If assistance in fully understanding the ethical problem or the process of ethical decision making is needed, then an ethics consultation should be considered.

KEY POINTS

- Ethical problem solving requires competency in a unique set of skills and knowledge that is distinct from competency within neurology or any other field of medicine.
- Ethical decisions are particularly difficult when stakeholders disagree about what is morally appropriate.
- In many circumstances, more than one decision is ethically permissible.
- An ethical dilemma is a problem in which fundamental ethical principles or values are in conflict and no decision can be made without violating one of them.
- Virtue ethics emphasizes the importance of the virtues of individual physicians and contends that the physician–patient relationship is unique, creating special ethical obligations for physicians.
- The ethics of care focuses on the unique ethical dimensions of close relationships, such as the professional relationship between patient and physician.

KEY WORDS

Beneficence—the active pursuit of the good of the patient.

Nonmaleficence—the avoidance or minimization of harm to the patient.

Respect for autonomy—respecting the right of persons to make informed, uncoerced healthcare decisions, or to have another person (surrogate) make those decisions on their behalf.

Justice—addresses the fair distribution of healthcare resources among patients or within society.

Respect for persons—treating all persons as unique individuals of worth; respecting their dignity, feelings, thoughts, and experiences; and treating them with consideration, courtesy, and civility.

NOTE

This chapter is adapted from the syllabus *The Landscape of Ethics* presented by Tyler Reimschisel, MD, as part of the course "Identification and Management of Ethical Issues in Neurological Practice" at the annual meeting of the American Academy of Neurology in Boston in 2007. Adapted with permission.

REFERENCES

1. American Academy of Neurology. Code of Professional Conduct. December 2009. Available at www.aan.com/globals/axon/assets/7708.pdf. Accessed April 25, 2012. [*PECN* appendix document A and available at www.aan.com/view/PECN].
2. American Medical Association. Code of Medical Ethics. Available at www.ama-assn.org/ama/pub/physician-resources/medical-ethics/code-medical-ethics.page#. Accessed April 25, 2012.
3. Dubler NN, Liebman CB. *Bioethics Mediation: A Guide to Shaping Shared Solutions*. New York: United Hospital Fund of New York, 2004.

4. Fletcher JC, Spencer EM, Lombardo P, eds. *Fletcher's Introduction to Clinical Ethics, 3rd ed.* Hagerstown, MD: University Publishing Group, Inc., 2005:58–60.
5. Bernat, 119–24, Ch. 5.
6. Bernat, 81, Ch. 4.
7. Pellegrino ED, Thomasma DC. *The Virtues in Medical Practice.* New York: Oxford University Press, Inc., 1993.
8. MacIntyre A. *After Virtue, 2nd ed.* Notre Dame, IN: University of Notre Dame Press, 1984.
9. Fletcher, et al. *Fletcher's Introduction to Clinical Ethics, 3rd ed.,* 15–6.
10. Swick HM. Toward a normative definition of medical professionalism. Acad Med 2000; 75:612–6.
11. Beauchamp TL, Childress JF. *Principles of Biomedical Ethics, 5th ed.* New York: Oxford University Press, Inc., 2001.
12. Bernat, 13–4, Ch. 1.
13. Bernat, 9–11, Ch. 1.
14. National Institutes of Health. Office of Human Subjects Research. The Belmont Report: Ethical principles and guidelines for the protection of human subjects of research. Available at http://ohsr.od.nih.gov/guidelines/belmont.html. Accessed April 17, 2012.
15. Gilligan C. *In a Different Voice: Psychological Theory and Women's Development.* Revised Edition. Boston, MA: Harvard University Press, 1993.
16. Miller FG, Fins JJ, Bacchetta MD. Clinical pragmatism: John Dewey and clinical ethics. In: Fletcher JC, Miller FG, eds. *Frontiers in Bioethics: Essays Dedicated to John C. Fletcher.* Hagerstown, MD: University Publishing Group, 2000.
17. Fletcher JC, Spencer EM, Lombardo PA, eds. *Fletcher's Introduction to Clinical Ethics, 3rd ed.* Hagerstown, MD: University Publishing Group 2005:339–47.

CLINICAL PRAGMATISM: A CASE METHOD OF MORAL PROBLEM SOLVING

ASSESSMENT

1. What is the patient's medical condition?
   a. Identification of medical problems and history
   b. Diagnosis/diagnostic hypotheses
   c. Predictions and uncertainties regarding prognosis (What are the prospects for full or partial recovery? Is the patient terminally ill?)
   d. Provisional formulation of goals of treatment and care
   e. Treatment recommendations and reasonable alternatives

2. What are the relevant contextual factors?
   a. Demographic factors (age, gender, education)
   b. Life situation and lifestyle of patient
   c. Family relationships
   d. Setting of care (home or institution)
   e. Socioeconomic factors (such as insurance coverage)
   f. Language spoken
   g. Cultural factors
   h. Religion

3. Is the patient capable of decision making?
   a. Legally incompetent (e.g., the patient is a child, or a court has determined the patient to be incompetent)
   b. Clearly incapacitated (e.g., patient is unconscious)
   c. Diminished capacity (e.g., patient is diagnosed with depression or other mental disorder that interferes with understanding or judgment)
   d. Fluctuating capacity
   e. Prospects for enhancing capacity

4. What are the patient's preferences?
   a. Understanding of condition
   b. Views on quality of life
   c. Values relevant to decision making about treatment
   d. Current wishes for treatment
   e. Advance directives
   f. Reasons for seeking treatment that is regarded as medically inappropriate or refusing treatment that is regarded as medically indicated

---

Adapted from Fletcher JC, Spencer EM, Lombardo PA, eds. *Fletcher's Introduction to Clinical Ethics, 3rd ed.* Hagerstown, MD: University Publishing Group, 2005, used with permission. All rights reserved.

5. What are the needs of the patient as a person?
   a. Psychic suffering and possible interventions for relief
   b. Interpersonal dynamics
   c. Resources and strategies for helping patient to cope
   d. Adequacy of home environment for care of patient
   e. Preparation for dying

6. What are the preferences of family/surrogate decision makers?
   a. Competence as surrogate decision maker
   b. Judgment and evidence of relevant patient preferences
   c. Opinions on quality of life of patient
   d. Opinions on best interests of patient
   e. Reasons for seeking treatment that is regarded as medically inappropriate or refusing treatment that is regarded as medically indicated

7. Are there interests other than, and potentially competing with, those of the patient?
   a. Interests of family (e.g., concerns about burdens of caring for patient or disagreements with preferences of patient)
   b. Interests of fetus
   c. Scarce resources and competing needs for their use
   d. Interests of healthcare providers (e.g., professional integrity)
   e. Interests of healthcare organization

8. Are there issues of power or conflict in the interactions of the key actors in the case that need to be addressed?
   a. Between clinicians and patient/family
   b. Between patient and family members
   c. Among family members/surrogates
   d. Between members of the healthcare team (e.g., between attending physicians and housestaff, between physicians and nurses)

9. Have all parties involved in the case had an opportunity to be heard?

10. Are there institutional factors that contribute to moral problems posed by the case?
    a. Work routines
    b. Fears of malpractice/defensive medicine/legal problems
    c. Biases favoring disproportionately aggressive treatment or neglect of treatable conditions
    d. Cost constraints/economic incentives

MORAL DIAGNOSIS

1. Examine how the moral problems in the case are being framed by the participants. Determine whether this framing should be reconsidered and replaced by an alternative understanding.

2. Identify and rank the range of relevant moral considerations.

3. Identify any relevant institutional policies pertaining to the case.

4. Consider ethical standards and guidelines, drawing on consensus statements of commissions or interdisciplinary or specialty groups.

5. Consider similar cases and discussions in the literature that might shed light on the analysis and resolution of moral problems in the case.

6. Identify the morally acceptable options for resolving the moral problems posed by the case.

GOAL SETTING, DECISION MAKING, AND IMPLEMENTATION

1. Consider or reconsider and negotiate the goals of treatment and care for the patient.

2. Consider ideas (hypotheses) for possible interventions to meet the needs of the patient and resolve moral problems.

3. Deliberate regarding merits of alternative options for resolving the moral problems.

4. Endeavor to resolve conflicts.

5. Assess whether ethics consultation is necessary or desirable.
   a. Is there persistent conflict between clinicians and patients/surrogates or among clinicians regarding how to resolve the moral problems posed by the case?
   b. Would ethics advice be helpful in understanding or providing guidance on moral issues presented by the case?

6. Negotiate acceptable plan of action.

7. If negotiations, including ethics consultation, fail to achieve satisfactory resolution, consider judicial review.

8. Implement plan of action.

EVALUATION

1. Current evaluation
   a. Is the plan of action working? If not, why not?
   b. Do the observed results of implementing the plan indicate the need for a modification of the plan?
   c. Have conditions changed in a way that suggests the need to rethink the plan?
   d. Are interactions between clinicians and the patient or surrogate helping to meet the needs of the patient, to respect the patient as a person, and to serve the goals of the plan of care?
   e. Are there relevant interests, institutional factors, or normative considerations that have not been adequately addressed in planning for the care of the patient?

2. Retrospective evaluation
   a. What opportunities for resolving the moral problem were missed?
   b. How did the care received by the patient match the standards of good practice?
   c. What factors contributed to a less-than-optimal resolution of the problems posed by the case?
   d. Was the process of problem solving satisfactory in this case?
   e. What might have been done to improve the care of the patient?
   f. What changes in institutional policy, feasible changes in the clinical environment, or educational interventions might help to prevent or resolve the moral problems posed by similar cases?

APPLYING THE CLINICAL PRAGMATISM MODEL TO CASE-BASED LEARNING IN THIS TEXT

The purpose of *PECN* is to help the learner to grasp the clinical application of ethics by using the clinical pragmatism model to assess and resolve the cases presented. Learning in ethics is best achieved by active learning rather than passive learning. If *PECN* is being used in group discussion, one approach is for the facilitator to assign each case and its questions to one or two learners, who will then present their thoughts to the group. If *PECN* is being used for self-directed study, the learner should consider his or her own answers and try to imagine the answers that others might offer.

- Read the cases in detail.
- Review and attempt to answer the questions posed for each case.
- Review the relevant AAN documents and relevant chapters in Bernat's 3rd edition to help formulate answers.
- Write your thoughts for each of the questions, even if it is only a few notes or key words.
- Compare your thoughts to the discussion provided by the author or other participants in the group discussion.
- Take the time to explore the reasons for any differences in thoughts and opinions. This exploration, and the self-reflection inherent to it, is foundational to ethical reasoning, as you may find that you hold different values, have different goals of therapy, have a different ranking of competing ethical principles involved in the case, or use a different moral framework or approach to solve the problem. You may also find that your perspective is changed or that you come to a better understanding and acceptance of the perspectives and values of others.
- Be cautious not to presume that the ethical recommendations for cases are universal and automatically apply to similar cases that you may encounter in practice. The cases presented in the text are concise, hypothetical, and paradigmatic for the purposes of teaching and learning, and the analyses, conclusions, and recommendations are specific to the context of the cases.

- If you have a case similar to one in the text, use the text case as a starting point and ascertain important differences in your case for comparison and contrast as you use the Clinical Pragmatism Model for your analysis.
- Lastly, take the opportunity to find and read key references for each of the chapters. For example, using PubMed or Google Scholar, readers can find either cited articles or similar articles to learn more about an individual topic.

2

MEDICAL STUDENT RELATIONSHIPS WITH PATIENTS, PEERS, AND TEACHERS

Lois Margaret Nora, MD, JD, MBA, FAAN

OVERVIEW

Ethical issues that arise in a student-training environment present particular challenges and opportunities. Clinical ethics cases provide both the opportunity and the requirement for teaching case analysis and ethics problem solving. The presence of learners in the clinical environment also creates distinct permutations of ethics issues, including truth telling, professional boundaries, and acting within the scope of one's abilities. In addition, the learning environment creates ethical responsibilities for teachers and the training institution related to professionalism toward students and the creation of an appropriate learning environment. The case presented in this chapter focuses on some of the professionalism and ethics challenges that can arise related to the teaching setting. Although the case and discussion are framed from the perspective of the medical student, residents and students of the other healthcare professions have similar experiences.

LEARNING OBJECTIVES

Upon completion of this chapter, participants will be able to:

1. Identify and discuss ethical issues presented in the case about medical student–patient relationships.
2. Analyze their own experiences as medical students, residents, or attending physicians in light of the ethical issues presented.
3. Discuss ways in which ethical issues may present differently for medical students than for attending physicians.
4. Explain how a senior resident or attending physician can inquire effectively into the professionalism issues that students encounter.
5. Use the opportunity of this case discussion to identify other ethical or professionalism issues encountered by medical students.

LEARNING RESOURCES

Key chapters in Bernat's third edition—3

Key relevant AAN documents available at www.aan.com/view/PECN

A

CASE

A professional development advising team, consisting of 5 third-year medical students and their faculty advisor, meet halfway through the academic year. The advisor asks the group about the most challenging patient-related issues they have encountered during the year. Initially, the students talk about their experiences with clinical conditions such as myocardial infarction, cerebral herniation, uncontrolled seizures, diabetic ketoacidosis, cardiac arrest, and surgical emergencies. The advisor then asks whether the students have encountered any issues in the areas of ethics, professionalism, interpersonal behaviors, or communication in the clinical-care or clinical-teaching setting. Among the many experiences that they had, the students related the following incidents.

One student, Abigail, laughs and says that she enjoyed her 4-week rotation at the Veterans Administration Hospital but expresses concern at the behavior of some patients toward women students. Besides tiresome flirty talk and extremely offensive "jokes," she encountered a few instances in which patients tried to grope her body. The residents and attendings whom she told about it laughed and said, "Welcome to the VA."

A second student, Bob Simmons, reports that a resident introduced him as "Dr. Simmons" to a patient before he was to perform a spinal tap. Previously, Bob had only practiced spinal taps on a patient simulator. The resident supervised and the tap went well, but Bob expresses concern that the patient kept calling him "doctor" throughout the procedure and subsequently introduced him to her family as her doctor.

A third student, Celia, had difficulty when a patient asked her the results of a biopsy. Celia had heard in rounds that the tissue was malignant, but neither the resident nor the attending had yet spoken to the patient. Celia did not want to lie and say "I don't know" but felt it was not her charge to impart the cancer diagnosis. Instead, Celia told the patient that she knew but could not tell her. The patient became frantic, and the resident berated Celia, causing her to lose confidence in her ability to relate to patients.

Danielle recounts that she participated in the care of a man with a wrist fracture and abrasions from a bicycle crash. Before he was discharged from the ED, the patient asked her out to dinner. Danielle found him attractive and shared his interest in cycling but indicated that she could not date a patient. When the patient asked if he would still be her patient in 2 weeks, she said that she did not think so. The patient suggested that he might "friend" Danielle on Facebook in the near future. Danielle is interested in a relationship but wonders if this is professionally appropriate.

Finally, Ed relates his discomfort on his surgery rotation, where the attending physician's technical brilliance was overshadowed by his boorishness and antagonistic attitude. He publicly berated the surgical team members and made derogatory comments about his patients while they were under anesthesia. He often made crude comments and jokes about obese patients.

QUESTIONS FOR GROUP DISCUSSION

GETTING STARTED

1. Did any of the experiences presented by the 5 students in the case resonate with experiences that you or your colleagues (medical students, residents, attendings) have had?

ASSESSMENT

2. What ethical and professionalism issues are presented in each scenario?
3. What issue is common to all of the scenarios?
4. To whom is the medical student ethically responsible—the patient, the resident, or the attending physician?
5. What are the power dynamics in each scenario? How does power affect ethical discussions and responsibilities?
6. Do patients' cultural backgrounds influence your reaction to their behavior? Do physicians' positions, prestige, or cultural backgrounds influence your reaction to their behaviors?
7. What are possible motivating factors for the various behaviors of patients, students, residents, and attending physicians in these scenarios? Is motivation relevant?
8. What ethical issues are created by the relationship between the medical student and the patient and the relationship between the medical student and the other members of the healthcare team?
9. How does the role of "medical student" affect the ethics discussion in each scenario? Are the issues that were presented by these students ethical or practical in nature?

MORAL DIAGNOSIS

10. Does your institution have policies regarding the role of medical students in patient care, professional behaviors for healthcare professionals, or physicians' and medical students' social involvement with patients?
11. Does your institution enforce existing professionalism policies in a nondiscriminatory manner, without regard for a physician's volume of service, billings, seniority, prestige, or special expertise?
12. Does your institution have a mechanism by which students, residents, and others can identify and discuss concerns about their experiences in a confidential manner with faculty members or administrators who can facilitate student learning and bring issues forward to appropriate decision makers?
13. What is the "hidden curriculum"? Discuss the impact of the hidden curriculum on the discussion of ethics in the medical student environment.
14. Have any professional organizations established guidelines for medical student professional behaviors?

(continued)

GOAL SETTING, DECISION MAKING, AND IMPLEMENTATION

15. Was the conduct for the medical student in each of the scenarios appropriate? If so, explain why. If not, is there a more appropriate conduct, and why? More than one answer for each student scenario may be possible.
16. What would be appropriate responses for the faculty advisor in the case?

EVALUATION

17. What evaluation mechanisms can be used to determine whether the learning environment is conducive to respectful and excellent patient care and to student learning?

COMMENTARY ON DISCUSSION QUESTIONS

GETTING STARTED

1. **Did any of the experiences presented by the 5 students in the case resonate with experiences that you or your colleagues (medical students, residents, attendings) have had?**

These scenarios are based on actual situations described by medical students; similar instances have been published in the medical literature.[1-6] Although it is likely that attending physicians and residents are aware that students encounter these issues, they may not know the degree to which the students are bothered by such encounters. Students hesitate to bring forward concerns about ethical issues, professionalism in the learning environment, or their own competence. Reasons for this hesitation include fear of retribution, uncertainty about whether their concern truly reflects an ethical issue, the desire not to look stupid or whiney, and concerns that they will communicate their question ineffectively. It is important to recognize that students are a vulnerable population in the clinical training setting. (Note: Residents, fellows and other healthcare professionals in learning roles can face similar issues, and many parts of the discussion in this chapter are as applicable to them as they are to medical students.)

The case also demonstrates that when asked about challenging patient care–related experiences, medical students may tend to focus on challenging clinical cases rather than on ethical and professionalism concerns. *It is important that faculty advisors, course directors, and others take the time to ask about issues beyond the purely clinical.* Among the ethical issues that arise in the clinical setting, those dealing with the medical student's own professionalism and the professionalism of others in the learning environment may be particularly difficult to confront and examine.

ASSESSMENT

2. **What ethical and professionalism issues are presented in each scenario?**

These scenarios present a number of ethical issues, including the appropriate management of harassing behaviors by patients, truth telling (correct identification of the student as a student, candor about the nature of the student's role on the clinical team, admissions of ignorance), personal relationships with patients, behaving professionally, and dealing with unprofessional behaviors of others on the healthcare team (HCT), including superiors. Some of these issues occur at the level of the medical student–patient relationship. Others relate to the more indirect student–teacher/supervisor–patient relationship. Still others relate to the student–teacher/supervisor relationship.

Student experiences in this case demonstrate that many ethical questions in the clinical training setting arise from communication issues or are exacerbated by them. For medical students, ethical issues are often complicated by differential power among members of the HCT and by concerns (sometimes well founded) that an angry supervisor can affect grades and career possibilities. The case also underscores the fact that the teaching members of the HCT (residents and attending physicians) have ethical obligations to students, as does the medical school leadership (institutional ethics).[7,8] Some medical organizations have incorporated in their ethical codes the responsibilities that physicians have to learners.

Bernat, 62, Ch. 3
Bernat, 112, Ch. 5

3. **What issue is common to all of the scenarios?**

The presence of one or more medical students in the patient-care environment is common among the scenarios. The medical student's role in the clinical setting is primarily that of learner, although students are also expected to carry out service obligations and often play an important therapeutic role with patients. A medical student learns through the generosity of patients and under the tutelage of attending and resident physicians and other health professionals. Ethical conduct and professionalism are requirements of medical practice for practicing physicians, residents, and medical students.[9] Ethics training is a mandatory aspect of medical education.[10]

A medical student has ethical responsibilities in the clinical setting, some of which can be identified through a review of leading ethical codes and statements. Three codes of particular interest are the AMA Code of Medical Ethics, the AAN Code of Professional Conduct, and the Professionalism Charter crafted in 2002 by the American Board of Internal Medicine (ABIM), the American College of Physicians–American Society of Internal Medicine (ACP–ASIM), and the European Federation of Internal Medicine (EFIM).[11–13] Differences between the roles of medical students and practicing physicians may affect the interpretation of these guidelines written with practicing physicians in mind. The American Medical Student Association (AMSA) Code of Student Medical Ethics specifically addresses medical students and their ethical obligations in the clinical setting.[14]

4. To whom is the medical student ethically responsible—the patient, the resident, or the attending physician?

The medical student has ethical responsibilities to all of these parties. Responsibilities specific to the patient include the obligations to identify oneself as a medical student, to participate in care activities at the level to which the student is capable, and to obtain informed consent for any procedures that the student performs (e.g., venipuncture, spinal tap). Students should ensure that patients are aware that students are unable to promise to keep confidences from other members of the HCT. Responsibilities to the resident and the attending physician include obligations of honesty, diligence, respect for the HCT, and support of the primary relationship that exists between the attending physician and the patient. Situations may arise in which the student's obligations are in conflict with the actions of a resident or attending physicians; for example, the student may be introduced as "doctor" or expected to independently carry out an activity (e.g., perform a procedure or obtain informed consent) that the student does not feel capable of carrying out.

Medical students have the dual responsibilities of carrying out directives of their superiors and questioning directives that the students believe are contrary to the wishes or best interests of their patients. Questioning is a natural and important activity in any clinical setting and particularly important in a teaching setting. Residents, attending physicians, and other HCT members should welcome questions from students, and students should maintain appropriate behavior in the teaching setting. These behaviors include questioning in a respectful manner and reserving sensitive or highly charged questions for venues outside of the immediate patient-care area, both to protect the patient from undue worry and to accord respect to the teacher.

Situations in which a student would need to directly disagree with a resident or attending physician in the presence of a patient are rare but might include situations in which the student is given orders that she believes may endanger the patient or in which the student is expected to participate in a procedure that he finds morally unacceptable (e.g., conscientious objection). In most situations, the student can ask questions in a private setting and should do so, thereby enabling learning, demonstrating respect for the more senior members of the HCT, and facilitating the physician–patient relationship.

5. What are the power dynamics in each scenario? How does power affect ethical discussions and responsibilities?

Issues of power exist in any clinical setting. The fundamental power inequality between the patient and members of the HCT—the inherent vulnerability of the patient—is the basis of many professional obligations expressed in ethics codes and professionalism statements. Another important power dynamic that exists within the clinical team is the power differential among learners and teachers. Many members of the clinical team have reporting relationships to other members of the team, or other members of the team report to them. These power dynamics can make identifying and addressing ethical conflicts and professionalism issues difficult. For example, a resident may concur with a student's concern about an attending physician's behavior but may hesitate to speak up because of concerns about the resident's own working and evaluation relationships with the attending physician.

The power differential among members of the HCT and the position of the medical students (and students of other health professions) as vulnerable members of the HCT underscore the need for teachers and education administrators to understand and meet their ethical obligations to provide a good learning environment for students. Actions that support this obligation include but are not limited to the following:

- Training about ethics, professionalism, and difficult patients should be part of any medical school curriculum.
- Communication skills training designed to help the learner communicate about sensitive issues—both with patients and with other members of the care team (including nurses and other health professionals)—should be part of the curriculum.
- Teachers should behave professionally around and toward students and recognize that respectful questioning is an important and legitimate form of learning.
- Students should have access to "safe harbors," where they can ask sensitive questions, receive help assessing their situation (e.g., a behavior that a student interprets as unprofessional may not be), or receive coaching in appropriate responses from personnel in the school of medicine, such as faculty advisors, who have the training to do so and will maintain confidentiality.
- Institutional officials should be willing to address professionalism issues when they arise.
- Institutional leadership should work to achieve concordance and coherence among the formal and hidden curricula that the students encounter.

Residents are important care providers in the clinical environment; at the same time, they are also learners. Many of the experiences described by the students in the case presented are similar to situations that residents may encounter. All institutions should have policies and practices that facilitate resident discussion of these issues and provide mechanisms for issue identification and resolution.

6. **Do patients' cultural backgrounds influence your reaction to their behavior? Do physicians' positions, prestige, or cultural backgrounds influence your reaction to their behaviors?**

Cultural background should be taken into account when a patient's verbal habits and other behaviors are being analyzed. Doing so can render certain behaviors more understandable and can help medical students and others to approach patients in a more therapeutic manner. Understanding patients' backgrounds (cultural and otherwise) may also help to identify ways in which a negative or harmful behavior can be addressed most effectively. Although patients' backgrounds do not excuse inappropriate behaviors directed at medical students and others, knowledge of backgrounds can make the behaviors more understandable and make interventions more successful. An additional consideration is that some patients may have neurologic or psychiatric disorders such as dementia, delirium, or psychoses (to name but a few) that cause them to make statements or have behaviors that are inappropriate but may not be within the patients' ability to control.

Cultural background can also affect the behavior of a student, resident, or attending physician, especially if the person has only recently arrived in the United States. Institutions have a responsibility to help new trainees and members of the medical staff to transition successfully by providing information about appropriate behavior toward patients, students, and other members of the HCT.

Inappropriate behavior and lack of professionalism must be addressed regardless of a person's role on the HCT or position in the hospital or medical school hierarchy. Systems that teach, expect, and reward professionalism may diminish negative behaviors. If negative behaviors continue after appropriate education interventions have occurred, progressive discipline within the procedures of the health system, hospital, and college may be necessary.

7. **What are possible motivating factors for the various behaviors of patients, students, residents, and attending physicians in these scenarios? Is motivation relevant?**

It is important to consider possible motivations behind the actions of different people in the medical students' examples, and it is difficult to correctly ascribe motivation without direct inquiry. Such inquiries can help to prevent the incorrect attribution of a motivation that is different from that actually involved. Understanding motivation can help to explain behaviors that would otherwise be incomprehensible and can point toward more effective interventions to alter those behaviors.

The motivating factors behind the *students'* behaviors in the case presented may include ignorance about expectations in the clinical settings (e.g., what is the appropriate way to be introduced? what patient behaviors are tolerated in the clinical setting? what degree of humor is appropriate with patients?), lack of knowledge and experience in dealing with difficult patients, and poor communication skills. Other factors may include learning the professional role, personal experience with sexism, and wanting to fit in and impress others.

Motivating factors behind the *residents'* actions in the case may include sexism, ignorance about how to handle difficult patients' behaviors, fear of being the target of humor or anger from others, embarrassment at being mistreated by an attending, pride in the student learner, and personal convictions about the optimal ways to teach.

Possible motivating factors behind the *attending physicians'* behaviors may include, among others, personal experiences as medical students, opinions about optimal teaching styles, displacement of personal issues onto others in the environment, and temperament. Generational differences may contribute to differing opinions about appropriate humor and teaching styles.

Possible motivating factors behind the various *patients'* reported behaviors may include attempts to be funny or important among other patients, discomfort with the patient role (possibly exacerbated by the presence of a female medical student authority figure), attraction to a caregiver, sexism, and attempts to conform behavior to the perceived requirements of the setting.

8. **What ethical issues are created by the relationship between the medical student and the patient and the relationship between the medical student and the other members of the healthcare team?**

The ethical issues in this chapter evoke the ethical principles of beneficence, nonmaleficence, and respect for patient autonomy and underscore the obligations of physicians (and medical students as physicians-to-be) to treat others with respect, act in the best interests of patients, maintain confidences, act within the bounds of their individual competence, and uphold the professional standards of medicine.[9] Furthermore, these cases lend themselves to consideration of the characteristics of the virtuous physician—among them, prudence, commitment to lifelong learning, honesty, and fidelity.[15,16]

Bernat, 9–15, Ch. 1

The ethical obligations of the medical student are related to the obligations of the profession and the student's progression toward being a full member of the profession. Although most of these obligations are not specifically related to their student status, some are. For example, these obligations include (a) not permitting others to identify a student in a manner beyond the student's level of training or competence and (b) correcting patients and their families if they do not understand that the student is, in fact, a student.[14] Students have affirmative obligations to ask for supervision and assistance when appropriate. A medical student's obligation to be honest includes not cheating on exams or plagiarizing material. A student's obligation to acknowledge errors may be particularly challenging in situations in which a student aspires to a particular specialty or residency program.

Students also have obligations to other members of the HCT, including other students. These obligations are oftentimes articulated in student codes of behavior formulated at the institutional level.[14,17] Examples of obligations include maintaining professional composure despite stress, treating other healthcare professionals with respect, and being trustworthy. Consistent with their status as professionals-in-training, students also have obligations to identify and assist other students who are impaired and to work to change unprofessional aspects of the training environment. Efforts such as these are most effectively accomplished with the assistance of professionals in the school environment.

9. How does the role of "medical student" affect the ethics discussion in each scenario? Are the issues that were presented by these students ethical or practical in nature?

In most cases, the role of medical student does not affect the ethical analysis of a case. Most ethics cases present issues related to a patient and the care of that patient. For example, the analysis of a patient's capacity, determination of medical futility, research ethics, and other issues are not affected by the presence of a medical student on the service. The determination of the appropriate course of action — clinically and ethically — is based on the patient's situation and targeted toward the patient's good.

However, the role of "medical student" can affect the ethics discussion of cases in 2 substantial ways. First, some ethical issues arise between the medical student and the patient. Medical students have specific responsibilities toward patients, similar to those of physicians. These include ensuring that the patient knows that the student is, in fact, a student; obtaining informed consent for any procedures that are performed by the student; and maintaining confidences. Some of these issues are discussed in the case presented. Second, the presence of learners in the teaching environment is associated with a set of professionalism issues that are linked to the appropriate relationships among students, residents, and attending physicians and to the responsibility of the institution to maintain a professional learning environment. Ethical issues can arise in these areas.

The presence of learners in the clinical setting also creates certain practical issues related to ethics decision making. How does a student interact with an ethics consultation service or ethics committee? Does a student have standing to disagree with an ethics care plan, and if so, how should that disagreement be voiced? How does a student inquire into whether a teacher's behavior is considered professional? How does an institution ensure that the environment is conducive to students' bringing ethical questions forward without fear of retribution? These are important issues that are practical in nature but demand attention if a training environment conducive to the ethical development of students is to exist.

MORAL DIAGNOSIS

10. **Does your institution have policies regarding the role of medical students in patient care, professional behaviors for healthcare professionals, or physicians' and medical students' social involvement with patients?**

    Students, residents, and attending physicians should be aware of the policies and procedures that exist at their schools and in the various clinical settings in which they train. The Joint Commission, the US federal government, the Liaison Committee on Medical Education, and other regulatory bodies have established standards for accreditation and rules for participation in certain federal programs, and some of these rules have the force of law. Some of these standards and rules establish or require institutional policies on a variety of topics, including physician–patient social relationships, confidentiality, and the role of students in the learning environment. Practices may differ from one institution to another, and these differences may have relevance for medical students who participate in rotations across a number of institutions.

11. **Does your institution enforce existing professionalism policies in a nondiscriminatory manner, without regard for a physician's volume of service, billings, seniority, prestige, or special expertise?**

    Institutions should enforce professionalism policies fairly, regardless of physician prestige, productivity, or revenues generated for the hospital or health system. Medical, academic, and hospital administrative leadership must ensure that the system does not encourage or tolerate unprofessional behavior toward patients or students.

    Physicians, administrators, nurses, and other healthcare personnel must be vigilant of practices, behaviors, policies, and personnel that negatively affect patients and create a hostile setting for students and other members of the HCT. Patients can be directly harmed by breaches in ethics and professional behavior, or indirectly harmed if members of the HCT communicate poorly with the attending, remain quiet about problems, or fail to ask care-related questions because they fear the attending physician. Professional standards that are enforced erratically or preferentially can be especially harmful to the culture of a neurology service, a hospital, or a learning environment.

12. **Does your institution have a mechanism by which students, residents, and others can identify and discuss concerns about their experiences in a confidential manner with faculty members or administrators who can facilitate student learning and bring issues forward to appropriate decision makers?**

    As the case suggests, situations in the clinical environment may raise ethics and professionalism concerns for medical students. Concerns that are strictly related to the clinical aspects of diagnosis and treatment are usually readily addressed in the teaching environment. However, other concerns, particularly those that deal with ethics questions or professionalism, are not so easily raised by students. Students (and residents) are concerned about looking foolish, wasting others' time, creating tension and conflict on a ward service, receiving poor evaluations, and negatively affecting their residency-selection process. These concerns often make questioning or disagreeing with a decision more difficult.

Medical students must be able to ask questions about decisions, difficult cases, professionalism issues, and ethical issues that arise in the clinical environment. Course directors of neurology clerkships, departmental leaders, and medical school administrators share the responsibility of ensuring that students have a supportive place where they can voice their questions and concerns. Tremendous learning can occur if these issues are raised at "teachable moments," as in the scenarios discussed in this chapter, which cover a variety of professional issues, including the use of humor in clinical care, interactions between teachers and medical students, dealing with attraction between student (or doctor) and patient, truth telling, and mistreatment in the teaching environment.

The value of providing a safe environment for these discussions extends well beyond optimizing the teachable moment, however. The environment can contribute to a learner-friendly atmosphere that improves patient care and may be an advantage in attracting residents. The discussions can serve as an important quality-assurance mechanism for departmental and medical school leadership. Even though it is extremely important that patient and student confidences be maintained, the concerns to which they call attention—particularly those voiced over a period of time by multiple students—can act as a warning system for problems.

13. What is the "hidden curriculum"? Discuss the impact of the hidden curriculum on the discussion of ethics in the medical student environment.

The term *hidden curriculum* describes the norms, values, and rules in an education setting that affect student learning—even if they are not part of the explicit curriculum.[18] Students' actual experiences differ, sometimes dramatically, from the explicit curriculum that the students are taught. The importance of treating patients with respect is emphasized in the classroom, but students may observe physicians and others treating patients disrespectfully on the basis of gender, sexual orientation, disease process, and physical characteristics. Furthermore, they experience training environments that tolerate, and sometimes encourage, mistreatment of students and residents. The "disconnect" between the explicit and the hidden curricula can create substantial tension for students.

14. Have any professional organizations established guidelines for medical student professional behaviors?

A number of medical schools have established codes of student professionalism.[17] Several organizations have established guidelines for medical students concerning professional behavior and interactions with patients. Of particular import are the AMA Code of Medical Ethics and the AMSA Code of Medical Student Ethics.[11,14] It is also useful to note that Papakakis and colleagues demonstrated that physicians who are disciplined by their state medical boards often have a history of unprofessional behavior in medical school.[19]

Other tools are available to medical students, including general ethics textbooks, neurology-specific ethics books, and materials focused on the medical student and resident experience; among them are *Ward Ethics: Dilemmas for Medical Students and Doctors in Training*, by Kushner and Thomasma,[20] and the AMA's *Virtual Mentor,* an electronic publication that analyzes cases that arise in the medical student environment or have specific implications for the student.[21] The MedEd Portal of the Association of American Medical Colleges offers a variety of teaching resources that address medical student professionalism.[22]

GOAL SETTING, DECISION MAKING, AND IMPLEMENTATION

15. Was the conduct for the medical student in each of the scenarios appropriate? If so, explain why. If not, is there a more appropriate conduct, and why? More than one answer for each student scenario may be possible.

Abigail—It is appropriate for Abigail to attempt to set boundaries with the patients. It is also appropriate for her to bring these patients' actions to the attention of her supervising residents and attendings. The experience with her friend may suggest that such action will not be fruitful, but an attempt is still merited. She also has an obligation to advise her medical school (e.g., through the student affairs office or potentially through course evaluation forms) of the situation. Medical students have an obligation to assist in creating appropriate learning environments. Although reporting such incidents may not positively affect Abigail, it may help to prevent a similar situation for other students.

Medical students may find it difficult to perceive patients as vulnerable in settings similar to that described by Abigail. Several authors have reported on patients who harass their caregivers, and surveys of medical students provide evidence of patients' behaviors and of the distress that these behaviors cause students.[3,5,23] It can be of value to help students understand that in some cases, patients' harassing behaviors may be a reaction to their fears and loss of control.

Bob—Bob is correct in being uncomfortable with a situation in which a patient and family have been misled to believe that he is a physician. Both Bob and his resident failed in their duty when they did not clearly identify

Bob as a student. Bob should introduce himself as a medical student and should ask others to do so as well. If introduced as "doctor," he should clarify his role with the patient. Although it is permissible to do so, Bob is not ethically required to advise patients of the level of his previous experience when he performs healthcare procedures. However, he has an obligation to perform these procedures with appropriate oversight, and because of the risk of error and harm to a patient, he should refuse to perform a procedure without supervision if he lacks the training and experience to do so safely. The maxim of "see one, do one, teach one" is no longer acceptable. If a patient asks a medical student about his experience, he must be truthful.

If Bob had been correctly identified as a student and the patient had agreed to his participation, no ethical principle would have been violated. Medical students commonly learn and refine clinical procedural skills with the help of willing patients. The opportunity to learn the basics of performing a lumbar puncture and first practicing the procedure on simulators is valuable to the creation of a learning environment that is supportive of both learning and ethical development.

Celia—Celia was correct in not giving such sensitive test results to the patient. As the AMSA Code points out, the physician–patient relationship is between the attending physician and the patient; students should do no more than that which is appropriate within their scope of involvement in the case.[14] Unfortunately, Celia was not skilled in communicating the limits of her capability to the patient, which caused the patient distress. Medical students and their faculty members have a joint responsibility to discuss what information should be conveyed to patients and the communication strategies most appropriate to situations such as the one Celia described. If Celia were more skilled in her ability to advise patients of her role and to comfortably state her inability to provide information in a manner that did not require her to lie and did not confuse the patient, this situation could have been avoided. Celia should discuss the situation with others and learn how to respond in similar situations.

The feelings of inadequacy expressed by Celia are not rare. Medical students (and physicians) confront personal feelings of inadequacy; virtuous medical students and physicians work to acquire competence while recognizing their own fallibility. Celia's current strategy of avoiding patients if she knows information that she cannot disclose is understandable, but it is problematic. Medical students are important components of the HCT; avoidance not only limits her development as a physician, but may also impair the functioning of the entire team. If avoidance becomes Celia's preferred mode for dealing with conflict or emotional stress in the patient care setting, it will become ethically problematic and will certainly interfere with her professional development and competence.

Danielle—Danielle's story highlights the fact that attractions between medical students and patients occur and should be anticipated. Sexual relationships between physicians and patients are prohibited by multiple ethical codes on the basis of the power differential and the abrogation of necessary boundaries.[11,12] Social relationships that may lead to or imply sexual relationships are also problematic. In all instances, physicians must not enter into sexual relationships with current patients. In some instances (e.g., a previous psychiatric therapeutic relationship), physicians are prohibited from ever entering into sexual relationships with patients.

Danielle is not the patient's physician. However, she did meet him in her role as a medical student. It would have been inappropriate for her to ask him out. It is possible that the patient was attracted to Danielle in part because of her role as a medical student, and it is even possible that some element of transference was at work in his invitation to her. She wisely did not agree when he asked her out. Danielle must analyze whether she is likely to become involved in the patient's care again (e.g., through a follow-up visit) and whether the medical student–patient relationship has ended. She may be wise (although it is not ethically required) to ensure that the patient has been released from all medical care for his injuries from the cycling accident before engaging in a social relationship. If she does begin to date the patient, she should tell him at the outset that she cannot participate in providing medical care to him as long as they are dating or have an intimate relationship.

Ed—Ed is appropriately concerned about the behaviors of the surgeon, including disrespectful behavior toward patients, misuse of humor, and mistreatment of subordinate members of the HCT. The use of humor in the clinical environment is fraught with difficulties. Physicians can appropriately use humor in a therapeutic manner that enhances communication and well-being. However, humor can also be hurtful to patients, and patients may be reticent to express their feelings about offensive humor to the physician.

Ed's situation highlights some of the tensions that can occur in the training environment. He is clearly and understandably troubled. He finds the attending abusive to the HCT and to patients. If Ed chooses to confront the attending, he should do so away from the immediate patient-care area. If Ed chooses not to confront the attending, he should make his concerns known to the course director, a trusted faculty mentor, or someone in the dean's office. Such a consultation can help Ed to test his reactions with someone familiar with the clinical setting. If Ed remains concerned about the lack of professionalism, the more senior advisor may be helpful in forwarding a complaint that maintains Ed's anonymity.

What should Ed do in the clinical setting when the patient is insulted or joked about? Even if unaware, patients should not be the objects of jokes or humor. Ed should not participate in activities that are insulting to a patient. If the attending physician attempts to involve Ed in the inappropriate joking, he should refrain from doing so, and remaining silent may be the most appropriate and least risky response. Ed may experience peer pressure to join in inappropriate joking or other behaviors that are insensitive to patients.

16. What would be appropriate responses for the faculty advisor in the case?

This faculty advisor has done the students a great service by creating the appropriate atmosphere for discussion of some of these difficult cases. Even so, the faculty advisor may be surprised at some of the issues raised by the students. The faculty advisor can lead students in guided reflection and provide resources and information to help them come to decisions about their own behaviors. In addition, the faculty advisor has specific ethical obligations related to the students' stories. The students should be referred to appropriate resources (ethics codes, textbooks, ethics faculty, institutional ethics committees) for help. The advisor should inform the appropriate offices and individuals (e.g., clerkship course directors, department chairmen, and personnel in the dean's office) in the hospital or school of medicine about the ethical issues that students are encountering. Although the faculty advisor may find it difficult to inform the administration about another faculty member's behavior, the situation cannot be ignored and should be reported.

EVALUATION

17. What evaluation mechanisms can be used to determine whether the learning environment is conducive to respectful and excellent patient care and to student learning?

In addition to considering anecdotal evidence, institutional officials may perform an environmental scan. Available resources include surveys that have been used at other institutions, the "Draw-the-Line" exercise developed by the Office of Student Representatives of the Association of American Medical Colleges (AAMC), and focus-group conversations.[24] Individual medical schools can obtain data about their learning environments via the student survey completed as part of the self-study process of the Liaison Committee on Medical Education and the annual Graduation Questionnaire of the AAMC.[25,26] Environmental scans performed collaboratively by the medical school, the hospital ethics committee, and institutional quality assurance offices may be of particular value.

TOPICAL SYNOPSIS

Medical students and residents encounter a host of ethical issues in the clinical environment. Many of these issues take on particular significance either because they represent the first time the student has confronted the issue in the clinical setting or because the issue has specific nuances related to the particular role of students. Ethics issues presented in this chapter that are commonly encountered by students include confidentiality, truth telling, objectifying the patient, social relationships with patients, informed consent, patient mistreatment, evaluating the professionalism of others, responding to unprofessional behaviors by others, and learning procedures by performing them on patients.

This chapter also highlights ethical issues associated with professionalism among members of the HCT. Mistreatment of students and residents can have direct and indirect harmful effects on patients and substantial negative effects on students, including impeded learning, depression, anger, cynicism, and mistreatment of others by students. Developing the appropriate environment for learning is the responsibility of senior members of the teaching team, hospital personnel, and medical school administration. Discussing professionalism issues is an ethical responsibility.

KEY POINTS

- Students often hesitate to raise concerns about ethical issues, professionalism, or their own competence. Reasons for this hesitation include fear of retribution, uncertainty about whether their concern truly reflects an ethical issue, the desire not to look stupid or whiney, and concerns that they will communicate their question ineffectively. It is important to recognize that students are a vulnerable population in the clinical training setting. It is also important that faculty advisors, course directors, and others take the time to ask about issues beyond the purely clinical.
- Power dynamics can make identifying and addressing ethical conflicts and professionalism issues difficult.
- Students must have access to "safe harbors" where they can ask sensitive questions.
- The medical student's role in the clinical setting is primarily that of learner. Attending physicians remain responsible for the ethical care of their patients, even as they allow trainees to participate in the care of those patients. Students, in turn, have obligations to the patient that are similar to those of the physician.
- Students should be identified as students—and not as doctors—when they are introduced to patients and families.
- The maxim of "see one, do one, teach one" is no longer acceptable.
- Patients should not be the objects of jokes or humor.

KEY WORDS

Hidden curriculum—the multiple unarticulated and sometimes unrecognized values, behaviors, and organizational structures that create a culture and describe ways of operating in the educational setting. In medical education, discussions of the hidden curriculum often focus on the clinical training environment. It can be very different from the explicit curriculum that is taught to students, and the "disconnect" between the explicit and the hidden curricula can create substantial tension for students.

Power dynamics—differential power among members of the HCT or between the patient and members of the HCT that can influence persons with lesser power to accept decisions or tolerate conduct that they would not otherwise accept. Power dynamics can make identifying and addressing ethical conflicts and professionalism issues difficult.

Professionalism—obligations by physicians to uphold the primacy of patients' interests, to achieve and maintain medical competency, and to abide by high ethical standards.

Role modeling—the deliberate and conscious effort of teachers to demonstrate by example correct conduct in the care of patients and interactions with other health professionals. Not all teachers who role model explicitly identify their role modeling to learners.

Student mistreatment—a range of behaviors that may occur in the training environment, including exploitation, breach of teacher–learner boundaries, and public belittlement and humiliation. In addition to raising concerns about professional ethics, episodes of student mistreatment can limit students' ability to learn and can produce other negative consequences for the clinical learning environment.

Teachable moment—a time at which learning a topic or concept is especially possible because of the situation, timing, and people present.

REFERENCES

1. Christakis DA, Feudtner C. Ethics in a short white coat: the ethical dilemmas that medical students confront. Acad Med 1993; 68(4):249–54.
2. Goldie J, Dowie A, Cotton P, et al. Teaching professionalism in the early years of a medical curriculum: A qualitative study. Med Educ 2007; 41(6):610–7.
3. Hundert EM, Hafferty F, Christakis D. Characteristics of the informal curriculum and trainees' ethical choices. Acad Med 1996; 71(6):624–42.
4. Swenson SL, Rothstein JA. Negotiating the wards: Teaching medical students to use their moral compass. Acad Med 1996; 71(6):591–4.
5. Witte FM, Stratton TD, Nora LM. Stories from the field: Students' descriptions of gender discrimination and sexual harassment during medical school. Acad Med 2006; 81(7):648–54.
6. Wear D, Aultman JM, Varley JD, et al. Making fun of patients: Medical students' perceptions and use of derogatory and cynical humor in clinical settings. Acad Med 2006; 81(5):454–62.
7. Bernat, 62, Ch. 3.
8. Bernat, 112, Ch. 5.
9. Larriviere D, Beresford HR. Invited article: Professionalism in neurology: The role of law. Neurology 2008; 71:1283–8.
10. Liaison Committee on Medical Education. Functions and Structure of a Medical School. Standards for Accreditation of Medical Education Programs Leading to the MD Degree. May 2012. (See Standard ED-23). Available at www.lcme.org/functions. pdf. Accessed July 9, 2012.
11. American Medical Association. Council on Ethical and Judicial Affairs. Code of medical ethics: Current opinions with annotations, 2012–2013. Chicago: AMA Press, 2008.
12. American Academy of Neurology. AAN Code of Professional Conduct. [*PECN* appendix document A and available at www.aan.com/view/PECN]

13. ABIM Foundation. American Board of Internal Medicine; ACP–ASIM Foundation (American College of Physicians–American Society of Internal Medicine). European Federation of Internal Medicine. Medical professionalism in the new millennium: A physician charter. Ann Intern Med 2002; 136(3):243–6.

14. American Medical Student Association. AMSA Constitution & Bylaws. 2011 Preamble, Purposes, and Principles. Page 59, Principles regarding student rights and responsibilities. Available at www.amsa.org/amsa/homepage/about/AMSAConstitution.aspx. Accessed March 26, 2012.

15. Pellegrino ED, Thomasma DC. *The Virtues in Medical Practice*. New York: Oxford University Press, 1993.

16. Bernat, 9–15, Ch. 1.

17. Dartmouth-Hitchcock Medical Center. Code of Professional Conduct. Available at http://geiselmed.dartmouth.edu/students/resources/conduct. Accessed July 9, 2012.

18. Hafferty FW. Beyond curriculum reform: Confronting medicine's hidden curriculum. Acad Med 1998; 73(4):403–7.

19. Papadakis MA, Teherani A, Banach MA, et al. Disciplinary action by medical boards and prior behavior in medical school. N Engl J Med 2005; 353(25):2673–82.

20. Kushner TK, Thomasma DC. *Ward Ethics: Dilemmas for Medical Students and Doctors in Training*. Cambridge, England: Cambridge University Press, 2001.

21. American Medical Association Journal of Ethics. Virtual Mentor. Available at http://virtualmentor.ama-assn.org/. Accessed March 11, 2012.

22. Association of American Medical Colleges. MedEd Portal. Available at www.mededportal.org/. Accessed July 9, 2012.

23. Baldwin DC, Daugherty SR, Eckenfels, EJ. Student perceptions of mistreatment and harassment during medical school: A survey of ten United States medical schools. West J Med 1991; 155:140–5.

24. Association of American Medical Colleges. Recent trends in the reporting of medical student mistreatment. Analysis in brief.   July 2006, Vol. 6, No. 4. Available at www.aamc.org/download/102340/data/aibvol6no4.pdf. Accessed March 11, 2012.

25. Liaison Committee on Medical Education. The Role of Students in the Accreditation of Medical Education Programs in the US and Canada. Appendix C. Sample student opinion survey for the independent student analysis. Washington, DC: LCME, 2011: 21–4. Available at www.lcme.org/roleofstudents2011.pdf. Accessed March 26, 2012.

26. Association of American Medical Colleges. The Medical School Graduation Questionnaire (GQ). Available at www.aamc.org/data/gq/. Accessed March 26, 2012.

TRUTH TELLING AND DECEPTION

Ann E. Mills, Msc(Econ), MBA • Patricia H. Werhane, PhD

LEARNING OBJECTIVES

Upon completion of this chapter, participants will be able to:

1. Differentiate various forms of truth telling, omission, and deception.
2. Discuss ethical principles that support truth telling.
3. Discuss ethical and legal principles that oppose deception or withholding information.

LEARNING RESOURCES

Key chapters in Bernat's third edition—2, 3, 4, 14

Key relevant AAN documents available at www.aan.com/view/PECN

A

CLINICAL VIGNETTES

CASE 1

A neurologist strongly suspects that Howard, her 42-year-old male patient, has amyotrophic lateral sclerosis (ALS), but further tests are required to confirm the diagnosis. If he has ALS, it is likely that he will die within 2–5 years after inexorable decline of motor and bulbar function but preserved mental function. As the disease progresses, the patient will have to depend on healthcare professionals for treatment of the ALS and its symptoms to prolong his life. The patient has a wife and very young children. The neurologist is preparing to speak with her patient. Should she disclose her suspicion of ALS *before* the confirmatory testing has been completed?

CASE 2

Greta, who has been diagnosed with Alzheimer disease (AD), has mild symptoms, but her son and daughter have reported that she is increasingly having difficulty performing routine tasks such as washing her clothes and paying bills. Greta's husband died a few years ago from complications of AD, and she is being treated by the same neurologist who treated her husband. The patient and her family were devastated financially and emotionally by the stress of caring for her husband, but they have great faith in the neurologist's judgment and abilities. The patient and her children are desperate for a "cure" and have asked if the neurologist is aware of any clinical trials in which Greta can enroll.

Although the neurologist knows that a nearby teaching hospital is enrolling patients into a clinical trial of a new vaccine for AD, he has misgivings because it is similar to a vaccine that was associated with meningoencephalitis,[1] and he doubts that it will have a significant effect on the progression of Greta's AD. Should he tell the family about the vaccine trial?

CASE 3

Blake has had migraines for several years that are not changing in quality or frequency but respond readily to abortive therapy. He requests an MRI of his brain because his neighbor, who recently died from a brain tumor, also had headaches. Neither Blake's history nor his physical examination raises concern for a tumor, and the neurologist reassures him that a scan is not indicated, according to the AAN Practice Parameter for migraines.[2] The neurologist tells Blake that his insurance company will probably not approve the MRI for the indication of migraine, but Blake argues that he has been very anxious and losing sleep because of his worry and asks the neurologist to write "possible brain tumor" on the requisition form so that the insurance company pays for the scan that he wants. What should the neurologist do?

QUESTIONS FOR GROUP DISCUSSION

GETTING STARTED

1. Have you ever faced issues similar to those illustrated in these cases? If so, how did you react or respond? Have you ever deliberately omitted medical information in a conversation with your patient? What were your reasons?

ASSESSMENT

2. In each case, what are the relevant contextual factors? Who is affected by withholding information or deceiving the patient, the family, or the insurer?

3. How could disclosing or not disclosing medical information change the physician–patient relationship?

4. Could a conflict of interest or conflict of commitment influence what a physician chooses to disclose to a patient or family?

MORAL DIAGNOSIS

5. What ethical principles create a strong obligation to tell patients the truth? Would other principles or considerations mitigate this obligation?

(continued)

6. When discussing medical information with patients, what is the ethical distinction between withholding information and lying? Is it ever ethically permissible to withhold information from a patient? What is the ethical justification?
7. Does your institution have any relevant policies pertaining to truth telling, lying, or withholding information from patients? What can you do to find relevant policies?
8. Which professional organizations have established guidelines regarding truth telling in the physician–patient relationship?

GOAL SETTING, DECISION MAKING, AND IMPLEMENTATION
9. Describe how you would disclose important information to a patient or family. What actions are preferable in each of the cases?
10. If you needed help in deciding whether or how to disclose information, where could you obtain it?

COMMENTARY ON DISCUSSION QUESTIONS

GETTING STARTED

1. **Have you ever faced issues similar to those illustrated in these cases? If so, how did you react or respond? Have you ever deliberately omitted medical information in a conversation with your patient? What were your reasons?**

ASSESSMENT

2. **In each case, what are the relevant contextual factors? Who is affected by withholding information or deceiving the patient, the family, or the insurer?**

In Case 1, confirmatory tests for ALS have not been completed. Therefore, the diagnosis is not yet confirmed. If confirmed, however, the diagnosis and its treatment will significantly impact Howard and his young family.

In Case 2, Greta knows that she has AD, and based on previous experience with her husband's AD, she and her children are eager to slow or halt the progression of the disease and are willing to accept substantial risk to achieve that goal. The physician, who knows the patient and family well because he cared for her husband with AD, surmises that the patient will want to enroll in the vaccine trial if she learns of it. The physician's concern is that their emotional response to her AD may compromise their ability to consider the risks of participating in the study.

In Case 3, Blake asks the physician to lie about the diagnosis on the MRI requisition so that the insurance company will pay for it. The neurologist has already documented a normal neurologic examination and the diagnosis of migraine. The patient is not reassured and is very anxious.

3. How could disclosing or not disclosing medical information change the physician–patient relationship?

Premature disclosure of clinical suspicion before a diagnosis is confirmed, as in Case 1, has the potential to cause emotional distress for the patient and family, as the uncertainty associated with the wait for the test results can heighten fears. Should the test result be negative for ALS, the patient and family could be understandably upset with the physician for the unnecessary distress.

In Case 2, the wishes or preferences of Greta and her family are clear. They want the opportunity to enroll in a clinical trial of possible treatment of AD. If the physician withholds this information and the patient later learns of the vaccine trial, her trust in the physician will probably be damaged. It is quite likely that the family *will* be looking for AD trials and will learn of the vaccine trial independently.

In Case 3, if the physician chooses not to order an MRI with a false indication of possible brain tumor, the patient could feel that the physician has abandoned him or that the physician is uncaring. On the other hand, if the physician complies with the patient's request, the physician could feel a sense of compromised integrity.

4. Could a conflict of interest or conflict of commitment influence what a physician chooses to disclose to a patient or family?

The AAN Code of Professional Conduct, Section 5.2, states that "the neurologist must avoid practices and financial arrangements that would, solely because of personal gain, influence decisions in the care of patients. Financial interests of the neurologist that might conflict with appropriate medical care should be disclosed to the patient."[3] It is important to note that simply having a conflict of interest or commitment is not inherently unethical.[4] It only becomes unethical when one acts on that conflict in a way that violates acceptable rules for sound medical decisions, that jeopardizes professional judgment, or that causes harm to the patient.[5,6]

In Case 1, no conflict of interest is apparent. In Case 2, the physician has no conflict of interest in disclosing the vaccine trial to the patient and her family; however, if the physician were to have a financial interest either in referring the patient to the trial or in the vaccine itself, then the physician would have a conflict of interest that he is obligated to disclose to the patient and family. Section 8.2 of the AAN Code of Professional Conduct indicates that "the neurologist who is paid for treating patients in a clinical research project should inform the patient of any compensation the neurologist receives for the patient's participation."[5]

In most practice settings, a physician who refrains from ordering a test that is not clinically indicated has no conflict of interest. Thus, in Case 3, no conflict of interest is apparent. However, if the physician's

Bernat, 57–61, Ch. 3

payment were capitated by the insurance company, then a conflict of interest may be created by the placement of the physician's financial interests above the patient's health concerns. A more likely scenario exists for practices that own or have an ownership interest in an MRI facility. A financial conflict of interest exists if the physician orders an MRI and directs the patient to the MRI facility in which the physician has a financial interest without disclosing the interest to the patient and offering the option to obtain the MRI at a facility of the patient's choice.

MORAL DIAGNOSIS

5. **What ethical principles create a strong obligation to tell patients the truth? Would other principles or considerations mitigate this obligation?**

   The physician's primary fiduciary obligation is to the patient. Fiduciary relationships entail trust and honesty and require that the fiduciary (the physician) act in good faith and in the best interests of the beneficiary (the patient).[7] The AAN Code of Professional Conduct, Section 1.2 states that "the neurologist has an ethical duty to consider the interests of the patient first."[8] Fiduciary obligations should not be confused with compassion, kindness, or loyalty to one's colleagues or institution. For example, in Case 1, compassion and empathy may be sufficient justification to delay telling the patient that ALS is suspected, but once the test results are known, compassion and empathy for the patient would not justify withholding the information from the patient.[9,10]

   Bernat, 51, Ch. 3

   The physician's responsibility to the patient also includes an obligation to try to prevent harm, an argument that might be advanced to justify a decision in Case 2 to not tell the patient and her family about the AD vaccine trial. Considering that the patient and family have asked directly about a clinical trial, to withhold knowledge of a trial would be tantamount to a lie and would undermine the patient's autonomy.[11,12]

   Bernat, 9–11, Ch. 1

   Fiduciary obligations to the patient do not include falsifying records, as the patient in Case 3 is requesting. In fact, physicians have an equally strong obligation to respect and uphold the law.[13]

6. **When discussing medical information with patients, what is the ethical distinction between withholding information and lying? Is it ever ethically permissible to withhold information from a patient? What is the ethical justification?**

   Ethicists often distinguish between the forms of truth telling as (a) "full disclosure" of all that you know, believe, or have evidence for; (b) "omission," when one withholds factual information, one's prognosis, or opinion; and (c) lying or deception, when one knowingly tells falsehoods.[9]

Telling the truth depends, in part, on *knowing* the truth; therefore, one must be circumspect about sharing suspicions or intuitions with a patient before confirmatory test results are known. Of course, physicians will often signal concerns to their patients without necessarily divulging the suspected diagnosis, for example, by saying, "I'd like to get an EMG to help us understand the nature of your weakness." In Case 1, waiting for test results before disclosing a suspected diagnosis is not equivalent to withholding information; however, the physician has an obligation to ensure that the test results are received and reviewed so that the patient can be informed in a timely manner and be referred for appropriate treatment or additional testing.

It is argued that some situations exist in which disclosure of a diagnosis might result in psychological or emotional harm to the patient, thereby justifying withholding the diagnosis (known as *the therapeutic privilege*). Is this practice ever justified? In Case 1, an argument might be advanced that withholding information about the *confirmed* diagnosis of ALS would be justified to prevent emotional harm to the patient. However, doing so could prevent the patient from being referred for specialty care at an ALS clinic, which would harm the patient. From a more practical standpoint, it would be virtually impossible to prevent the patient from eventually learning of the diagnosis, as such information would be on medical records and insurance forms, and it would not be possible to prevent inadvertent disclosure of the diagnosis by other healthcare professionals involved in the patient's care. The use of the therapeutic privilege to justify withholding relevant medical information sets up a conflict in the physician–patient relationship, a relationship that relies on honesty and truthfulness. Some organizations, including the AMA, now hold the position that the therapeutic privilege cannot be ethically justified.[14]

Bernat, 38, Ch. 2

Physicians cannot and should not rely on the therapeutic privilege to withhold information from patients.[15]

Occasionally, patients clearly state that they do not wish to know details of their medical condition, and they assign decision-making authority to a family member or another surrogate.[16] In such circumstances,

Bernat, 92–1, Ch. 4

it may be ethically permissible to honor patients' requests and withhold information; however, this scenario is controversial.[17] Nevertheless, in most circumstances, patients should be given information about their condition.

In Case 3, to honor the patient's request to put the diagnosis of "possible brain tumor" on an MRI requisition, when the neurologist has already documented a normal neurologic examination and an established diagnosis of migraine, would put the neurologist at risk for charges of falsifying medical records. The patient's future insurability could also be at risk because of the appearance of the "possible brain tumor" diagnosis on the insurance records.

7. **Does your institution have any relevant policies pertaining to truth telling, lying, or withholding information from patients? What can you do to find relevant policies?**

In line with standards suggested by The Joint Commission,[18] many hospitals provide patients with a document about their rights and responsibilities.[19] Generally, these documents begin with a statement that patients have the right to know about their illnesses and proposed treatments and that they have the right to participate in the development of any plans of care. Many hospitals have additional policies that address ethical issues, and it can be helpful for practitioners to be familiar with these policies and with the institutional process for obtaining advice from an ethics committee.

8. **Which professional organizations have established guidelines regarding truth telling in the physician–patient relationship?**

Bernat, 9–11, Ch. 1

Bernat, 24, Ch. 2

Most professional organizations, including the AMA,[12] the American Hospital Association,[20] and the American Nurses Association,[21] as well as American tradition and law have addressed issues associated with patient autonomy, including information sharing or omission.[11] The position taken by these organizations is that the physician–patient relationship is based on trust, truth telling, and informed consent.[22] The AAN Code of Professional Conduct maintains that neurologists "should disclose information that the average person would need to know to make an appropriate medical decision,"[23] and although it makes no specific statement about truth telling or deception, the Code does indicate that neurologists should treat patients with "respect, honesty, and conscientiousness."[24]

GOAL SETTING, DECISION MAKING, AND IMPLEMENTATION

9. **Describe how you would disclose important information to a patient or family. What actions are preferable in each of the cases?**

Although styles and approaches to sharing information with patients abound, we offer the following recommendations:

- Gather and confirm all facts of the case and have the test results and medical records available so that, if necessary, they can be reviewed in response to any questions.
- Try to ascertain the social context of the case, such as family relationships, religious or cultural traditions, and community ties.
- Assess the patient's decision-making capacity and psychological state.
- Consider the institutional, professional, and legal constraints that must be considered for the particular situation.
- As much as possible, understand the patient's preferences so that they might be honored.

- Ensure that disclosure is timely.
- Allow enough time during the discussion to respond to concerns or fears of the patient and family, make recommendations, and answer questions associated with a plan of care.
- Ensure that disclosure takes place in an appropriate setting, with special attention to privacy.
- Ensure that meetings with the patient and family to discuss such issues are not interrupted.
- Use language that a patient can understand.
- Observe and be sensitive to the patient's responses. If it is clear that a patient does not understand current status and if a family member is not present, ask if a family member can be contacted.
- Avoid evasive language or omissions that may extend false hope or false pessimism.
- Ensure that the patient knows that support and help will be available throughout the course of the patient's illness.

In Case 1, it is ethically justifiable for the neurologist to defer telling the patient about the suspected ALS diagnosis until the test results are received. If the patient asks directly what the physician suspects, the physician can indicate the desire to delay the discussion until the test results are known, but if the patient is insistent, the physician should provide an answer about the clinical suspicion that is both truthful and compassionate and emphasizes that the diagnosis is not confirmed until the test results are known.

Nothing in Case 2 justifies withholding information about the vaccine trial, and the physician should provide the information to the patient and her family. However, the physician may also caution her against enrolling in the trial, explaining his understanding of the potential risks.

In Case 3, the physician has no obligation to accommodate the patient's request, but other issues must still be addressed. The patient is not sleeping well because of worry about a brain tumor. The physician is confident that the patient does not have a brain tumor and could thus reassure the patient; however, as this strategy has not been effective thus far, the physician could suggest that the patient return in a few weeks for re-evaluation.

10. If you needed help in deciding whether or how to disclose information, where could you obtain it?

The most frequently cited reason for an incomplete or misleading disclosure is inadequate communication, which can occur because of the many components of the healthcare system, the teams that function within the system, inadequate documentation of pertinent information, or poor communication skills on the part of an individual. However, a physician might find herself in a situation in which it is clear that a patient or family is not being told what they need to know in a timely fashion.

If delays are occurring (for instance, if the healthcare organization is asking physicians and others to withhold information from the family for legal reasons or because it is not clear who has the authority to tell the family members), then a physician might seek the advice of the ethics consultation service.

Each of the 3 cases presented contains a possible role for an ethics consultation, e.g., to help the physician to work through the ethical issues of the case and choose the best course of action or to provide a formal consultation, as might be needed if a family were insisting that a patient not be informed about a medical diagnosis.

KEY POINTS

- Fiduciary relationships entail trust and honesty and require that the fiduciary (the physician) act in good faith and in the best interests of the beneficiary (the patient).
- The use of the therapeutic privilege to justify withholding relevant medical information sets up a conflict in the physician–patient relationship, a relationship that relies on honesty and truthfulness.
- Patients have the right to be told the truth about their condition, illness, and plan of care.

KEY WORDS

Full disclosure—(in truth telling) telling all that is known, believed, or evidenced.
Lying or Deception—knowingly telling falsehoods.
Omission—withholding factual information, one's prognosis, or opinion.

ACKNOWLEDGMENTS

Donna Chen, MD, and Brad Worrall, MD, supplied 2 cases for this chapter. In addition, we are grateful for their advice and comments in the preparation of this manuscript.

REFERENCES

1. Orgogozo JM, Gilman S, Dartiques JF, et al. Subacute meningoencephalitis in a subset of patients with AD after AB42 immunization. Neurology 2003; 61:46–54.
2. Silberstein SD. Practice parameter: Evidence-based guidelines for migraine headache (an evidence-based review). Neurology 2000; 55:754–62.
3. American Academy of Neurology. Code of Professional Conduct. Section 5.2, Avoidance and Disclosure of Potential Conflicts. [*PECN* appendix document A and available at www.aan.com/view/PECN]
4. Bernat, 57–61, Ch. 3.
5. American Academy of Neurology. Code of Professional Conduct. Section 8.2, Disclosure of Potential Conflicts. [*PECN* appendix document A and available at www.aan.com/view/PECN]

6. Spencer EM, Mills AE, Rorty MV, Werhane PH. *Organization Ethics in Health Care.* New York: Oxford University Press, 2000:73–6.
7. Bernat, 51, Ch. 3.
8. American Academy of Neurology. Code of Professional Conduct. Section 1.2, Fiduciary and Contractual Basis. [*PECN* appendix document A and available at www.aan.com/view/PECN]
9. Boyle RJ. Communication, truth-telling and disclosure. In: Fletcher JC, Spencer EM, Lombardo PA, eds. *Fletcher's Introduction to Clinical Ethics, 3rd ed.* Fredericksburg, MD: University Publishing Group, 2005:99–116.
10. Marzanski M. Would you like to know what is wrong with you? On telling the truth to patients with dementia. J Med Ethics 2000; 26:108–13.
11. Bernat, 9–11, Ch. 1.
12. American Medical Association. Council on Ethical and Judicial Affairs. Code of Medical Ethics. Opinion 10.01, Fundamental Elements of the Patient–Physician. Available at www.ama-assn.org/ama/pub/physician-resources/medical-ethics/code-medical-ethics/opinion1001.page? Accessed March 20, 2012.
13. American Academy of Neurology. Code of Professional Conduct, Section 4.2, Respect for Agencies and the Law. [*PECN* appendix document A and available at www.aan.com/view/PECN]
14. American Medical Association. Council on Ethical and Judicial Affairs. Code of Medical Ethics. Opinion 8.082, Withholding Information from Patients (therapeutic privilege). Available at www.ama-assn.org/ama/pub/physician-resources/medical-ethics/code-medical-ethics/opinion8082.page? Accessed March 1, 2012.
15. Bernat, 38, Ch. 2.
16. Bernat, 92–7, Ch. 4.
17. Pellegrino ED. Is truth telling to the patient a cultural artifact? JAMA 1992; 268:1734–5.
18. Joint Commission on Accreditation of Healthcare Organizations: Individual rights and organization ethics. In: Fletcher JC, Spencer EM, Lombardo PA, eds. *Fletcher's Introduction to Clinical Ethics, 3rd ed.* Fredericksburg, MD: University Publishing Group, 2005:329–38, Appendix 1.
19. University of Virginia. Patient rights and responsibilities. Available at www.healthsystem.virginia.edu/medcntr/depts/patient-ed/pt-rights.html. Accessed March 20, 2012.
20. American Hospital Association. Privacy Policy. Available at www.aha.org/help/privacy.shtml. Accessed March 20, 2012.
21. American Nurse Association Committee on Ethics. Code of Ethics for Nurses, with Interpretive Statements. Section 1.4 maintains the right of patients to self-determination. Available at www.nursingworld.org/MainMenuCategories/EthicsStandards/CodeofEthicsforNurses/Code-of-Ethics.pdf. Accessed March 1, 2012.
22. Bernat, 24, Ch. 2.
23. American Academy of Neurology. Code of Professional Conduct, Section 1.4, Informed Consent. [*PECN* appendix document A and available at www.aan.com/vlew/PECN]
24. American Academy of Neurology. Code of Professional Conduct, Section 4.1, Respect for the Patient. [*PECN* appendix document A and available at www.aan.com/view/PECN]

4 CONFIDENTIALITY

Don W. King, MD, JD, FAAN
Michael A. Williams, MD, FAAN

LEARNING OBJECTIVES

Upon completion of this chapter, participants will be able to:

1. Describe the ethical and legal issues involved in maintaining the confidentiality of patient information.
2. Define the ethical and legal issues that arise when it becomes necessary to disclose confidential patient information.
3. Identify the steps used to resolve the conflict between one's duty to maintain patient confidentiality and one's duty to warn others of risks.

LEARNING RESOURCES

Key chapters in Bernat's third edition—3
Key relevant AAN documents available at www.aan.com/view/PECN

A J K

CLINICAL VIGNETTES

CASE 1

A 75-year-old gentleman with complex partial seizures comes to the office for a follow-up visit. Each seizure, which consists of staring spells and mouthing movements, lasts 30–60 seconds. The patient has had no generalized tonic-clonic seizures. When the diagnosis was first made, the neurologist discussed the risks of driving and the state laws that govern driving and epilepsy. The patient agreed to refrain from driving until he had been seizure-free for at least 3 months. At his previous visit, the patient reported that he was tolerating the medication well but was having approximately 3 seizures per month. The neurologist increased the anticonvulsant dose and again counseled the patient to refrain from driving.

At the present visit, the patient states that the frequency of his seizures has improved. He has had only 2 seizures in the past 3 months and, as a result, has resumed driving. He states that because many of his friends need him to drive for errands and appointments, it is essential for him to drive. He asks the neurologist to keep all information about his condition strictly confidential and, specifically, not to tell his grown children, who live nearby.

CASE 2

A neurologist's nurse receives a telephone request for medical records from the nurse of another physician who is treating one of the neurologist's patients. The neurologist's nurse insists that it would be a violation of both ethical principles and HIPAA for the records to be released without the patient's consent. The requesting physician's nurse becomes upset at this response, and the nurse turns to the neurologist and asks, "Am I correct that I can't send the information without the patient's okay?"

CASE 3

A neurologist is treating a local elected official who was hospitalized following a seizure that occurred during a public event. The event was covered by the media, and as a result, the seizure and hospitalization are public knowledge. An internist colleague who was not involved in the patient's care tells the neurologist that she accessed the official's electronic medical record, and the MRI showed a large frontal meningioma. The hospital has a clearly stated policy that only professionals with a need to know should access medical records.

QUESTIONS FOR GROUP DISCUSSION

ASSESSMENT
1. What ethical duties does a physician have to maintain a patient's confidentiality?
2. What legal duties does a physician have to maintain a patient's confidentiality?
3. In what circumstances may a physician ethically breach a patient's confidentiality?
4. In what circumstances does the law require a physician to breach a patient's confidentiality?

MORAL DIAGNOSIS
5. What are the ethical issues in each case?
6. What factors should be considered when choosing whether to breach a patient's confidentiality?
7. What options are available in each case?
8. What factors should one consider in choosing the best option?

GOAL SETTING, DECISION MAKING, AND IMPLEMENTATION
9. In Cases 1 and 2, should the neurologists breach the patients' confidentiality?
10. In Case 3, how should the neurologist respond to a colleague's breach of patient confidentiality?

(continued)

EVALUATION
11. What type of follow-up should the physician schedule for the patient in Case 1?
12. What responsibility does the physician have to ensure that the patient in Case 1 is not driving?

COMMENTARY ON DISCUSSION QUESTIONS

ASSESSMENT

1. What ethical duties does a physician have to maintain a patient's confidentiality?

Bernat, 52–3, Ch. 3

Physicians have an ethical duty to maintain their patients' confidentiality because of the special relationship that physicians have with their patients.[1-4] To enable physicians to provide care, patients frequently disclose personal information that they would not disclose to anyone else, and they allow physicians to examine them in ways that they would not tolerate from others. The duty of confidentiality includes both maintaining the security of medical records and refraining from disclosing patient information to unauthorized persons.

Patients must be able to trust that physicians will limit the disclosure of personal information to those situations in which disclosure is medically necessary or legally required. Inappropriate disclosure of personal health information may be embarrassing and, in some situations, harmful. For example, disclosure that a person has epilepsy, as in Case 1, may have a harmful effect on a person's personal life or employment. In addition, if patients cannot trust physicians to maintain confidentiality, patients are less likely to seek medical care and may not reveal information that would be necessary for quality patient care.[5]

The AAN Code of Professional Conduct, Section 1.2, states that a neurologist has a duty "…to respect patients' autonomy, confidentiality, and welfare,"[6] and Section 2.3 states that "the neurologist must maintain patient privacy and confidentiality. Details of the patient's life or illness must not be publicized."[1] Similarly, the AMA Principles of Medical Ethics, Section IV, states that "a physician shall respect the rights of patients . . . and shall safeguard patient confidences and privacy within the constraints of the law."[7]

Bernat, 52–3, Ch. 3

In addition, physicians have an ethical duty to refrain from accessing information about patients if they do not have a need to know the information.[4] Neither the fact that a patient is an elected official nor the fact that the elected official's seizure occurred in public is justification for a physician or hospital employee to look at a patient's medical records, unless the physician or employee has a need to know the information.

Finally, an important tenet of professionalism is the duty to "abide by high ethical standards," which includes a "duty to sanction colleagues whose conduct violates ethical or other professional norms."[8] Similarly, Section 6.3

of the AAN Code of Professional Conduct states that "neurologists should not knowingly ignore a colleague's...professional misconduct."[9]

2. What legal duties does a physician have to maintain a patient's confidentiality?

Physicians also have a legal duty to maintain patient confidentiality.[10–13] In response to lawsuits, many state courts have found physicians liable for disclosing patients' health information.[11] In addition, the US Congress and many state legislatures have passed statutes that require confidentiality for specific conditions such as HIV/AIDS and alcohol or drug abuse.[11] Finally, based on authorization granted by HIPAA, the US Department of Health and Human Services has developed detailed regulations that govern the privacy (Privacy Rule) and security (Security Rule) of personal health information.[14,15]

Bernat, 52–3, Ch. 3

HIPAA regulations are complex and frequently misunderstood.[4] For example, in Case 2, the neurologist's nurse incorrectly believes that a patient's written authorization is required before releasing records for patient care. In fact, HIPAA regulations specifically state that "protected health information" may be shared with another healthcare provider without the patient's consent *for the purposes of treatment*.[16]

At the same time, the Privacy Rule does allow a physician's office or a hospital to have a higher standard, stating, "A covered entity is permitted, *but not required* [emphasis added], to use and disclose protected health information, without an individual's authorization" for the purpose of treatment.[17] As a result, a neurologist may decide to require written authorization before releasing patient records. However, if the neurologist decides to require written authorization, it would be wise for the neurologist to make an exception in case of an emergency.

Finally, sometimes a neurologist may have a legal duty to report a colleague who accesses medical information inappropriately. Inappropriate access of patient information, as in Case 3, represents a potential liability for the hospital if such misconduct becomes widespread. In 2011, the University of California-Los Angeles Health System was fined more than $850,000 because "...employees repeatedly and without permissible reason looked at the electronic protected health information" of celebrity patients.[18]

3. In what circumstances may a physician ethically breach a patient's confidentiality?

Although a physician's primary responsibility is to his or her patient, occasional situations arise in which a physician faces a conflict between 2 ethical duties—a conflict sometimes called an *ethical dilemma*. For example, a physician caring for a patient with epilepsy, as in Case 1, may occasionally face a conflict between the duty to maintain confidentiality and the duty to protect third parties known to be at imminent risk of harm because of the physician's patient.[19] The duty to warn others

Bernat, 64–6, Ch. 3

Bernat,
64–6,
Ch. 3

arises from a physician's general duty to prevent harm to others and from a physician's professional duty to protect the safety and improve the health of all members of society.[3,19] Thus, to prevent harm to another person, a physician may sometimes ethically disclose specific, limited information about a patient.[2–4,19,20]

4. In what circumstances does the law require a physician to breach a patient's confidentiality?

Laws vary from state to state. However, a number of state courts have held that if, while caring for a patient, a physician or other health professional becomes aware that the patient poses a risk to a specific, identified third party, the professional has a legal duty to warn that third party of the risk. In a 1976 case, Tarasoff v. Regents of the University of California, a patient told a psychologist of his plans to kill his girlfriend, whom the patient identified by name. Even though the psychologist notified the police, the patient later carried out his plans.[21] The victim's parents sued the psychologist, and the court held that the psychologist had a duty not only to inform authorities, but also to warn a potential victim of the imminent risk of harm.

In addition to a physician's duty to warn, federal and state laws require a physician to report certain conditions (e.g., substance abuse and some sexually transmitted diseases) to appropriate authorities, regardless of the patient's wishes.[11] Courts also have held that physicians have a legal duty to warn a patient's spouse of certain risks[22] and to "protect the public" from the dangers of a patient with uncontrolled epilepsy who continues to drive.[23]

As of 2012, 7 states (California, Delaware, Maine, Nevada, New Jersey, Oregon, and Pennsylvania) required treating physicians to report a patient's epilepsy to the state's department of motor vehicles (DMV).[24,25] However, most states do not mandate the reporting of epilepsy, and in most states, if a physician reports a patient's epilepsy to the appropriate authorities in good faith, the physician is not liable for violating confidentiality.

The HIPAA Privacy Rule contains a number of mandatory and permissible exceptions to the duty of confidentiality.[26] For example, physicians must disclose certain health information if the patient requests that it be disclosed or if the US Department of Health and Human Services requests the information to monitor regulation compliance. In addition, the Privacy Rule permits physicians to disclose information without fear of liability if disclosure is necessary for treatment, payment, or healthcare operations.

MORAL DIAGNOSIS

5. What are the ethical issues in each case?

In Case 1, the duty of confidentiality to one's patient conflicts with the duty to warn others of potential harm. Thus, the primary issue is, should the confidentiality of the patient be breached in an attempt to prevent harm to the patient, his family and friends, and other unidentified persons?

In Case 2, the primary issues are (a) is the need for the patient's medical records for patient care (i.e., beneficence) sufficient to override the patient's interests in privacy and confidentiality? and (b) is the potential harm from a delay that results from requiring signed authorization (i.e., non-maleficence) sufficient to override the patient's interests in privacy and confidentiality?

In Case 3, the primary ethical issue is, how should a neurologist handle a colleague's inappropriate access of a patient's medical record?

6. What factors should be considered when choosing whether to breach a patient's confidentiality?

Bernat, 52–3, Ch. 3

A physician should consider a number of factors in determining whether to breach a patient's confidentiality.[3,4] Potential factors include the probability and severity of harm that would occur to either the patient or other persons if confidentiality *is not* breached, the probability of preventing the harm to others through disclosure, the severity of harm to the patient if confidentiality *is* breached, the policies of the institution in which one practices, guidelines from professional organizations, and applicable state and federal laws.

To determine the probability and severity of harm, knowledge of clinical studies is often necessary. For example, with respect to Case 1, Taylor and Chadwick found that drivers with epilepsy had no greater risk of accidents than did drivers without epilepsy.[27] However, drivers with epilepsy had an approximate 40% greater risk of accidents that resulted in serious physical injury. Krauss et al. compared patients with epilepsy who had had seizure-related automobile accidents to patients with epilepsy who had not.[28] They found that drivers who had had seizure-free intervals greater than 12 months and those who had reliable auras before their seizures had a lower risk of seizure-related accidents than did drivers with epilepsy who did not have these features.

In addition, evidence based guidelines, such as those developed by the AAN, the American Epilepsy Society, and the Epilepsy Foundation of America, should be considered.[24,29] These guidelines recommend that patients with epilepsy not operate motor vehicles until they have been seizure-free for at least 3 months. The guidelines also recommend that if a patient refuses to report the information and the patient poses a threat to others by continuing to drive, states should allow physicians the option of reporting such a patient's epilepsy to the DMV without fear of liability. Finally, physicians must consider the laws of the state in which the patient is licensed to drive. Most states prohibit individuals with epilepsy from driving until they have been free of seizures for some designated period of time.[28,30,31]

In Case 2, the neurologist must consider the benefit to the patient of disclosing the medical records to the requesting physician against the harm that may result from disclosure of such information. In Case 3, the neurologist should consider both the hospital's policy on privacy and confidentiality and the national standards for professionalism and ethics.

7. **What options are available in each case?**

A neurologist can approach Case 1 in a number of ways. Initially, the neurologist could discuss with the patient the potential danger that continued driving poses to both the patient and to others. After a complete discussion of the risks, most patients will agree to refrain from driving until the seizures are controlled. If the patient voluntarily refrains from driving, a conflict no longer exists between the physician's duty of confidentiality and the duty to prevent harm to others. However, if the patient has recurrent seizures and continues to drive, or if the neurologist cannot be certain that the patient is not driving, the following options are available: (a) preserve the patient's confidentiality; (b) notify the DMV, which can suspend the patient's driver's license; (c) notify the patient's children, who may be able to prevent the patient from driving; or (d) notify the patient's friends to warn them of the risk of riding with the patient. Depending on the law in the state where the patient is licensed to drive, some of these options may not be available.

In Case 2, the neurologist could correctly tell the nurse that sending the medical records to the treating physician is both ethically and legally permissible, provided that the nurse is reasonably certain that the caller is from the physician's office. The neurologist could also tell the nurse to ask for a faxed request for the records that can be attached to the neurologist's patient record, documenting the request for the records and its purpose.

In Case 3, the neurologist could decide to do nothing related to this matter, talk directly with the colleague concerning the inappropriate access of patient information, or inform the hospital of a potential breach of hospital policy.

8. **What factors should one consider in choosing the best option?**

In Case 1, a number of questions must be considered, including (a) which option is most likely to prevent harm to others? (b) which option (violating the patient's confidentiality or restricting the patient's driving and mobility) is least likely to harm the patient? and (c) which option complies with the institutional policies, professional guidelines, and laws of the state in which one is practicing?[3,4,19]

Bernat, 52–3, Ch. 3

Bernat, 64–6, Ch. 3

In Case 2, the neurologist should consider the benefit to patients when records are shared expeditiously with other health professionals for the purposes of treatment, as opposed to the small and unlikely risk that doing so would compromise patient confidentiality.

In Case 3, the neurologist should consider whether the colleague's breach was a one-time event or something that occurs frequently, the potential harm to the patient and to the hospital if inappropriate access of medical records becomes widespread, and the potential harm to the relationship with a colleague if it becomes necessary to report the colleague's violation of patient confidentiality.

GOAL SETTING, DECISION MAKING, AND IMPLEMENTATION

9. In Cases 1 and 2, should the neurologists breach the patients' confidentiality?

A physician's first duty is to the patient, and breaching confidentiality carries a risk of seriously damaging a physician–patient relationship and of harming patient care. In Case 1, it is essential that the physician advise the patient that continued driving poses a serious risk of harm to himself, to those who ride with him, and to others. It may be helpful to discuss other options for transportation and to describe how other patients with epilepsy have managed the loss of driving privileges. The physician should also discuss the state laws that are related to epilepsy and driving and should advise the patient that he may face liability if he has a seizure-related accident after being warned against driving. This discussion should be documented in the chart. In most cases, patients will agree to stop driving until they have been seizure-free for the period applicable in their state.

In addition, a neurologist has both an ethical and legal duty to notify a third party of potential danger if a patient poses a risk to a third party. Because the patient in Case 1 is not seizure-free and drives frequently for other people, the probability that continued driving would cause harm to others is significant. Because the patient is retired and family members live nearby, the potential harm to the patient from not driving is less than if he were the sole support of a family and had no other options for transportation. Also, disclosing the information to either the patient's children or the DMV is likely to be very effective in preventing the patient from driving until he is no longer a threat to others. Based on each of these considerations, if the patient will not willingly refrain from driving, breaching his confidentiality is ethically permissible.

If the neurologist decides to breach the patient's confidentiality, it is important to discuss the matter with the patient and explain the reason. The patient may prefer that the neurologist notify his children rather than the DMV. If the neurologist lives in a state that does not require reporting of a patient with epilepsy, this may be a viable option. Also, if the children are able to provide transportation, the patient may be more willing to refrain from driving. However, if notifying the children does not result in the restriction of driving, notifying the state may be necessary.

The neurologist also could consider notifying the patient's friends. However, notifying the family or the DMV is more likely to completely eliminate the risk of harm to others, and attempting to notify all potential victims would be impossible. A duty to notify a potential victim arises primarily when a specific, identified victim is at risk.

In Case 2, as long as the neurologist knows that the requesting physician is seeing the patient whose records are being requested and unless the patient has specifically requested that records not be sent, a significant ethical issue does not really exist. Sending records to referring physicians is standard practice, and the probability of benefit to the patient is greater than the risk of harm from disclosing the information without written authorization. Also, the harm from delaying the disclosure of the information to the treating physician is likely to be greater than any benefit to the patient from withholding the information.

10. In Case 3, how should the neurologist respond to a colleague's breach of patient confidentiality?

Case 3 is more difficult. Because discussion of cases among physician colleagues is very helpful for patient care, patient information often becomes widespread among physicians. However, it is a breach of professional ethics to look up information about a specific patient, unless there is a need to know the information. If it is clear that the colleague specifically looked up the information out of curiosity, the ethically preferable approach would be to inform the colleague that his or her actions represent a breach of professional ethics and a violation of hospital policy. Depending on the emphasis that the hospital has placed on similar breaches, it may be worthwhile to work with the hospital to help educate members of the medical staff concerning the importance of refraining from accessing the medical records of a patient if the physician is not involved in that patient's care. If a colleague repeatedly violates the policy, it may become necessary to report the colleague to the hospital.

EVALUATION

11. What type of follow-up should the physician schedule for the patient in Case 1?

In Case 1, the physician would undoubtedly schedule follow-up visits to reassess the occurrence of seizures and medication side effects. If the patient continues to have seizures, the physician should continue to counsel the patient concerning the risks to himself and to others of continued driving. As noted earlier, it may be helpful to talk with the patient concerning ways to deal with his transportation problems. If the patient continues to drive while having seizures, additional steps may be necessary to prevent harm to the patient and to others.

12. What responsibility does the physician have to ensure that the patient in Case 1 is not driving?

Although the neurologist has a clear duty to inquire about driving and to warn both a patient and potential victims concerning the risks of continued driving, the neurologist has no ethical or legal duty to investigate or monitor whether a patient is driving or whether a patient is taking appropriate precautions.

KEY POINTS

■ Physicians owe patients an ethical duty of confidentiality because of the special relationship they have with their patients.

■ Although rare, situations do occur in which a physician's duty to maintain confidentiality conflicts with a physician's duty to warn others of potential harm.

■ HIPAA regulations specifically state that for the purposes of treatment, "protected health information" may be shared with other healthcare providers without a patient's consent.

KEY WORDS

Confidentiality—the principle in medical ethics that the information a patient reveals to a physician or other health professional is private and has limits on how and when it can be disclosed to a third party.

Disclosure—the act of revealing private information to one who did not previously know the information.

Health Insurance Portability and Accountability Act (HIPAA)—act of the US Congress passed in 1996 that, among other things, authorized the Department of Health and Human Services to develop regulations that govern the privacy and security of confidential health information.

REFERENCES

1. American Academy of Neurology. Code of Professional Conduct. Section 2.3, Confidentiality. [*PECN* appendix document A and available at www.aan.com/view/PECN]
2. American Medical Association. Council on Ethical and Judicial Affairs. Code of Medical Ethics. Opinion 5.05, Confidentiality. Available at www.ama-assn.org/ama/pub/physician-resources/medical-ethics/code-medical-ethics/opinion505.page? Accessed March 20, 2012.
3. Beauchamp TL, Childress JF. Professional–patient relationships. In: Beauchamp TL, Childress JF. *Principles of Biomedical Ethics, 5th ed.* Oxford: Oxford University Press, 2001.
4. Bernat, 52–3, Ch. 3.
5. Salinsky MC, Wegener K, Sinnema F. Epilepsy, driving laws, and patient disclosure to physicians. Epilepsia 1992; 33:469–72.
6. American Academy of Neurology. Code of Professional Conduct. Section 1.2, Fiduciary and Contractual Basis. [*PECN* appendix document A and available at www.aan.com/view/PECN]
7. American Medical Association. Principles of Medical Ethics, Section IV. Available at www.ama-assn.org/ama/pub/physician-resources/medical-ethics/code-medical-ethics/principles-medical-ethics.page? Accessed March 20, 2012.
8. Larriviere D, Beresford HR. Professionalism in neurology: The role of law. Neurology 2008; 71(16):1283–8.
9. American Academy of Neurology. Code of Professional Conduct. Section 6.3, Criticism of a Colleague. [*PECN* appendix document A and available at www.aan.com/view/PECN]
10. Beresford HR. Legal aspects of ethical dilemmas. In: Beresford HR. *Neurology and the Law: Private Litigation and Public Policy*. Philadelphia: F.A. Davis Co., 1998.
11. Furrow BR, Greaney TL, Johnson SH, et al. *Health Law, 2nd ed.* St. Paul: West Group, 2000, 4:95–143.

12. Hall MA, Bobinski MA, Orentlicher D. The treatment relationship: Confidentiality, consent, and conflicts of interest. In: Hall MA, Bobinski MA, Orentlicher D. *Health Care Law and Ethics, 6th ed.* New York: Aspen Publishers, 2003.
13. Rutberg MP. Medical records confidentiality. Neurol Clin 1999; 17(2):307–13.
14. Public Law 104–191; 110 Stat. 1936 (1996). Available at http://library.clerk.house.gov/reference-files/PPL_HIPAA_HealthInsurancePortabilityAccountabilityAct_1996.pdf. Accessed July 19, 2012.
15. 45 CFR Parts 160 and 164. Available at www.wedi.org/snip/public/articles/45cfr160&164.pdf. Accessed July 19, 2012.
16. Code of Federal Regulations. Title 45, Volume 1. (45 CFR 164.506, page 700–2). Public Welfare. Security and Privacy. Privacy of Individually Identifiable Health Information. Consent for uses or disclosures to carry out treatment, payment, or health care operations. Available at http://edocket.access.gpo.gov/cfr_2002/octqtr/45cfr164.506.htm. Accessed March 20, 2012.
17. US Department of Health & Human Services. Summary of the HIPAA Privacy Rule. Available at www.hhs.gov/ocr/privacy/hipaa/understanding/summary/index.html. Accessed March 20, 2012.
18. US Department of Health & Human Services. University of California settles HIPAA privacy and security case involving UCLA Health System facilities. Available at www.hhs.gov/news/press/2011pres/07/20110707a.html. Accessed March 20, 2012.
19. Bernat, 64–6, Ch. 3.
20. American Academy of Neurology. Code of Professional Conduct. Section 5.5, Conflicting Ethical Duties. [*PECN* appendix document A and available at www.aan.com/view/PECN]
21. Tarasoff v. Regents of the University of California, 17 Cal. 3d 425 (1976).
22. Bradshaw v. Daniel, 854 S.W. 2d 865 (Tenn. 1993).
23. Harden v. Dalrymple, 883 F. Supp. 963 (1995).
24. Bacon D, Fisher RS, Morris JC, et al. American Academy of Neurology position statement on physician reporting of medical conditions that may affect driving competence. Neurology 2007; 68:1174–7.
25. American Medical Association, National Highway Traffic Safety Administration. State licensing and reporting laws, Ch. 8. In: *AMA Physician's Guide to Assessing and Counseling Older Drivers, 2nd ed.* Chicago: AMA, 2010. Available at www.ama-assn.org/ama1/pub/upload/mm/433/older-drivers-chapter8.pdf. Accessed March 20, 2012.
26. 45 CFR § 164.502.
27. Taylor J, Chadwick D. Risk of accidents in drivers with epilepsy. J Neurol Neurosurg Psychiatry 1996; 60:621–7.
28. Krauss GL, Krumholz A, Carter RC. Risk factors for seizure-related motor vehicle crashes in patients with epilepsy. Neurology 1999; 52:1324–9.
29. American Academy of Neurology, American Epilepsy Society, and Epilepsy Foundation of America. Consensus statements, sample statutory provisions, and model regulations regarding driver licensing and epilepsy. Epilepsia 1994; 35:696–705.
30. Drazkowski JF, Fisher RS, Sirven JI. Seizure-related motor vehicle crashes in Arizona before and after reducing the driving restriction from 12 to 3 months. Mayo Clin Proc 2003; 78:819–25.
31. Berg AT, Engel J. Restricted driving for people with epilepsy. Neurology 1999; 52:1306–7.

SUGGESTIONS FOR FURTHER READING

American Medical Association, National Highway Traffic Safety Administration. *AMA Physician's Guide to Assessing and Counseling Older Drivers, 2nd ed.* Chicago: AMA, 2010. Available at www.ama-assn.org/ama/pub/physician-resources/public-health/promoting-healthy-lifestyles/geriatric-health/older-driver-safety/assessing-counseling-older-drivers.page. Accessed March 20, 2012.

5 RESPONDING TO MEDICAL ERRORS

Michael A. Williams, MD, FAAN

LEARNING OBJECTIVES

Upon completion of this chapter, participants will be able to:

1. Describe the differences between ethics-based and compliance-based approaches to patient safety and medical errors.
2. Outline essential steps in identifying and responding to medical errors.
3. Describe when and how to apologize to patients and families when a medical error occurs.

LEARNING RESOURCES

Key chapters in Bernat's third edition—2, 3, 5

Key relevant AAN documents available at www.aan.com/view/PECN

A   B   C

CLINICAL VIGNETTES

CASE 1

Keshawn Robinson, a 27-year-old postgraduate student with known epilepsy is brought to the ED for a generalized seizure that occurred in the classroom. When first seen by the neurologist, she is confused but improving. Her tongue was bitten, and she is wet from incontinence. A CT scan has already been performed. Her antiepileptic blood level is therapeutic. The neurologist is talking to the patient and her husband when suddenly another generalized seizure starts. The neurologist has the husband leave the room and asks the nurse to give IV lorazepam. When the nurse asks how much, the neurologist, who is used to 1 mL vials with 2 mg/mL solution, states, "Give one vial over 1–2 minutes. I'll be back right after I see her CT scan." The nurse takes a vial from the medication cart and administers it as instructed. The neurologist returns a moment later to find that the patient is apneic and unresponsive. She asks the nurse how much lorazepam he gave, and he holds up a 10 mL multiple-dose vial of 2 mg/mL solution and says, "One vial, just like you said." The neurologist groans and mutters, "You just gave her 10 times the dose. Let's get her intubated and up to the ICU." After the patient is transferred out of the ED, the nurse reports the medication error and its circumstances to the hospital's error-reporting system.

In addition to the ICU admission, the patient also requires another head CT to rule out the possibility of an intracranial event and continuous EEG monitoring to rule out subclinical seizures. The next day, the neurologist receives a call from the ICU, advising her that Keshawn has been extubated and will be transferred to the neurology service. She is then contacted by an administrator about the medication error and, when first asked, starts to blame the nurse for giving the wrong dose. When the administrator relates the nurse's report, the neurologist relents and acknowledges that she told him a dose of "one vial" and was away from the bedside when the dose was given. The administrator tells the neurologist that they must inform the patient and her husband of the error, to which the neurologist responds, "Are you nuts?! They'll sue us all for malpractice. Nobody needs to know. Patients with seizures get intubated all the time."

CASE 2

A new patient, Mrs. White, is referred to a neurologist for a lumbar puncture (LP) to evaluate CSF pressure for possible pseudotumor cerebri. Per practice protocol, the patient's weight, brain imaging scans, and laboratory results (i.e., PT, INR, CBC) are reviewed in advance, and the referring physician completes the lab requisitions for CSF testing. When the patient arrives for the outpatient LP, the neurologist explains to her the nature of the procedure, its rationale, risks, benefits, and alternatives. The patient indicates her understanding and, as she is getting ready to sign the consent form, asks whether her baclofen pump is a problem for the LP. The neurologist re-reviews the documentation sent over for the LP referral and finds no indication that the patient had the baclofen pump. Inspection of the back shows a healed midline lumbosacral scar at the level where the LP would normally be performed. The catheter is not palpable, and no images of the spine are available to show the entry level of the catheter in relation to the iliac crests. The neurologist steps out of the room to telephone the referring physician, who comments, "I wasn't aware that was an issue for the LP. Why can't you just go above or below the scar?"

CASE 3

A first-year neurology resident is on rotation in the ICU. A patient, James Cooper, is admitted to the neurosurgery service for a right thalamic hemorrhage with right-to-left shift, intraventricular extension, and obstructive hydrocephalus. The third-year neurosurgery resident comes to insert the intraventricular catheter (IVC) and offers to teach the neurology resident how to insert it, even though neurology residents do not perform this procedure in this hospital. The patient is comatose, with extension posturing on the left and flexion or possible localization on the right; however, because the patient has been fully draped for the IVC insertion, the motor deficits and posturing are not visible. While prepping the head for the procedure, the neurosurgery resident asks the neurology resident to retrieve the CT scan to determine an appropriate trajectory to insert the IVC. The neurology resident in error retrieves the scan of another patient, Jane Hooper, who was admitted the same evening with a similar left thalamic hemorrhage (i.e., on the opposite side) with left-to-right shift. The neurology resident turns the computer monitor so that they can see the scan from behind the head of the bed while inserting the IVC, but the patient's name is not clearly visible at that distance. Consequently, based on the displayed scan that shows the hemorrhage on the left, the 2 of them erroneously agree to insert the IVC on the wrong side. They both scrub for the procedure. After 5 failed attempts by the neurologist to find the ventricles, the neurosurgeon asks the neurologist to look at the scan again, and the neurologist immediately spots the error and tells the neurosurgeon. The neurosurgeon shrugs, "Well that happens sometimes. We'll just re-drape, and I'll insert it on the other side. This patient isn't going to have a good outcome anyway." The IVC is finally inserted, and when the family asks how the procedure went, the neurosurgeon tells them that it was difficult because of the size of the hemorrhage but does not tell them about the wrong-side procedure. The head dressing conceals the wrong-side attempted insertion site. Mr. Cooper's neurologic exam worsens, with bilateral extension. A CT scan shows that the hydrocephalus is decompressed; however, several obvious linear tracks are visible in the thalamus from the IVC attempts on the wrong side. The neurology resident insists that they need to tell the attending physician and then the family, and the neurosurgery resident responds, "No way! It's your fault anyway because you pulled up the wrong patient's scan, and you're the one who couldn't hit the ventricles. Nobody needs to know."

QUESTIONS FOR GROUP DISCUSSION

GETTING STARTED
1. Have you ever been involved in the care of a patient when a medical error occurred? How did you feel? Was the error reported to hospital leadership? Was the error disclosed to the patient and family?

ASSESSMENT
2. In each case, what is the patient's medical condition?
3. What are the relevant contextual factors of each case?
4. What are the needs of the patients as persons?
5. Are interests other than those of the patients involved?
6. Have all parties involved in the cases had an opportunity to be heard?

MORAL DIAGNOSIS
7. Identify and rank the range of relevant moral considerations in each case.
8. Identify any relevant institutional policies and national standards and guidelines that pertain to the case.

(continued)

GOAL SETTING, DECISION MAKING, AND IMPLEMENTATION

9. Consider ideas (hypotheses) for possible interventions to meet the needs of the patients and resolve the moral problems.
10. Implement plans of action.

EVALUATION

11. Might desirable changes in institutional policy, feasible changes in the clinical environment, or educational interventions help to prevent or resolve the moral problems posed by similar cases?

COMMENTARY ON DISCUSSION QUESTIONS

GETTING STARTED

1. **Have you ever been involved in the care of a patient when a medical error occurred? How did you feel? Was the error reported to hospital leadership? Was the error disclosed to the patient and family?**

It has been more than a decade since the Institute of Medicine published its report, "To Err is Human,"[1] which resulted in extensive media coverage, creation of Joint Commission Standards and patient safety committees, and establishment of countless policies with the intent of promoting patient safety and reducing the harm that results from medical errors. The AAN has a Patient Safety Committee and holds a Patient Safety Colloquium at its annual meeting. A new AAN Patient Safety Award that recognizes research or care improvement projects designed to meet The Joint Commission's National Patient Safety Goals was first presented in 2012.

The estimated direct cost (excluding indirect costs such as malpractice insurance premiums) of medical errors that harm patients in the US in 2008 was $17.1 billion, of which two-thirds was attributable to the top 10 errors (e.g., postoperative infection and pressure ulcers).[2] In 2012, The Joint Commission identified 15 patient safety goals for hospitals in 6 categories: (1) identify patients correctly, (2) improve staff communication, (3) use medicines safely, (4) prevent infection, (5) identify patient safety risks, and (6) prevent mistakes in surgery.[3] Even though the goals of reduced errors and patient safety are unassailable, the realization that errors will nonetheless occur is widely accepted. As a consequence, physicians, nurses, healthcare administrators, and other healthcare professionals (HCPs) bear the responsibility for responding to errors when they occur.

The HCPs involved in a medical error often feel like second victims and harbor guilt or shame.[4] Many are reluctant to disclose the error to patients or families, or they do not know how to do so.

ASSESSMENT

2. In each case, what is the patient's medical condition?

In the context of these cases, the patients' medical condition at the time of presentation is arguably less important than their medical condition after the medical error or procedural misadventure; however, this is not to suggest the baseline condition is irrelevant.

In Case 1, Mrs. Robinson was harmed by a medication error—an overdose of lorazepam. As a result, she was intubated, admitted to the ICU, had an additional CT, and continuous EEG monitoring. She was placed at risk of complications associated with intubation and ICU stay, the hospital length of stay was prolonged, and the costs of the hospitalization were increased. Fortunately, she recovered quickly and appears to have suffered no enduring harm.

In Case 2, Mrs. White was not harmed because the error was avoided, but this "near-miss" will result in the patient having to return on another day to have the LP performed. Thus, although no physical harm resulted from the near-miss, the patient was inconvenienced and will have to again mentally prepare herself for the procedure and miss another day of work.

In Case 3, Mr. Cooper's baseline condition is critical, with coma, a large intracerebral hemorrhage, and obstructive hydrocephalus. Although it might be tempting to claim, as the neurosurgeon did, that the patient "isn't going to have a good outcome anyway," the change in clinical condition from unilateral extension posturing to bilateral extension with CT evidence of injury from the IVC insertion on the wrong side is clearly evident that the patient was harmed. The patient's chances for recovery with predominantly unilateral deficits are now much reduced, and the bilateral injury will most likely result in a worse degree of impairment after recovery and may even result in a less robust recovery of consciousness.

3. What are the relevant contextual factors of each case?

Case 1 takes place in an ED, where patient condition can rapidly change and where the urgent administration of medication on the basis of verbal orders is common. Factors that contributed to the error include (a) the assumption on the part of the neurologist that all vials of lorazepam are the same (i.e., 1 mL vial of 2 mg/mL solution) and her stating the dose in an unclear fashion ("Give one vial"); (b) the failure of the nurse to clarify the dose before administering it and, possibly, his lack of knowledge regarding correct and incorrect dosages, as usually no more than 4 mg of lorazepam is administered IV; and (c) a pharmacy system that stocks multiple-dose vials in the ED, when a safer practice would be to have single-dose vials.

Case 2 takes place in a more controlled setting and involves an elective procedure to be performed by a neurologist in private practice. Appropriate screening and preparations for the LP were all followed.

However, the patient had a contraindication to the LP that had not been contemplated in the screening process and which the referring physician either did not anticipate as being problematic or did not think of at all.

Case 3 takes place in the ICU, where multiple patients may have similar conditions and one patient's condition or scan might easily be mistaken for that of another. Case 3 is also encumbered with a sense of urgency, as treatment of hydrocephalus with an IVC can prevent secondary injury to the brain. In addition, Case 3 takes place in a teaching setting, where residents are often eager to teach each other new skills and knowledge. In this instance, the teaching and learning are unsupervised and occur at night. Lastly, because the patient is both comatose and beneath surgical drapes for the procedure and because the CT scan is viewed from across the room, the patient identifiers and physical exam cues regarding the side of the hemorrhage are not present. The circumstances that led to this error match the so-called "Swiss cheese" scenario for medical errors in which a series of small individual errors or lapses line up in such a way that a major error can occur.[5]

The nature of an error is context-dependent. The Patient Safety Primer on Safety Culture published by the Agency for Healthcare Research and Quality (AHRQ) emphasizes, "In a just culture, the response to an error or near-miss is predicated on the type of behavior associated with the error, and not the severity of the event."[6] Several different behavioral categories can be found in error investigations:

- **Human error** occurs when individuals should have done something other than what they did, and the action that they took inadvertently caused or possibly caused an undesirable outcome.
- **Negligence** is the failure to exercise the skill, care, and learning expected of a reasonably prudent HCP.
- **Reckless conduct**, also known as gross negligence, involves a conscious disregard of a visible, significant risk.
- An **intentional rule violation** occurs when a person knowingly violates a rule while performing a task regardless of whether the rule violation is associated with risk taking.[7]

Examples of rule violations include taking shortcuts and ignoring required safety steps. The AHRQ Safety Culture Primer further explains, "A just culture focuses on identifying and addressing systems issues that lead individuals to engage in unsafe behaviors, while maintaining individual accountability by establishing zero tolerance for reckless behavior."[6] Cases 1 and 3 include examples of reckless behavior.

4. What are the needs of the patients as persons?

In Case 1, Mrs. Robinson and her family are unaware of the error, as it has not been disclosed to them yet. One could argue that they have no "need" to know about the error and that disclosing the error without a "need" could cause them unnecessary emotional turmoil and lack of trust in the hospital and the doctors and nurses involved in the error. However, as a result of the error, Mrs. Robinson was harmed and had additional tests, exposure to complications, and a prolonged hospital stay. Additionally, depending on the nature of her insurance, she may incur out-of-pocket expenses related to the error. Further, even though they may not realize it, the Robinsons, like all patients and families, expect and need physicians to meet all of their fiduciary responsibilities, which includes telling the truth and making reparations for harm.[8,9]

Bernat, 51, Ch. 3
Bernat, 67–9, Ch. 3

In Case 2, Mrs. White needs reassurance that her disclosure regarding her baclofen pump was helpful in preventing a potential error from occurring (as an LP without fluoroscopic guidance could result in damage to the intrathecal catheter by the LP needle) and, more likely than not, wants or needs an apology for the miscommunication that led to the near-error. Some patients may want or need an act of "service recovery," but few will ask for it outright. An excellent response would be to anticipate this need and offer, in addition to the apology, a refund of any copay that may have been paid and, perhaps, a parking pass for the inconvenience.

In Case 3, Mr. Cooper is comatose; however, his family needs accurate information regarding his condition, response to treatment, and prognosis. They need support and reassurance, and to make informed treatment decisions on the patient's behalf, they also need to know about the procedural misadventure that appears to have led to substantial injury to the patient that will adversely affect the outcome. Families in these situations want to know the truth when an error occurs, and they want assurances that an investigation will be conducted and that the hospital will take steps to prevent similar errors from occurring to other patients in the future. As in Case 1, the family also needs to be told about the error and should be made an offer of reparations.

5. Are interests other than those of the patients involved?

In Case 1, the neurologist's expressly stated interest is in avoiding a malpractice lawsuit from Mrs. Robinson. The hospital also has an interest in avoiding a malpractice lawsuit. However, its policy regarding error disclosure may be based on the presumption that by telling the truth about the error, the likelihood of a malpractice lawsuit is reduced and that the total costs to the hospital by offering reparations are lower than the costs involved in a lawsuit.[10] The hospital also has an interest in being seen as reputable, responsible, responsive, and truthful. The nurse and other staff involved in the error may have needs related to feelings of guilt regarding the error.[4]

In Case 2, the neurologist who was asked to perform the LP has an interest in preventing future errors from happening.

In Case 3, the neurosurgery and neurology residents may perceive an interest in preserving their reputations and avoiding embarrassment or disciplinary action for their errors. Fear of legal ramifications and the inexperience of residents with hospital culture and patient-safety efforts are among the most common barriers to resident engagement in those efforts.[11] It appears that the residents realize that their errors were acts of recklessness and intentional rule violation, as the neurosurgery resident wishes to conceal the act or blame it on the neurology resident, and the neurology resident feels the need to inform the attending physician. Each of these residents is now a so-called "second victim" of the medical error[4,12] and is susceptible to intense emotional response that can last for weeks or longer.

Moreover, in Case 3, the hospital and the residency program directors have an interest in investigating the cause of the error and creating policy or system changes to prevent such an error from recurring. Although errors in learning are inherent to the training of students and residents in medicine and are generally identified or addressed through appropriate supervision, errors in judgment by residents performing procedures independently and unsupervised could also be the result of poor policy or guidance from hospital leadership, in which case a system error exists in addition to the residents' error in judgment.

6. Have all parties involved in the cases had an opportunity to be heard?

In Case 2, Mrs. Rogers is aware of the near-miss, has had the opportunity to be heard, and will most likely have her needs met by the neurologist.

In Cases 1 and 3, the patients and families have not had an opportunity to hear the truth regarding the respective medical errors and, as a result, have not had the opportunity for their reaction to the error to be heard. The deliberate withholding of this information serves only to intensify any reaction the family may have when they eventually learn of the error and exacerbates the liability from the level of error in Case 1 or reckless misconduct in Case 3 to one of conspiracy or cover-up, which puts the hospital and all involved HCPs at even greater risk. In Case 3, the neurology resident has not had a chance to be heard and is in a serious bind because any disclosure of his own involvement in the error automatically implicates the neurosurgery resident, which sets up the potential for the neurology resident to be labeled by peers as disloyal or as a tattler.

MORAL DIAGNOSIS

7. Identify and rank the range of relevant moral considerations in each case.

In these 3 hypothetical cases, the facts of the errors have been clearly described. However, in actual cases, the nature of the circumstances is rarely as evident. The events must be investigated to determine whether an error occurred, whether the causes of the error are attributable to a so-called systems error, whether misconduct (i.e., negligence, recklessness, or rule violation) by a physician or other HCP contributed to the error, whether the patient was harmed by the error, and whether reparations should be made to the patient and family. Such investigations stem from the fiduciary relationships owed by physicians, nurses, other HCPs, and hospital leadership to patients, and from the supportive relationship that hospital leadership owes to physicians, nurses, and other HCPs who may be involved in errors.[8]

Bernat, 51, Ch. 3

As mentioned previously, distinguishing adverse events that are the result of misconduct from errors that are "true" errors that perhaps have contribution from the system or environment is an important moral consideration. The systems approach to analysis of medical errors and patient safety has rightly moved medicine away from a culture of blame and shame. Nevertheless, all HCPs possess individual responsibility and accountability for the creation of an environment that promotes patient safety.[9] A hospital's safety mission is to create a safe, protected environment for reporting and responding to errors. Less often appreciated is the responsibility of hospitals to ensure that all staff and leadership uphold their responsibility and accountability toward the safety mission, which means that circumstances exist (e.g., negligence or incompetence) in which disciplinary action is appropriate.[13]

Bernat, 67–9, Ch. 3

Although 2 of the 3 cases in this chapter illustrate misconduct as a contribution to error, most errors in hospitals are the result of systems issues rather than misconduct. Therefore, HCPs should feel comfortable participating in investigations of errors. However, a 2012 AHRQ survey of HCPs about their hospital's response to error showed that most HCPs "believe their organizations are still more interested in punishing missteps and enforcing hierarchy than in encouraging open communication and using adverse-event reports to learn what's gone wrong."[14,15]

The primary moral consideration in most medical errors, as shown in all 3 cases presented, relates to honesty and disclosure. In ethics, honesty is often described as the principle of truth telling, and in patient safety, it immediately raises the issue of disclosure. Honesty is applicable in the context of errors and patient safety in 2 ways: (a) the obligation to disclose errors to patients and their families if the errors involve immediate harm or could put the patient at risk of harm later and (b) honesty in safety reporting, prevention, and surveillance activities.

In Case 1, the primary moral considerations are whether to disclose the error to Mrs. Robinson and her family and whether the costs of the hospitalization should be forgiven. No justifiable reason supports concealment of the facts of the error from the patient and family. The physician will need support from the hospital through the disclosure process, and the physician has an obligation to participate in the investigation of the error. If the investigation confirms the errors as described in the case, the neurologist and nurse involved may merit disciplinary action.

In Case 2, the neurologist and the patient become aware of the near-miss error simultaneously. Here, although the neurologist has avoided blaming the referring physician for the error, one could argue that the referring physician made a human error, best described as a lapse in communication regarding the patient's baclofen pump.

In Case 3, the neurosurgery resident tells the neurology resident that they do not need to disclose the error, but the neurology resident feels otherwise. As in Case 1, no ethical or legal justification exists for deliberately not disclosing the error first to the attending physician and subsequently to the patient and family. Physicians are ethically obligated to take precautions to prevent harm to patients (i.e., nonmaleficence), and they are further bound by the physician–patient relationship to disclose the truth.[8,9] The question is when and how to disclose the error and to whom. In this instance, because the circumstances of the injury to the patient include multiple errors (failure to confirm that the identity of the patient and the scan match and inappropriate teaching of a neurosurgical procedure [IVC insertion] to a neurology resident without authorization or approval by the residency directors), many of which are known to be associated with wrong-side craniotomy,[16] the residents should first disclose the error to the attending physician, who can then consult with appropriate administrators or attorneys for guidance on formulating a plan of action to disclose the error and offer reparation to the patient's family. The neurology resident might argue that they disclose the error themselves directly to the family; however, evidence suggests that such disclosures are high-stakes conversations with families that should be conducted by a highly experienced HCP or administrator who should coordinate the disclosure with the hospital attorneys or risk-management department.

The reckless behavior and rule violation by the neurology and neurosurgery residents must be addressed. As described in Case 3, they bypassed important safeguards for patient identification, attempted to conceal the error from their supervisors, and were involved in unauthorized and unsupervised teaching of a neurosurgical procedure to a neurology resident. Combined, these represent serious lapses in judgment, negligence, and recklessness for which disciplinary action is warranted after appropriate investigation. A discussion of the nature of the disciplinary action is beyond the scope of this chapter; however, the discipline should be proportionate to the severity of the transgression and should include educating these residents to prevent their future misconduct. The residency program director may also need to respond by educating all of the residents regarding the risks associated with such misconduct.

8. **Identify any relevant institutional policies and national standards and guidelines that pertain to the case.**

As of 2012, nearly all hospitals, state and national medical societies, and specialty societies had endorsed efforts to promote patient safety, and nearly all hospitals had developed protocols for responding to

Bernat, 51, Ch. 3
Bernat, 67–9, Ch. 3

medical errors, investigating them, and disclosing them or apologizing to patients and families. The AAN provides numerous resources on its website in the area of patient safety.[17] The AHRQ Patient Safety Network website provides access to an extensive repository of resources and references in "The Collection," which the AHRQ truthfully (but not immodestly) describes as the "world's most robust collection of patient safety information."[18]

In regard to disclosure of errors and apology for errors, Section 4.1 of the AAN Code of Professional Conduct states that "the neurologist must treat patients with respect, honesty, and conscientiousness,"[19] which would support an obligation on the part of neurologists to disclose errors to patients. An overview of the legal and ethical issues involved in medical errors is provided in the syllabus for the course, "Practical Legal Issues for Neurologists," which was presented at the annual meeting of the AAN in 2012.[20] Additional detailed guidance regarding the legal and ethical issues in medical errors, disclosure, and apology can be found in the book *Sorry Works! 2.0.*[21]

GOAL SETTING, DECISION MAKING, AND IMPLEMENTATION

9. Consider ideas (hypotheses) for possible interventions to meet the needs of the patients and resolve the moral problems.

10. Implement plans of action.

The art and practice of disclosing errors to patients and families is complex. The book *Sorry Works! 2.0* distinguishes between expressions of empathy (i.e., saying "sorry"), disclosure, and apology.[21] Saying "sorry" or expressing empathy to the patient and family is always appropriate after an error or adverse event. A *disclosure* is a statement made to the patient, family members, or both to inform them that an error or event has occurred, and it should include an expression of empathy. Disclosure is always appropriate; however, because the initial disclosure generally occurs very soon after the error and before the investigation is complete, the status of an HCP's responsibility for the error is usually unknown, and an apology is not yet appropriate. An *apology* is a communication or disclosure that also expresses responsibility for the error. An apology should only be offered after investigation has shown that the standard of care has been breached and is causally related to the injury and that, therefore, the HCP or hospital is responsible for the error.[21]

The responses to questions 9 and 10 for Cases 1 and 3 are similar and will be discussed together. When an error occurs, the first task—always— is to take care of the patient. Once the patient is stable, the second task is to get help from a physician or nurse leader (preferably both). Then, the error must be investigated, which may take time. Important questions to ask are whether there was a departure from a standard of care and whether the patient was harmed. After the physician and nurse leader have met with appropriate administrators or members of the hospital committee for responding to errors, they should arrange to sit with the patient and family to discuss events. An investigation need not be completed by the time of the first meeting, as the delay would be so long that it would amount to little more than avoidance. It is perfectly acceptable—in fact, advisable—to state the known events, to describe that an investigation is ongoing, and to inform the patient and family that as more information becomes available, they will be updated.[22,23]

What are the Components of a Disclosure Conversation?

Conducted properly, the disclosure conversation consists of a number of components.[24–26] The persons who disclose should be highly skilled and in positions of responsibility. In teaching hospitals, this means the attending physician—and not the intern, resident, or fellow.[22] It is permissible for a trainee to observe such a conversation, but it is not appropriate to have a trainee conduct the conversation. Ideally, for hospital-based errors, a nurse (preferably, the nurse manager) should also be present. The conversation should be planned in advance, and advice can and should be obtained from the hospital counsel, an ethics consultant, or both. The principle of respect for persons engenders an obligation on the part of hospital leadership to provide physicians and nurses with the assistance necessary to respond to medical errors, investigate them, and disclose them to patients and families, which *Sorry Works! 2.0* describes as a formal "event management process."[21] *Event management* is a process in which "support can be given after an adverse event occurs in an effort to ensure that good communication and appropriate documentation occur and that patients and families are kept informed."[21]

The most important aspects of disclosure to patients and families are an honest and earnest expression of regret or empathy, an explanation of the facts and events as best as they are understood from the investigation, and a promise to investigate and prevent future errors.[21,24–26] In disclosing an error, staff members should be prepared for an emotional response from the patient and family. Anger and distrust are naturally occurring emotions in this context; it is usually best that the staff not respond to the emotions (and certainly not become defensive) and that, instead, they be supportive, understanding, and empathetic. Many of the same emotional-handling skills used in breaking bad news are necessary for disclosing errors.

Error disclosure is not a single event. Rather, it is a series of meetings and discussions with the family to update them on the patient's condition and the progress of the investigation. If the investigation ultimately reveals no breach in the standard of care and, thus, no responsibility or liability on the part of the HCP or hospital, the family should be informed and an apology should not be offered.[10,21] On the other hand, if the investigation reveals a breach in the standard of care and reveals responsibility for the error, as illustrated in Cases 1 and 3, then an apology should be offered. *Sorry Works! 2.0* maintains that an effective, meaningful apology has 4 basic elements:

a. Empathy or "sorry"
b. Admission of fault
c. Explanation of what happened and how it will be prevented from happening again
d. As necessary, an offer of compensation or some sort of fix to the problem that has been created[21]

EVALUATION

11. **Might desirable changes in institutional policy, feasible changes in the clinical environment, or educational interventions help to prevent or resolve the moral problems posed by similar cases?**

Most errors, once investigated, will lead to changes in institutional policy and practice. An investigation in Case 1 should look at practices related to verbal orders in the ED and ICU and at the pharmacy's practice of stocking multiple-dose vials. In Case 2, the neurologist may need to modify the screening procedures for LPs to ask specifically whether the patient has a baclofen pump, or perhaps more generally, whether the patient has had any surgical procedures or devices implanted that could affect the LP procedure.

An investigation in Case 3 should look to changes in policy regarding the teaching of neurosurgical procedures only to appropriate trainees and hospital procedures for time-outs and matching of patient identifiers on neuroimages to patient identifiers on the patient.

Nationally, evidence is accumulating that proper investigation, disclosure, apology, and remediation of errors is a best practice. Experience at the University of Michigan Health System (UMHS), which in 2001 began admitting fault and offering compensation to patients and families whenever an internal investigation revealed a medical error, shows that the total number of claims that resulted in lawsuit significantly diminished, that the time to resolution of cases fell from 1.36 to 0.95 years, and the average cost per lawsuit fell from $406,000 to $228,000.[10] UMHS also found that mean legal expenses decreased by 61%.[10] They suggest that because of their transparency, "patients (and their lawyers) may also be less likely to seek compensation if they believe that they are getting the 'real story' when UMHS denies that an error occurred. The UMHS's stance not to settle nuisance claims may also decrease the number of paid claims."[10] Similarly, the University of Illinois Medical Center at Chicago has preliminary evidence of "no increase in lawsuits and no increase in payouts from our self-insurance fund related to full disclosure."[27]

KEY POINTS

- A just culture focuses on identifying and addressing systems issues that lead individuals to engage in unsafe behaviors, while maintaining individual accountability by establishing zero tolerance for reckless behavior.
- Disclosure is always appropriate when an error occurs; however, because the initial disclosure generally occurs before the investigation is complete, the status of an HCP's responsibility for the error is usually unknown, and an apology is not yet appropriate.
- An apology should only be offered after investigation has shown that the standard of care has been breached and is causally related to the injury and that, therefore, the HCP or hospital is responsible for the error.

KEY WORDS

Apology—a communication or disclosure that also expresses responsibility for the error.

Disclosure—a statement made to a patient, family, or both to inform them that an error or event has occurred; it should include an expression of empathy.

Human error—occurs when individuals should have done something other than what they did, and the action that they took inadvertently caused or possibly caused an undesirable outcome.

Intentional rule violation—when a person knowingly violates a rule while performing a task, regardless of whether the rule violation is associated with risk taking.

Negligence—the failure to exercise the skill, care, and learning expected of a reasonably prudent HCP; i.e., the failure to recognize a risk that should have been recognized.

Reckless behavior—action that carries substantial and unjustifiable risk for an adverse event. A person who acts recklessly recognizes the risk but does not intend or expect the adverse consequence to occur. Recklessness entails a *conscious disregard* of a visible, significant risk.

NOTE

The content of this chapter borrows from the syllabus prepared for the course, "Practical Legal Issues for Neurologists," presented at the 2012 AAN Annual Meeting. The discussion has been modified. We wish to thank the AAN for permission to reuse the case.

REFERENCES

1. Kohn LT, Corrigan JM, Donaldson MS, eds. *To err is human: Building a safer health system*. Washington, DC: National Academy Press, 2000.
2. Van Den Bos J, Rustagi K, Gray T, et al. The $17.1 billion problem: The annual cost of measurable medical errors. Health Aff (Millwood) 2011; 30:596–603.
3. National Patient Safety Goals. Available at www.jointcommission.org/standards_information/npsgs.aspx. Accessed April 12, 2012.

4. Wu AW. Medical error: The second victim. The doctor who makes the mistake needs help too. BMJ 2000; 320:726–7.

5. Reason J. Human error: Models and management. BMJ 2000; 320(7237):768–70.

6. Agency for Healthcare Research and Quality. Patient safety primer: Safety culture. Available at www.psnet.ahrq.gov/printviewPrimer.aspx?primerID=5. Accessed April 12, 2012.

7. Marx D. *Patient Safety and the "Just Culture": A Primer for Health Care Executives.* New York: Trustees of Columbia University in the City of New York, 2001.

8. Bernat, 51, Ch. 3.

9. Bernat, 67–9, Ch. 3.

10. Kachalia A, Kaufman SR, Boothman R, et al. Liability claims and costs before and after implementation of a medical error disclosure program. Ann Intern Med 2010; 153:213–21.

11. Padmore JS, Jaeger J, Riesenberg LA, et al. "Renters" or "owners"? Residents' perceptions and behaviors regarding error reduction in teaching hospitals: A literature review. Acad Med 2009; 84(12):1765–74.

12. Scott SD, Hirschinger LE, Cox KR, et al. The natural history of recovery for the healthcare provider "second victim" after adverse patient events. Qual Saf Health Care 2009; 18(5):325–30.

13. Wachter RM, Pronovost PJ. Balancing "no blame" with accountability in patient safety. N Engl J Med 2009; 361:1401–6.

14. Sorra J, Famolaro T, Dyer N, et al. Hospital survey on patient safety culture: 2012 user comparative database report. Rockville, MD: Agency for Healthcare Research and Quality, 2012.

15. O'Reilly KB. Fear of punitive response to hospital errors lingers. Available at www.ama-assn.org/amednews/2012/02/20/prl20220.htm. Accessed February 22, 2012.

16. Cima RR. Wrong-site craniotomy. J Neurosurg 2010; 113(3):458–9.

17. American Academy of Neurology. Patient Safety. Available at www.aan.com/go/practice/patientsafety. Accessd April 11, 2012.

18. AHRQ Patient Safety Network. The Collection. Available at www.psnet.ahrq.gov/collection.aspx. Accessed April 12, 2012.

19. American Academy of Neurology. Code of Professional Conduct. Section 4.1, Respect for the Patient. [*PECN* appendix document A and available at www.aan.com/view/PECN]

20. Williams MA. Legal issues in medical errors, disclosure, and apology. Presented as a section in the course Practical Legal Issues for Neurologists at the 64th Annual Meeting of the American Academy of Neurology. New Orleans, LA, 2012.

21. Wojcieszak D, Saxton JW, Finkelstein MM. *Sorry Works! 2.0: Disclosure, Apology, and Relationships Prevent Medical Malpractice Claims.* Bloomington, IN: AuthorHouse, 2010.

22. Conway J, Federico F, Stewart K, et al. *Respectful Management of Serious Clinical Adverse Events, 2nd ed.* IHI Innovation Series white paper. Cambridge, MA: Institute for Healthcare Improvement, 2011.

23. Gallagher TH, Denham CR, Leape LL, et al. Disclosing unanticipated outcomes to patients: The art and practice. J Patient Saf 2007; 3:158–65.

24. Boyle D, O'Connell D, Platt FW, et al. Disclosing errors and adverse events in the intensive care unit. Crit Care Med 2006; 34:1532–7.

25. Massachusetts Coalition for the Prevention of Medical Errors. When things go wrong: Responding to adverse events. A consensus statement of the Harvard Hospitals. Available at www.macoalition.org/documents/respondingToAdverse Events.pdf. Accessed April 12, 2012.

26. Wojcieszak D, Banja J, Houk C. The Sorry Works! Coalition: Making the case for full disclosure. Jt Comm J Qual Patient Saf 2006; 32:344–50.

27. McDonald TB, Helmchen LA, Smith KM, et al. Responding to patient safety incidents: The "seven pillars." Qual Saf Health Care 2010; 19:e11.

6 GIFTS FROM INDUSTRY

Jacqueline J. Glover, PhD • Steven P. Ringel, MD, FAAN • Mark Yarborough, PhD

LEARNING OBJECTIVES

Upon completion of this chapter, participants will be able to:

1. Describe the ethical issues associated with accepting gifts from industry, including pharmaceutical companies, medical device manufacturers, and medical service companies.
2. Identify factors that can be used to determine whether accepting a particular gift from industry is ethically permissible or impermissible.
3. Describe current professional guidelines and standards for accepting gifts.
4. Apply a process of ethical analysis to cases that raise questions about appropriately accepting and declining various gifts from industry.

LEARNING RESOURCES

Key chapters in Bernat's third edition—1, 3, 19

Key relevant AAN documents available at www.aan.com/view/PECN

A   D   E   F

CLINICAL VIGNETTES

The medical director of an epilepsy-monitoring unit (EMU) in a regional medical center and 4 other neurologists are in a group practice that treats patients of all ages who have epilepsy. Consider the 2 cases below in which the medical director is offered gifts from industry. For each situation, decide if the medical director should accept or decline the gift and consider your rationale for your decisions.

CASE 1

Part A. The medical director enjoys a relationship with Pat Jones, a sales representative for a pharmaceutical company that manufactures 2 antiepileptic medications—one has been widely used for many years; the other is new. The medical director had participated in the clinical trial that established the efficacy of the new medication and its approval by the FDA for adjunctive therapy for refractory partial complex seizures. At the weekly

CHAPTER 6: GIFTS FROM INDUSTRY

epilepsy conference, Pat provides lunch, distributes educational materials about the products, and restocks the free-sample cupboard with new antiepileptic medication.

Part B. Pat has also given gifts to the practice's administrative assistant, including a bouquet of flowers for a birthday and a basket of treats for a holiday. At a meeting scheduled by the administrative assistant, Pat brings a copy of a new epilepsy textbook and invites the medical director to speak about her experience using the company's antiepileptic medication at an industry-sponsored meeting at a resort. Pat's company would cover travel, lodging, and meal expenses and would provide the neurologist an honorarium for speaking.

Part C. At the speaking engagement, Pat and the medical director talk about the epilepsy program and plans to expand it. Pat is concerned that the hospital has not added the new antiepileptic medication to its formulary and wonders if the medical director could speak to the pharmacy and therapeutics committee. Pat also suggests that one reason that the new medicine has not been added to the formulary is that, based on physician-specific prescribing data available to Pat, the other neurologists in the practice are not using the drug as much as the medical director is.

CASE 2

Part A. A neurologist has both a business relationship and a social relationship with Joe Schmidt, a regional sales representative for a company that makes epilepsy-monitoring equipment. The neurologist uses equipment that the sales representative sells. Their wives are in the same book club, they both have teenage children, and they both enjoy going to sporting events. The sales representative suggests that he and his wife host the neurologist and his wife at a country club for golf and dinner.

Part B. Because of increasing patient volumes, the neurologist has been urging the hospital to add 2 EMU rooms. The hospital agrees and begins to explore options for equipment purchases. Joe schedules a meeting with the neurologist to inquire about the needs for the expanded unit and, during the visit, mentions that he has 2 tickets for the NCAA Final Four and offers to take the neurologist to the games with him.

QUESTIONS FOR GROUP DISCUSSION

GETTING STARTED

1. Have you ever been offered a gift from a pharmaceutical company or medical-device manufacturer? Did you ever consider whether you should or should not accept the gift? What reasons did you consider?

ASSESSMENT

2. Who are the stakeholders in cases that involve gifts?

(continued)

MORAL DIAGNOSIS

3. What ethical values are in tension for these stakeholders?
4. What ethical considerations are most relevant?
5. Are gifts from industry ever acceptable? Discuss the characteristics that make gifts acceptable or unacceptable.
6. Using the framework from the previous question, compare and contrast the various gifts in the cases.
7. Does your institution have policies that pertain to accepting gifts from industry?
8. Have any professional organizations established guidelines for accepting gifts from industry?

GOAL SETTING, DECISION MAKING, AND IMPLEMENTATION

9. What is the justification for your decision about gifts from industry?
10. If you thought that a gift was inappropriate according to guidelines, how would you respond?

COMMENTARY ON DISCUSSION QUESTIONS

GETTING STARTED

1. **Have you ever been offered a gift from a pharmaceutical company or medical device manufacturer? Did you ever consider whether you should or should not accept the gift? What reasons did you consider?**

Physicians regularly interact with pharmaceutical companies and medical-device manufacturers, beginning in medical school and continuing throughout their careers.[1–3] These representatives' companies sponsor CME conferences and provide free meals, gifts, and drug samples.[1–4] Typically, third-year medical students attend industry-sponsored activities or receive gifts from industry as often as once per week,[5] and residents receive an average of 6 gifts per year from pharmaceutical companies.[4] Some research suggests that most medical students and residents feel that they are entitled to these gifts.[5,6] Trainees surveyed recognized that the information that they received was biased but still believed that their exposure to it would not affect their future prescribing behavior.[5–7] Paradoxically, they were concerned about how the same exposure would affect their colleagues' behavior.[5–7] Other research suggests that most medical students at one institution, both preclinical and clinical, did not agree that it is appropriate to receive gifts.[8]

The pharmaceutical industry provides financial support to the medical profession by defraying the cost of medical journals through advertisements, sponsoring educational programs, providing gifts, and sponsoring clinical pharmacological research.[9] A 2001 Kaiser Family Foundation survey found that 92% of physicians who had completed training received drug samples and that 61% received free meals and tickets for entertainment or free travel. Financial incentives to participate in clinical trials were accepted by 12% of physicians.[10]

Bernat,
58–60,
Ch. 3

Many reasons are proffered for accepting gifts. Industry wants contact with physicians to promote the use of their products. Such industry–physician exchanges provide opportunities to educate physicians about the benefits of products, a clearly favorable goal. Additionally, physicians want to be able to provide free samples for their patients, particularly for those who cannot afford to pay for medications.[11]

ASSESSMENT

2. Who are the stakeholders in cases that involve gifts?

Bernat, 57–61, Ch. 3

Bernat, 481–4, Ch. 19

Patients, physicians, other healthcare professionals, hospitals, professional societies, universities, researchers, industries, government, and other payers of healthcare each have a stake in the important ethical issues involved in the complex relationship between healthcare professionals and the healthcare industry.[9,12]

MORAL DIAGNOSIS

3. What ethical values are in tension for these stakeholders?

Bernat, 51–2, Ch. 3

All stakeholders have an interest in the well-being of patients and communities and in the preservation and promotion of their own institutions, but it is the individual healthcare professionals who promise an historic and defining commitment to the ethical value of putting their patients' interests first when those interests are in tension with other values. Professionals have promised to do what they can to benefit their patients, keep them from harm, and treat them fairly and with respect. Trust is at the heart of the patient–healthcare professional relationship.[13] Healthcare institutions and industries also value patient welfare and the good that their products and services will accomplish. Healthcare has become a major sector of the economy, and much good has been accomplished by the development of new drugs, devices, and services. However, a conflict arises when these patient-centered goals are in tension with financial goals.[14] Thompson defines a financial conflict of interest as "a set of conditions in which professional judgment concerning a primary interest (such as a patient's welfare or the validity of research) tends to be unduly influenced by a secondary interest (such as financial gain, publication in peer-reviewed journals, and academic promotion)."[15] Patients are concerned about the effects of financial incentives,[16] and the role that the healthcare industry plays in the increasing costs of healthcare engenders ever-increasing concern.[17]

4. What ethical considerations are most relevant?

Bernat, 57–61, Ch. 3

Although healthcare has become an important business, it should always be viewed primarily as a profession, and business practices should be viewed through the lens of professional obligation. Even though in this complex relationship between the professions and industry all conflicts of interest cannot be eliminated, they should always be managed in such a way so as to preserve the overall confidence that patients and the public have in the medical profession.[9] Patient welfare and trust in the integrity of medical decision making are the most relevant ethical considerations in a discussion regarding the acceptability of gifts.

5. Are gifts from industry ever acceptable? Discuss the characteristics that make gifts acceptable or unacceptable.

Physicians differ widely on whether they consider gifts acceptable or unacceptable.[18] Similarly, institutions, professional societies, and regulatory bodies vary significantly in their recommendations. Some academic leaders call for a complete ban on all gifts, free meals, and payments for attending meetings; urge physicians to reject free drug samples; and recommend restricting all consulting relationships to those that deal with scientific issues—not marketing efforts.[19,20] This total ban is based largely on social science research that demonstrates a strong impulse to reciprocate for even small gifts.[21,22]

In its Opinion on Gifts to Physicians from Industry, the AMA empha-sizes that many gifts serve an important and socially beneficial function, and its guidelines allow for the acceptance of gifts that entail a benefit to patients, are not of substantial value, and are related to the physician's work (e.g., pens and notepads).[23] The AMA position was developed in association with the 2002 code of the Pharmaceutical Research and Manufacturers of America (PhRMA), and they were very similar in their approach to gifts. PhRMA has recently updated their Code on Interactions with Healthcare Professionals, and it no longer allows the gifting of non-educational materials, such as clipboards, pens, mugs, or similar practice-related items.[24] In its most recent Code of Ethics, the Advanced Medical Technology Association (AdvaMed) joins PhRMA in such a ban.[25]

Because of the growing expense of medications, physicians increasingly seek ways to provide drugs to patients who cannot afford to purchase them. In being able to give patients free samples, a physician can determine if a patient will tolerate a medication before the patient has to purchase it. Free drug samples fit within both the AMA and PhRMA guidelines.[23,24] An alternative approach is that many pharmaceutical companies have programs to assist patients who cannot afford the full cost of drugs.[26]

Perhaps the most beneficial contribution to patient welfare is funding for educational programs provided by pharmaceutical companies and medical-device manufacturers. No standards currently exist to argue against such underwriting altogether, but various guidelines have been put in place to manage conflicts and to erect firewalls between marketing and CME grant-making offices[27] and between the funding and the content of educational programming.[28]

6. **Using the framework from the previous question, compare and contrast the different gifts in the cases.**

In Case 1, the gifts that pharmaceutical representative Pat Jones provided ranged from inexpensive to costly. Two of them—lunch at the noon epilepsy conference and an epilepsy textbook—were directly related to physician education. The flowers and treats that Pat gave to the administrative assistant served no educational purpose. The free medication samples allow physicians to gain experience in using a new drug and to treat patients who cannot afford the medication. According to most but not all guidelines, the educational gifts are acceptable and the flowers and treats are not.

The expense-paid trip to speak at an industry-sponsored meeting, coupled with an honorarium, has both positive and negative features. As the medical director had participated in a clinical trial using the antiepileptic medication, her expertise was valuable for educating other physicians, but some evidence suggests that participation in clinical trials affects physicians' guideline adherence and drug preferences.[29] If the meeting were sponsored by a professional society, current guidelines would not permit this type of gift. The AAN, ACCME, AMA, and PhRMA guidelines all require unrestricted funds to be paid directly to the society (or university) that is sponsoring the meeting.[23,24,27,28] The physician could receive no direct reimbursement from the industry representative. This practice is in keeping with the ethical guidelines to clearly separate the marketing from the educational programming. When industry is present at professional meetings at exhibit halls, the guidelines require clear separation between the two—including clear signage, separate spaces with no required passage through the exhibit halls to get to the educational meeting, and no presence of influential professionals at the marketing events to blur the distinction between marketing and education.[30] At this writing, some debate the appropriateness of industry-sponsored satellite symposia, where industry sponsors a program as an adjunct to a professional society meeting and the society receives a payment. Rothman et al. argue against all such activities,[31] and the AAN has voted not to offer corporate-sponsored satellite symposia at AAN annual meetings.[30] Critical to the acceptability of any such industry-sponsored program are the requirements of the certified CME-granting organization and the strict firewall between marketing and education.

In Case 1, the medical director is asked to talk with the pharmacy and therapeutics committee and with other physicians about increasing their usage of the drug. Some evidence suggests that interactions with industry representatives increase requests for additions to hospital formularies.[32] In Case 2, a dual relationship exists between Joe Schmidt and the epileptologist. Their wives are social friends; thus, it felt quite natural for the epileptologist and his wife to be entertained by Joe and his wife at a country club. However, at a time when the epileptologist had influence over the decision by his hospital to purchase epilepsy-monitoring equipment, Joe's offer to spring for a trip to the NCAA Final Four tournament could be viewed as a means to influence the neurologist's recommendation to the hospital regarding the new equipment purchase. Such entertainment is not acceptable by the guidelines discussed thus far. It is neither educational nor aimed at patient welfare, and it appears to come with "strings attached" (the language in the AMA opinion).[23]

In both cases, research results that find that gift recipients feel a need to reciprocate a gift giver's generosity suggest that acceptance of Joe Schmidt's and Pat Jones' gifts will influence the future behavior of the physician in ways that will ultimately be beneficial to the pharmaceutical company and device manufacturer. So long as the companies, through their representatives, provide something of value to the physician, the physician will be motivated to act in ways that will preserve those beneficial relationships.[21]

At the heart of the disagreement about whether even small gifts are acceptable are whether and how these gifts are influential and the effect that these gifts have on patient welfare. Some would point out the general harm to the trust relationship between physicians and patients and to the integrity of the medical profession.[13] If the trust in physicians and professional societies is eroded, patients may not trust research results, health information publications or practice guidelines, professional advocacy on health issues, or the truthfulness of professional public statements.[12,30] Others would point to the real potential effects on patient welfare when the integrity of medical decision making is affected and first-line medications are not used; when patients are given samples that may not be best and may last for only a short period of time, and then patients no longer have access[33,34]; and when general harms occur because of the increased costs of medications and devices to cover such marketing expenses.[35] Evidence also suggests that drug samples are not primarily used for patients who cannot afford to buy the drugs.[33] The core ethical principles of beneficence, nonmaleficence, and justice are involved in the debate about accepting gifts.[36]

Bernat, 51–2, Ch. 3

Bernat, 481–4, Ch. 19

Bernat, 8–14, Ch. 1

7. Does your institution have policies that pertain to accepting gifts from industry?

An increasing number of institutions have developed policies that forbid accepting any gifts from industry.[19] For example, Stanford University,[37] the University of Michigan and Dartmouth-Hitchcock Medical Center,[19] and The University of Colorado Anschutz Medical Campus[38] ban all gifts to physicians (and others). None of the gifts in Cases 1 and 2 (lunches, country club golf outings with dinner, or college basketball play-off tickets) would be acceptable. Most institutions do not have a total ban but have policies that more closely follow the AMA guidelines, which set limits on the types and amounts of gifts. Generally, institutions include guidelines for addressing conflicts of interest as part of their institutional codes of conduct, their policies directing the pharmacy and therapeutics committees, and their policies governing continuing-education sponsorships. Many institutions also have policies that provide specific guidelines for interactions with pharmaceutical representatives, such as rules governing activities within the hospital and clinic (e.g., where representatives can meet with staff, the need for appointments), patient confidentiality, and drug samples. In Case 1, the lunches, educational materials, and free samples might be permitted, but direct payment for the trip to the resort for the meeting and the honorarium are not permitted. These gifts are also not permitted by ACCME, PhRMA, and AdvaMed guidelines. Also, the neurologist would have to disclose any conflicts of interest when she submitted a request to the pharmacy and therapeutics committee for any formulary addition requests. In Case 2, tickets to the basketball play-off would not be permitted, as they are not related to patient care.

Those who are uncertain or unclear about whether their institutions have policies governing interactions with the healthcare industry should contact the compliance office or the organizational ethics committee at their institutions; these resources should be able to provide the relevant policies.

8. Have any professional organizations established guidelines for accepting gifts from industry?

Several professional organizations have established guidelines for accepting gifts from industry, and stipulations range from a total ban to trying to manage conflicts of interest by setting limits. The American Medical Student Association favors a total ban and has an active campaign that calls on medical students to educate themselves and others and to take a "Pharm Free Pledge."[39] The American College of Physicians in its 2012 Ethics Manual also strongly discourages physicians from accepting individual gifts, hospitality, trips, and subsidies of all types from the healthcare industry, but it also sets out guidelines for accepting some gifts, provided that they are inexpensive and intended solely for office use, education, or patient care.[40] The AMA Council on Ethical and Judicial Affairs has issued ethical guidelines for physicians based on the premise that gifts that primarily serve the interests of patients are acceptable, but those that primarily serve the interests of physicians (cash, junkets, tickets to events, expensive meals) are unacceptable.[23] The PhRMA and AdvaMed guidelines that govern the interaction of pharmaceutical sales representatives and healthcare professionals are stricter in some ways than the AMA opinion, in that they do not allow non-educational small gifts such as pens and notepads.[24,25]

Much attention has been directed to the relationship between industry and professional medical societies, and many have developed guidelines.[31] It is problematic when physicians are subject to restrictions in their clinical practices by their academic institutions, hospitals, and state regulations, but their professional medical societies continue to be supported to a large degree by industry. In 2010, the AAN accepted a Report of the Task Force on Academy-Industry Relations that surveyed industry funding of the AAN and applied the AAN Policy on Conflicts of Interest to its own governance. The task force made recommendations for handling conflicts of interest that include the application of 4 general principles to remedy conflicts of interest—avoidance, separation, disclosure, and regulation. The 8 special guidelines includes policies such as the AAN will not involve itself in the production, sale, endorsement, or marketing to consumers of products that claim a health benefit; relationships between the AAN and external sources of support must not permit or encourage influence by the external source of support on AAN policies, priorities, or actions; no external funding can be accepted for core governance activities; and a clear separation must be made between corporate-sponsored activities and education.[30]

Many of these guidelines have been developed to emphasize the need for professionals to voluntarily manage the conflicts of interest that arise from relationships with industry, but legal mechanisms to address conflicts of interest are increasing. Many states have enacted their own laws that require reporting, open access to such reports, and a range of consequences from fines to effects on licensure.[41] The federal Health Care Reform law passed in 2010 also includes a so-called "sunshine provision" to mandate disclosure.[42] The consequences to ignoring the ethical and legal issues associated with gifts from industry can be great.

GOAL SETTING, DECISION MAKING, AND IMPLEMENTATION

9. What is the justification for your decision about gifts from industry?

The strongest arguments in support of refusing all gifts from industry include concern for a trusting patient relationship, professional integrity, and justice concerns related to increasing costs. Conflicts of interest can put at risk the primary commitment to patient well-being through the loss of the objectivity necessary to practice evidence-based medicine. The strongest arguments in support of receiving some gifts include (a) some gifts offer a valuable benefit for patients and (b) physicians are able to manage conflicts and not be affected by the gift relationship. A concern for patient well-being (beneficence) is used to support both sides of the question of gifts. The difference rests on the empirical claim about whether physicians are influenced. Research supports the presence of such influence.[21]

10. If you thought that a gift was inappropriate according to guidelines, how would you respond?

The first step is to engage in the kind of ethical analysis modeled in this chapter, but this skill of ethical analysis does not necessarily translate into the skill of implementing decisions. The cases presented here involve 2 aspects of inappropriate gift giving—the types of gifts offered and dual relationships with industry representatives. A response to an inappropriate gift offer of the first type could include reference to existing institutional, professional, or state policies, guidelines, or laws. A response to an inappropriate gift offer of the second type can be more complicated. A rich dialogue about dual relationships with patients and appropriate professional boundaries can be found in the family medicine, psychiatry, and rural healthcare literature.[43] A key feature is self-awareness and intentional discussion to set specific boundaries. In the dual relationship in Case 2, the neurologist should have a discussion with Joe Schmidt about where the lines are drawn between their professional and social relationships, including where and when professional discussions occur, what information is shared, and who pays for social events. Adapting guidelines that are intended to address multiple relationships between professionals and patients in the rural context, listed below are some keys to anticipating and preventing ethics conflicts.

- Be aware of ethical standards guiding patient–industry relationships.
- Communicate with industry representatives about professional responsibilities.
- Expect ethics conflicts, owing to multiple roles.
- Be able to recognize when boundaries are being crossed.
- Recognize potential fallout from the professional realm to the interpersonal one.
- Analyze ethics conflicts and generate multiple potential responses—there is rarely only one solution.
- Identify and use colleagues to discuss patient–industry conflicts.
- Identify and seek support from ethics resources regarding clinician–industry conflicts.[44]

KEY POINTS

- Gifts to physicians from the healthcare industry raise ethical concerns because of the impact on building a trusting physician–patient relationship, professional integrity, and justice related to increasing costs.
- Conflicts of interest can put at risk the primary commitment to patient well-being through the loss of objectivity necessary to practice evidence-based medicine.
- An increasing body of social science and psychological research has provided evidence of the influence of gifts on physician behavior.
- Physicians should be aware of the various guidelines, policies, and laws for managing financial conflicts of interest in clinical care that have been developed by professional societies, institutions, and state and federal governments.

KEY WORDS

Conflict of interest—a set of conditions in which professional judgment concerning a primary interest (such as a patient's welfare or the validity of research) tends to be unduly influenced by a secondary interest (such as financial gain).

Gift relationship—the social rule of reciprocity that imposes on the recipient an obligation to repay for favors, gifts, invitations, etc. Calling various medical marketing tools by the label "gifts" seeks to capitalize on this often-times subtle phenomenon of reciprocity.

REFERENCES

1. Martin JB. The pervasive influence of conflicts of interest: A personal perspective. Neurology 2010; 74:2016–21.
2. Campbell EG, Gruen RL, Mountford J, et al. A national survey of physician–industry relationships. N Engl J Med 2007; 356:1742–50.
3. Blumenthal D. Doctors and drug companies. N Engl J Med 2004; 351(18):1885–90.
4. Wazana A. Physicians and the pharmaceutical industry: Is a gift ever just a gift? JAMA 2000; 283:373–80.
5. Sjerles FS, Brodkey AC, Cleary LM, et al. Medical students' exposure to and attitudes about drug company interactions. A national survey. JAMA 2005; 294:1034–42.
6. Sah S, Lowenstein G. Effect of reminders of personal sacrifice and suggested rationalizations on residents' self-reported willingness to accept gifts. JAMA 2010; 304:1204–11.
7. Steinman MA, Shlipak MG, McPhee SJ. Of principles and pens: Attitudes and practices of medicine housestaff toward pharmaceutical industry promotions. Am J Med 2001; 110:551–7.
8. Hyman PL, Hochman ME, Shaw JG, et al. Attitudes of preclinical and clinical medical students accepting gifts from pharmaceutical industry. Acad Med 2007; 82:94–9.
9. Bernat, 57–61, Ch. 3.
10. The Kaiser Family Foundation. National Survey of Physicians. Part II: Doctors and prescription drugs. Washington, DC: The Henry J. Kaiser Family Foundation, March 2002.
11. Chren MM. Interactions between physicians and drug company representatives. Am J Med 1999; 107:182–3.
12. Bernat, 481–4, Ch. 19.
13. Bernat, 51–2, Ch. 3.
14. Lo B. Serving two masters—conflicts of interest in academic medicine. N Engl J Med 2010; 669–71.
15. Thompson DF. Understanding financial conflicts of interest. N Engl J Med 1993; 329:573–6.
16. Licurse A, Barber E, Joffe S, et al. The impact of disclosing financial ties in research and clinical care. Arch Intern Med 2010; 675–82.
17. Kaiser Family Foundation. Prescription drug trends. Washington, DC: The Henry J. Kaiser Family Foundation, June 2007.
18. Korenstein D, Keyhani S, Ross JS. Physician attitudes toward industry: A view across specialties. Arch Surg 2010; 145:570–7.
19. Brennan TA, Rothman DJ, Blank L, et al. Health industry practices that create conflicts of interest. A policy proposal for academic medical centers. JAMA 2006; 295:429–33.
20. Rothman DJ, Chimonas S. Academic medical centers' conflict of interest policies. JAMA 2010; 304:2294–5.
21. Dana J, Loewenstein G. A social science perspective on gifts to physicians from industry. JAMA 2003; 290:252–5.

22. Chimonas S, Brennan TA, Rothman DJ. Physicians and drug representatives: Exploring the dynamics of the relationship. J Gen Intern Med 2007; 22:184–90.
23. American Medical Association. Code of Medical Ethics. Opinion E-8.061, Gifts to physicians from industry. Available at www.ama-assn.org/ama/pub/physician-resources/medical-ethics/code-medical-ethics.shtml. Accessed March 21, 2012.
24. Pharmaceutical Research and Manufacturers of America. Company interactions with healthcare professionals contribute to patient care. Available at www.phrma.org/valueofinteractions. Accessed March 21, 2012.
25. Advanced Medical Technology Association. Code of Ethics on Interactions with Health Care Professionals, 2009. Available at www.AdvaMed.com. Accessed March 21, 2012.
26. Partnership for Physician Assistance. Available at www.pparx.org. Accessed March 21, 2012.
27. American Academy of Neurology. Code of Professional Conduct. Section 7.3 and Section 8.2, Disclosure of Potential Conflicts. [PECN appendix document A and available at www.aan.com/view/PECN]
28. Accreditation Council for Continuing Medical Education. ACCME Standards for Commercial Support: Standards to Ensure the Independence of CME Activities. Available at www.accme.org/requirements/accreditation-requirements-cme-providers/standards-for-commercial-support. Accessed March 21, 2012.
29. Andersen M, Kragstrup J, Sondergaard J. How conducting a clinical trial affects physicians' guideline adherence and drug preference. JAMA 2006; 295:2759–64.
30. Hutchins JC, Rydell CM, Griggs RC, et al. American Academy of Neurology policy on pharmaceutical and device industry support. Neurology 2012; 78:750–4.
31. Rothman DJ, McDonald WJ, Berkowitz CD, et al. Professional medical associations and their relationships with industry: A proposal for controlling conflict of interest. JAMA 2009; 301:1367–72.
32. Chren MM, Landefeld CS. Physicians' behavior and their interactions with drug companies. A controlled study of physicians who requested additions to a hospital drug formulary. JAMA 1994; 217:684–9.
33. Cutrona SL, Woolhandler S, Lasser KE, et al. Characteristics of recipients of free prescription drug samples: A nationally representative analysis. Am J Public Health 2008; 98:284–9.
34. Cutrona SL, Woolhandler S, Lasser KE, et al. Free drug samples in the United States: Characteristics of pediatric recipients and safety concerns. Pediatrics 2008; 122(4):736–42.
35. Alexander GC, Zhang J, Basu A. Characteristics of patients receiving pharmaceutical samples and association between sample receipt and out-of-pocket prescription costs. Med Care 2008; 46:394–402.
36. Bernat, 8–14, Ch. 1.
37. Policy and guidelines for interactions between the Stanford University School of Medicine, the Stanford Hospital and Clinics, and Lucile Packard Children's Hospital with the Pharmaceutical, Biotech, Medical Device, and Hospital and Research Equipment and Supplies Industries ("Industry"). Available at www.med.stanford.edu/coi/siip/policy.html. Accessed March 21, 2012.
38. University of Colorado. Conflicts of Interest and Commitment. Available at www.ucdenver.edu/academics/research/AboutUs/regcomp/conflictofinterest/COI%20Documents/Conflict%20of%20Interest%20and%20Commitment%20Policy%201-7-10.pdf. Accessed March 21, 2012.
39. American Medical Student Association. PharmFree Pledge. Available at www.pharmfree.org/. Accessed March 21, 2012.
40. Snyder L for the American College of Physicians Ethics Professionalism, and Human Rights Committee. Ann Intern Med 2012; 156:73–104.
41. Studdert DM, Mello MM, Brennan TA. Financial conflicts of interest in physicians' relationships with the pharmaceutical industry—self-regulation in the shadow of federal prosecution. N Engl J Med 2004; 351:1891–900.

42. Physician Payments Sunshine Act Guide. Available at www.prescriptionproject.org/sunshine_act. Accessed March 21, 2012.
43. Rourke JTB, Smith LFP, Brown JB. Patients, friends, and relationship boundaries. Can Fam Physician 1993; 30:2557–64.
44. Pomerantz A. Ethics conflicts in rural communities: Overlapping roles. In: Nelson W, ed. *Handbook for Rural Health Care Ethics: A Practical Guide for Professionals.* Lebanon, NJ: Dartmouth, 2011.

SUGGESTIONS FOR FURTHER READING

Association of American Medical Colleges. In the interest of patients: Recommendations for physician financial relationships and clinical decision making: Report of the task force on financial conflicts of interest in clinical care. Washington, DC: AAMC, 2010. Available at www.aamc.org/download/157030/data/coi_in_clinical_care.pdf. Accessed March 16, 2012.

Association of American Medical Colleges and Baylor College of Medicine. The scientific basis of influence and reciprocity: A symposium. Washington, DC: AAMC, 2007. Available at www.aamc.org/download/157014/data/new_document.pdf. Accessed March 16, 2012.

Dana J. *How Psychological Research Can Inform Policies for Dealing with Conflict of Interest in Medicine, Conflict of Interest in Medical Research, Education and Practice.* Washington, DC: The National Academies Press, 2009.

Katz D, Caplan A, Merz J. All gifts large and small: Toward an understanding of the ethics of pharmaceutical industry gift giving. Am J Bioeth 2003; 3(3):39–46.

Pew Prescription Project. Available at www.prescriptionproject.org. Accessed March 22, 2012.

7 GIFTS FROM PATIENTS

Tyler Reimschisel, MD

LEARNING OBJECTIVES

Upon completion of this chapter, participants will be able to:

1. Describe the ethical issues associated with accepting gifts from patients.
2. Identify the factors that make the acceptance of a gift from a patient either ethically permissible or impermissible.
3. Incorporate into their practices methods for appropriately accepting and declining various gifts.

LEARNING RESOURCES

Key chapters in Bernat's third edition—1, 2, 3

Key relevant AAN documents available at www.aan.com/view/PECN

A

CLINICAL VIGNETTES

Because of a shortage of child neurologists in his area, an adult epileptologist for a large regional medical center also provides care to children with epilepsy. Consider the cases below in which he is offered various types of gifts from patients. For each case, decide if he should accept or decline the gift and consider the rationale for your decisions.

CASE 1

Adam, a 6-year-old boy with absence seizures, returns to clinic for a routine follow-up appointment. Over the course of several months, he has grown to enjoy his visits. When the physician walks into the room, Adam runs up, hugs him, and hands him a picture that he drew of the physician.

CASE 2

Adam's mother, Mrs. Stockdale, always attends clinic with him. She is a prominent local artist whose work is highly valued. She is thrilled that the epileptologist has been able to control Adam's seizures with only a single medication. He is no longer "day dreaming" throughout the day, and he is doing very well in school. At the end of each visit, she always expresses her appreciation. However, after the current visit, she states that she wants to demonstrate in a more tangible way the depth of her appreciation and unwraps a large picture that she painted and offers it to the physician as a gift.

CASE 3

For several years, the epileptologist has provided care to Mrs. Clevenger, a 74-year-old widow who has a well-controlled focal seizure disorder. Her routine follow-up visits every 6 months are usually brief. However, the physician enjoys having the opportunity to catch up on her recent travels and the activities of her children and grandchildren, and she enjoys coming to clinic and spending time talking with the physician, nurses, and staff. At a recent visit, she hands the physician a container of cookies that she made herself that morning. After the visit, she mentions that she has scheduled a meeting with her lawyer and that she is planning to include the physician as a beneficiary in her will.

CASE 4

Mr. Leighton is a 41-year-old man with generalized seizures who is a prominent businessman in the community. The epileptologist recently assumed Mr. Leighton's care because Mr. Leighton became frustrated with his previous neurologist and heard about the superb reputation that the epileptologist has in the community. He gave the physician two bottles of wine at his last visit and, since then, has called the office repeatedly to get a return visit that is sooner and fits into his ever-changing schedule. Mr. Leighton has also mailed to the office physical examination forms that he wants the physician to complete as part of his application for a new health insurance policy. Although the physician explained that Mr. Leighton should have his internist complete the forms, the patient states that he does not have time to go to more than one doctor and asks, "What's the matter, don't you know how to listen to my heart?" When the physician enters the exam room today, Mr. Leighton presents 2 more bottles of wine.

QUESTIONS FOR GROUP DISCUSSION

GETTING STARTED
1. Have you ever been offered a gift from a patient? If yes, how did it make you feel? Did you consider the ethical implications of accepting or rejecting the gift?

ASSESSMENT
2. Compare and contrast the cases. What distinguishes the gifts in each case from one another?
3. What are the possible motivating factors for gift giving?
4. Should institutions mandate a complete prohibition of accepting gifts from patients? Justify your answer.

(continued)

5. How could *not accepting* a gift change the physician–patient relationship? Are there situations in which not accepting a gift could cause more harm than would accepting the gift? Describe the characteristics of those situations. Do those characteristics apply to any of the cases presented?
6. How could *accepting* a gift change the physician–patient relationship?
7. Lyckholm has suggested that gift giving is an example of the patient manifesting his or her autonomy.[1] If it is, then declining a gift is an indirect refusal to honor the autonomy of the patient. In which of the cases presented do you think it would be ethically permissible to decline the gift? Provide ethical justification for not honoring the patients' autonomy in those cases.
8. How could the physician–patient relationship change for patients who have not given gifts but learn that their physicians have accepted gifts from other patients?
9. Should a patient's cultural background influence a physician's decision to accept or decline a gift from the patient?

MORAL DIAGNOSIS
10. Does your institution have any relevant policies pertaining to accepting gifts from patients? If you do not know, what would you do to determine if your institution has any relevant policies?
11. Have any professional organizations established guidelines for accepting gifts from patients?

GOAL SETTING, DECISION MAKING, AND IMPLEMENTATION
12. If you think that a gift is *appropriate*, describe the process that you would use to accept the gift.
13. If you think that a gift is *inappropriate*, describe the process that you would use to decline the gift.

COMMENTARY ON DISCUSSION QUESTIONS

GETTING STARTED

1. Have you ever been offered a gift from a patient? If yes, how did it make you feel? Did you consider the ethical implications of accepting or rejecting the gift?

If you have only recently begun practicing medicine, you may not yet have been offered a gift from a patient or family, but it is just a matter of time because gift giving from patients is commonplace. A survey of more than 300 British physicians showed that 20% received gifts from patients in the preceding 3 months.[2] The most common gifts were alcohol, chocolate, and money.

The primary question regarding the ethics of gift giving from patients is whether and how the physician–patient relationship is influenced when physicians accept gifts. Does a conflict of interest arise when a physician

Bernat, 57, Ch. 3

accepts a gift from a patient?[3] How does accepting a gift affect the physician–patient relationship with other patients who have not offered gifts? These questions and many others will be addressed in this chapter as we discuss the process for considering the ethical aspects of gift giving from patients, as well as potential responses to patients who offer gifts.

ASSESSMENT

2. Compare and contrast the cases. What distinguishes the gifts in each case from one another?

Most gifts offered to physicians have modest value and serve as a token of appreciation and gratitude. Adam's picture and Mrs. Clevenger's homemade cookies are examples of these types of gifts.

On the other hand, some gifts may be more costly, such as Mrs. Stockdale's painting or Mrs. Clevenger's making the physician a beneficiary in her will. These expensive gifts could also be simple expressions of gratitude. However, their value raises concern. Accepting gifts that have more than a modest value creates a potential conflict of interest because the physician may feel an obligation to repay the patient. Alternatively, expensive gifts could be an attempt to garner special treatment or to change the professional relationship between the patient and the physician. Therefore, gifts that have more than a modest value should be graciously and diplomatically declined. Because patients may not appreciate the unique aspects of the physician–patient relationship, physicians should explain how accepting these types of gifts could compromise the unique fiduciary responsibility that physicians have toward all of their patients.[4]

Bernat, 51, Ch. 3

Lastly, some gifts are only slightly veiled attempts to gain preferential treatment, such as Mr. Leighton's repetitive gifts of wine associated with recurrent and bold expectations of special treatment. From his perspective, this may simply be the approach that successful businessmen take to business transactions. Therefore, it would be helpful to explain to Mr. Leighton that the culture of healthcare and the physician–patient relationship is different from the business culture and that his gifts will be declined because it is ethically impermissible for physicians to provide preferential care to select patients.

3. What are the possible motivating factors for gift giving?

Patients or their families may offer gifts to their physicians for multiple reasons. Anderek suggests 3 main motives: pure beneficence, appreciation, and influence.[5] Many individuals simply enjoy giving gifts, and they do not expect or want anything in return. Others may give gifts merely as a token of their appreciation, especially on special occasions or during the holiday seasons. Anderek contends that, in general, it is ethically permissible for physicians to accept gifts in these situations. However, if the gift is being offered to influence an outcome or to garner special treatment, then the gift is a form of a bribe that should not be accepted.[5]

Drew and colleagues studied this issue by having internists in a single group practice keep a diary of the gifts that they received.[6] When the internists were interviewed about their experiences and the reasons that they ascribed to the gift giving, they offered several motives. For example, they suggested that the gifts may serve as "tips" to promote personalized service, continued interest, and tolerance of the patient. They also perceived that sometimes the gifts were given to address the unequal balance of power that exists between the physician and the patient. For example, they noted that patients may be trying to redeem the loss of status that occurs when one assumes the sick role.

Gift giving may also serve an underlying need for the patient or family. For example, "gifts may provide a way for patients to satisfy their own sense of worth and need for relationships."[7] Mrs. Clevenger's gift of cookies may have been offered for this reason. Additionally, a gift offered in the name of a loved one who has passed away may be a token of appreciation and an important aspect of the grieving process.[8] Gifts may also be offered to honor a physician, nurse, or other healthcare professional. In fact, honoring another person is a common motivational factor for institutional gift giving. For the patient or family who expresses an interest in institutional giving, the physician can recommend that they work together with the institution's development office to best honor the patient's wishes.

During your discussion of these cases, you may identify additional motivating factors. However, it is unlikely that a physician will be able to discern all of the motivating factors that prompted a patient to offer a gift. Therefore, it is helpful to consider motivating factors for gift giving when it occurs, but it is more prudent to focus primarily on whether accepting the gift could create a potential conflict of interest. It is ethically permissible to accept modest gifts because they are most likely simple expressions of gratitude and are unlikely to alter the relationship. However, gifts that are costly, extravagant, or personal may unduly influence a physician or could change the professional nature of the relationship. These types of gifts should be declined because such gifts may compromise the physician–patient relationship.[1]

4. **Should institutions mandate a complete prohibition of accepting gifts from patients? Justify your answer.**

Most ethicists and physicians do not advocate a complete prohibition on accepting gifts from patients. However, Weijer points out quite cogently that multiple reasons exist for declining all gifts, regardless of their value.[9] He argues that accepting gifts violates the fiduciary nature and erodes the moral character of the physician–patient relationship. Further, despite the discussion in Question 3 on the motivations behind gift giving, Weijer states that physicians cannot definitely determine or "divine" the various motivations of gifts. Because the gift *could be* to receive preferential treatment even though that motivation may not be evident, he believes that the most prudent standard is to refuse all gifts. Ultimately, he thinks that accepting gifts of any kind and value diminishes the true value of the care given.[9]

It is axiomatic that gifts that are costly, extravagant, or personal in nature could certainly violate and erode the physician–patient relationship. However, modest gifts of gratitude such as Adam's hand-drawn picture and Mrs. Clevenger's homemade cookies do not threaten the physician–patient relationship.[1,5] Though an individual physician may decide to decline all gifts regardless of their nature or value, most ethicists and professional organizations (see discussion at Question 11) contend that it is not ethically imperative to decline all gifts from patients.[1,5,8,10]

5. **How could *not accepting* a gift change the physician–patient relationship? Are there situations in which not accepting a gift could cause more harm than would accepting the gift? Describe the characteristics of those situations. Do those characteristics apply to any of the cases presented?**

For modest gifts that are merely tokens of appreciation and gratitude, as characterized in the situations exemplified by Adam's gift of a hand-drawn picture and Mrs. Clevenger's offer of homemade cookies, refusing to accept the gifts can appear petty or insincere and could insult, alienate, or embarrass the patient or family member. For situations in which the patient or family has offered a modest gift that is very unlikely to change the physician–patient relationship, refusing to accept the gift could be perceived by the patient or family as a personal rejection.[11] In these cases, a refusal demonstrates a lack of respect for the patient and could worsen the underlying power differential between the physician and patient.[12] Therefore, in situations in which the gift is a modest token of appreciation or gratitude, will not unduly influence or impact the physician–patient relationship, and does not cross professional boundaries, it is ethically permissible to accept it.

6. **How could *accepting* a gift change the physician–patient relationship?**

Bernat, 51, Ch. 3

Depending on the gift, accepting it could create a conflict of interest for the physician, cause the physician to lose objectivity in the patient's care, engender a sense of special obligation to the patient, undermine the fiduciary nature of the physician–patient relationship,[4] or make the relationship more personal and less professional. In all of these situations, it is ethically permissible to decline the gift and refuse to honor the patient's autonomy because accepting a gift should not change the professional nature of the physician–patient relationship.

7. **Lyckholm has suggested that gift giving is an example of the patient manifesting his or her autonomy.[1] If it is, then declining a gift is an indirect refusal to honor the autonomy of the patient. In which of**

the cases presented do you think it would be ethically permissible to decline the gift? Provide ethical justification for not honoring the patients' autonomy in those cases.

Honoring patient autonomy is one of the ethical pillars of clinical practice in Western medicine, but it is not absolute. Physicians also possess autonomy and cannot be required to offer care or treatment that violates their moral code or would be illegal or unprofessional.[13] Similarly, physicians do not have to honor patient wishes if doing so would jeopardize the professional nature of the physician–patient relationship.

Bernat, 52, Ch. 3

Mr. Leighton's repeated gift giving in Case 4 is an attempt to change the nature of the relationship. He is attempting to acquire special treatment through gift giving, but physicians ought to treat all patients without preference. Therefore, it is ethically permissible to decline his repeated gifts. In this situation, the physician should decline the gift and explain that Mr. Leighton cannot receive preferential treatment, regardless of whether he offers gifts. As such gift giving may be common in business, confrontation with Mr. Leighton can be avoided by explaining that the physician–patient relationship is different from business relationships, and accepting gifts in exchange for preferential treatment is unacceptable in the context of the physician–patient relationship. Sharing the institution's policy on gift giving may also be helpful.

Though not as explicit as Mr. Leighton's gift giving, the hand-painted picture from Mrs. Stockdale in Case 2 and being named a beneficiary in Mrs. Clevenger's will in Case 3 should also be declined. These gifts have more than a modest value and could create a conflict of interest for the physician. Regardless of the motivation of the patients, accepting gifts like these could easily change the nature of the physician–patient relationship by engendering a sense of obligation in the physician to recompense the patient through preferential treatment.

Because outright refusal of gifts can be hurtful or perceived as being disrespectful, the physician should discuss alternative forms of gifting with the patient. For example, when Mrs. Stockdale offers the expensive painting, the physician could thank her for her gracious offer, explain the rationale for declining the gift, and suggest that she donate it to the hospital. Similarly, when Mrs. Clevenger offers to make the physician a beneficiary in her will, the physician can suggest that she could make a charitable donation to the organization of her choice in the physician's name or make a bequest to the physician's clinic or research efforts.

8. **How could the physician–patient relationship change for patients who have not given gifts but learn that their physicians have accepted gifts from other patients?**

The response from patients who do not offer gifts will quite likely depend on the type of gift that was accepted. A modest gift that appears to be merely a token of gratitude is unlikely to impact the relationship that the physician has with other patients. However, accepting gifts that are costly, extravagant, or personal may make other patients feel obligated to also give gifts to the physician, as they may perceive that the giver is receiving better treatment.[1] Alternatively, the physician's apparent materialism may cause patients to lose respect for the physician who accepts these types of gifts.

9. **Should a patient's cultural background influence a physician's decision to accept or decline a gift from the patient?**

In Western culture, giving gifts to physicians is neither expected nor required,[7] but in some cultures, gift giving is a sign of respect to the physician.[8] If a physician has a patient who is from a culture in which gift giving is expected as a demonstration of respect, then declining a gift could be an affront to the patient's customs or culture.[8] In these situations, it is probably preferable to accept the gift unless it is costly, extravagant, intimate, or could otherwise create a conflict of interest. When a physician thinks that he or she may be in such a situation, it can be helpful to discuss with the patient whether unique cultural factors are influencing the gift giving.

MORAL DIAGNOSIS

10. **Does your institution have any relevant policies pertaining to accepting gifts from patients? If you do not know, what would you do to determine if your institution has any relevant policies?**

Most hospitals and universities have a formal policy on accepting gifts from patients; therefore, you should take the time to determine the policy at your institution. If a formal policy has not been developed or if you have questions about the policy, you could contact your institution's ethics committee, legal-affairs office, or chief-of-staff office. Physicians who work in private practice should also have a policy on gift giving so that they are prepared to respond to patients when gifts are offered.

11. **Have any professional organizations established guidelines for accepting gifts from patients?**

Though gift giving is common, very few professional organizations have established guidelines for accepting gifts from patients. In a policy statement on managing boundaries in pediatrician–family–patient relationships, The American Academy of Pediatrics has a single paragraph on gift giving from parents:

> Patients or parents sometimes give pediatricians gifts, especially after providing help for a complex or troubling health-related problem. Under most circumstances, gifts have a far more symbolic than material value. For most pediatricians,

accepting modest gifts does not involve a serious conflict; in fact, refusal of a gift may constitute a social or cultural affront. As the monetary worth of the gift increases, however, so does the psychological and ethical difficulty in maintaining appropriate boundaries in the professional relationship. When the pediatrician feels uncomfortable with a gift that a family insists on delivering, he or she must voice the concern and suggest acceptable alternatives, such as a charitable donation in the pediatrician's name. Highly valued gifts may indicate that these boundaries have been crossed. The patient or loved one may have misinterpreted the pediatrician's earlier behavior or may be inviting the pediatrician to engage in a relationship that could compromise medical judgment and action.[10]

The most comprehensive publication by a professional organization on gift giving from patients is the AMA's Report of the Council on Ethical and Judicial Affairs, entitled "Gifts from Patients to Physicians."[8] The Council notes that it is ethically permissible to accept modest gifts from patients that are simply "...an expression of appreciation and gratitude."[8] However, gifts that signal psychological needs or that are given to secure preferential treatment should be declined because they could damage the integrity of the physician–patient relationship. In all cases, they recommend using the rule of transparency—a gift should only be accepted if the physician would be comfortable disclosing acceptance of the gift to the physician's colleagues or the public. Finally, for gifts bequeathed in the context of a will, the Report states that "...the physician should consider declining the gift if the physician believes that its acceptance would present a significant hardship (financial or emotional) to the family."[8]

GOAL SETTING, DECISION MAKING, AND IMPLEMENTATION

12. If you think that a gift is *appropriate*, describe the process that you would use to accept the gift.

Once a physician has decided that it is ethically permissible to accept a gift from a patient or family, the physician should accept it by being gracious but brief. For example, you could simply say, "Thank you for your generous gift. It is a privilege to provide medical care for you." As Andereck suggests, "provided that patients are not trying to influence their relationship with their physician, the doctors should accept the gift with a smile, send a thank-you note, and move on."[5] Gifts of food or other items that can be shared can be accepted on behalf of the clinic personnel,[11] but caution should be exercised so that gifts are not displayed where other patients can see them, as this may make other patients feel like they should also offer gifts.

13. If you think that a gift is *inappropriate*, describe the process that you would use to decline the gift.

If a gift is costly, extravagant, too personal or intimate, or appears to be an attempt to influence or change the physician–patient relationship, then it should be declined. Again, this should be done graciously and succinctly. After politely declining a gift, a physician should provide a brief explanation of why it is being declined.[7] For example, the physician can appeal to a general rule that he or she always declines gifts unless they are modest tokens of appreciation. If the gift is costly, the physician can recommend that the patient donate to a charity in the physician's name. Regardless of the precise words used, it is imperative that the patient understand that nonacceptance of a gift is not a rejection of the patient and that the patient will continue to receive the same quality of medical care.[12]

CONCLUSION

The principle ethical questions regarding gifts from patients are whether accepting the gift will alter the physician–patient relationship and how the physician can respond in a way that is in the best interest of that relationship.[11] Prior to accepting a gift, it is prudent to consider whether accepting the gift will create a potential conflict of interest and whether motivating factors other than appreciation might be prompting the gift giving. Consider using the "rule of transparency" when deciding whether a gift should be accepted—if you would feel embarrassed or uncomfortable discussing the gift with a colleague, then you should decline the gift. However, if the gift is modest, will not create a potential conflict of interest, and appears to be motivated purely by gratitude, then it is ethically permissible to accept the gift.

KEY POINTS

- Gift giving to physicians is common.
- The primary ethical issue regarding gift giving is whether accepting the gift would create a conflict of interest for the physician.
- It is ethically permissible to accept modest gifts of appreciation.
- Gifts that are extravagant or expensive, cross professional boundaries, or are interpreted as an attempt to receive special treatment should be declined because they are likely to create a conflict of interest.

KEY WORDS

Conflict of interest—a set of conditions in which professional judgment concerning a primary interest (such as a patient's welfare) tends to be unduly influenced by a secondary interest (such as financial gain).

Cultural competence—a set of congruent behaviors, knowledge, attitudes, and policies that come together in a system, organization, or among professionals that enables effective work in cross-cultural situations.

Gift—anything given willingly without payment.

Physician–patient relationship—the unique fiduciary relationship that exists between physicians and their patients.

Professional boundaries—limitations on appropriate interactions between physicians and their patients that are based on the fiduciary nature of the physician–patient relationship.

REFERENCES

1. Lyckholm LJ. Should physicians accept gifts from patients? JAMA 1998; 280:1944–6.
2. Levene M, Sireling L. Gift giving to hospital doctors—in the mouth of the gift horse. BMJ 1980; 281:1685.
3. Bernat, 57, Ch. 3.
4. Bernat, 51, Ch. 3.
5. Andereck W. Point-counterpoint: Should physicians accept gifts from their patients? Yes: If they are given out of beneficence or appreciation. West J Med 2001; 175:76.
6. Drew J, Stoeckle JD, Billings JA. Tips, status, and sacrifice: Gift giving in the doctor–patient relationship. Soc Sci Med 1983; 17:399–404.
7. Capozzi J, Rhodes R. Gifts from patients. J Bone Joint Surgery 2004; 86A:2339–40.
8. American Medical Association. Report of the Council on Ethical and Judicial Affairs. CEJA Report 4-A-03, Gifts from patients to physicians, June 2003. Available at www.ama-assn.org/resources/doc/ethics/4a03.pdf. Accessed March 25, 2012.
9. Weijer C. Point-counterpoint: Should physicians accept gifts from their patients? No: Gifts debase the true value of care. West J Med 2001; 175:77.
10. American Academy of Pediatrics. Committee on Bioethics. Policy Statement: Pediatrician-family-patient relationships: Managing the boundaries. Pediatrics 2009; 124:1685–8.
11. Gaufberg E. Should physicians accept gifts from patients? Am Fam Physician 2007; 76:437–8.
12. Spence SA. Patient bearing gifts: Are there strings attached? BMJ 2005; 331:1527–9.
13. Bernat, 52, Ch. 3.

8 TERMINATION OF THE PHYSICIAN–PATIENT RELATIONSHIP

Jill Conway, MD, MA

LEARNING OBJECTIVES

Upon completion of this chapter, participants will be able to:

1. Identify important elements of the physician–patient relationship.
2. Define patient abandonment and understand the ethical and legal implications of sudden withdrawal of care.
3. Indicate the conditions under which physicians may terminate a relationship with a patient.
4. Describe the steps that must be taken before a physician can terminate a relationship with a patient.

LEARNING RESOURCES

Key chapters in Bernat's third edition—2, 3

Key relevant AAN documents available at www.aan.com/view/PECN

A

CLINICAL VIGNETTES

CASE 1

A neurology resident sees patients in an outpatient clinic one afternoon each week, and the clinic has a 6-month waiting list for new patient visits. Miss Stanley is a 25-year-old woman with pseudotumor cerebri who has been seen by residents in clinic for the last 8 years. She has appeared for only 5 of her last 30 clinic appointments. During her initial appointment with this resident, which was 15 months ago, her prescriptions were refilled. She has not arrived for any follow-up appointments, despite rescheduling 6 times.

CASE 2

A neurologist practicing in a large multispecialty group has cared for Mrs. McCaslin, a 55-year-old woman with myasthenia gravis, for many years. Recent financial pressures have led the group to adopt a policy to decline public health insurance because the fee structure does not cover expenses, and physicians have been asked by the practice managers to stop seeing patients who are on public assistance within 3 months' time. Mrs. McCaslin has public insurance and advises that she cannot find another physician within a 3-month period.

CASE 3

A general neurologist in a suburban office has been providing care to Mr. Meeland, a 60-year-old man with chronic headache, for the last 10 years. He and his wife divorced 5 years ago, and since then, he has increased the frequency of his contact with the neurologist in office visits and phone calls. Although he schedules visits for neurologic chief complaints, he seems more interested in having a personal conversation than in discussing his medical issues. He behaves in an increasingly familiar manner more appropriate to a social relationship than a relationship between doctor and patient: he addresses the physician and staff by their first names, asks detailed questions about their personal relationships, and steers discussion away from medical concerns and toward general topics. He asks for details about the doctor's personal life and offers to "fix him up" with a family member. In his latest visit, he invited the doctor to dinner at a restaurant.

CASE 4

Mrs. Backer, a 40-year-old woman with multiple sclerosis, has been seen by a neurologist for 5 years. The relationship has always been strained, and she frequently seems angry with physician and staff. Mrs. Backer's rude and angry comments during phone calls have caused the receptionist to cry on multiple occasions, and the nurse who returns most of the phone calls has requested to have no further contact with the patient. During today's clinic visit, Mrs. Backer becomes angry about waiting for her appointment and begins screaming in the waiting room. While staff members attempt to reason with her, she threatens, "You will all be sorry for treating me this way!" Security is called, which further aggravates Mrs. Backer. She leaves the premises as requested by the security guard, screaming more threatening remarks as she goes.

QUESTIONS FOR GROUP DISCUSSION

GETTING STARTED
1. What obligations do physicians have toward their existing patients? Are there circumstances in which these obligations can be ended?

ASSESSMENT
2. What obligations does a physician have to patients on a waiting list for care? Does a physician's responsibility to existing patients take precedence over responsibility to future patients?
3. Why might a patient miss many clinic appointments or not follow-up on recommended treatment and monitoring? Are some reasons more acceptable or justifiable than others? Why?

(continued)

4. Do physicians owe patients medical care even if their practices will not be fully reimbursed?

5. Does patient noncompliance change the physician's obligations to a patient? How so? Does providing care to a noncompliant patient increase exposure to malpractice liability?

6. If caring for a patient makes a physician uncomfortable for any reason (e.g., patient use of racist or sexist language, sexually explicit comments), is the physician still obligated to provide care? Under what circumstances can a physician terminate a relationship because of personal distress?

7. Consider alternative methods of dealing with the "difficult" patient. What steps might allow a physician to negotiate a more effective relationship with a "difficult" patient?

GOAL SETTING, DECISION MAKING, AND IMPLEMENTATION

8. If you decide to maintain a strained relationship with a patient, how can you establish clear boundaries and common goals to work toward a more effective therapeutic relationship?

9. What threshold or degree of disruptive conduct by a patient is sufficient to make terminating the relationship with that patient ethically permissible?

10. What steps should be taken by a physician who has decided to terminate a physician–patient relationship to ensure that all ethical and legal obligations to the patient have been met?

COMMENTARY ON DISCUSSION QUESTIONS

GETTING STARTED

1. What obligations do physicians have toward their existing patients? Are there circumstances in which these obligations can be ended?

The physician–patient relationship forms the cornerstone of medical practice. Patients enter into this relationship seeking help for medical problems. Medical ethical codes have long recognized patients' vulnerability and required that the physician–patient relationship be conducted with the highest standards of interpersonal interaction, including professionalism, honesty, and respect for the patient's rights and interests.[1–3] The physician–patient relationship confers a fiduciary duty on the physician to act on behalf of patients' best interests, to use their knowledge of patients' personal details only for the patients' benefit, and to subjugate their own self-interest and hold the patients' interests as paramount, superceding physicians' desires for career advancement or financial gain. Ideally, physicians and patients have mutual respect and confidence in each other, with patients trusting physicians to act in patients' best interests.

Conceiving of the physician–patient relationship as based on trust distinguishes the practice of medicine from business practices that rely on formal contracts and "marketplace relationships."[4] This ethical framework for the physician–patient relationship would make financial concerns secondary, if not tertiary. However, medical practices in the United States routinely face financial constraints and "market pressures" influenced by contracts with third-party payers.

Although physicians have obligations to patients, they retain certain rights about managing their practices. Physician autonomy allows physicians to make choices about the type of practice they join, the diseases they treat, and within certain restrictions, the types of patients they treat.[5] The AMA Code of Ethics states that a physician's prerogative to enter into the physician–patient relationship is overridden only in a few situations, such as medical emergencies, when there are contractual agreements to provide care, or when the reason for refusal of care is discriminatory.[6] Both the AMA and the AAN prohibit discrimination against patients on the basis of race, religion, nationality, sexual orientation, gender, or other similar criteria.[7,8] However, physicians may refuse new patients if the physicians are ill or plan to retire, or if they are unable to meet obligations to current patients (i.e., the practice is full). Doctors may choose to stop performing certain procedures or providing care for certain diseases. They may limit a practice to a particular area of expertise and interest and refuse patients with conditions that are outside their specialty.

Bernat, 51–2, Ch. 3

Once physician and patient have agreed to enter a relationship, the presumption in many but not all circumstances is that the relationship will continue, with exceptions such as ED physicians and hospitalists, who have no obligation to continue the therapeutic relationship after the patient leaves their practice setting. As the physician–patient relationship develops over time, shared history allows physicians to provide better patient care with more understanding of the nuances and particularities of individual patients. Exceptions do exist when a relationship has a predetermined course, as when the patient seeks a procedure and follow-up care only. Sometimes the relationship has a finite duration, as in residency clinics.[9]

ASSESSMENT

2. **What obligations does a physician have to patients on a waiting list for care? Does a physician's responsibility to existing patients take precedence over responsibility to future patients?**

Physicians have a higher obligation to care for existing patients than they do for future patients; however, when multiple appointments are missed, the needs of both prospective and existing patients may have aggregate weight. Physicians' time to see patients is finite, and repeated missed appointments can adversely affect the quality of care given to other patients. In Case 1, a patient makes repeated appointments but fails to keep them. Missed appointments are typically not reimbursed, and each appointment represents lost revenue or lost opportunity for another patient to see the physician; therefore, the result is both an economic impact on the practice and an impact on patients who are waiting for new-patient openings.

3. **Why might a patient miss many clinic appointments or not follow-up on recommended treatment and monitoring? Are some reasons more acceptable or justifiable than others? Why?**

Physicians should explore the reasons behind patients' missed appointments and try to find solutions. Many neurologic conditions make it difficult for patients to maintain independence or to drive, leaving them to rely on public transportation, medical transport vans, or friends and family. Inability to keep appointments may reflect failure of transportation beyond the patient's control. Patients may have cognitive impairment that makes it more difficult for them to manage appointments or remember phone conversations, although arguably, neurologists should be aware of these patients' limitations and be certain that the patients' families or support systems are contacted regarding appointments.

In many cases, the patient and physician (or the physician's staff) can identify the impediments to clinic visits and find workable solutions. For example, patients might be called with reminders of their appointments, or appointments can be scheduled when transportation would be most reliable.

4. **Do physicians owe patients medical care even if their practices will not be fully reimbursed?**

Practice failure because of economic stressors serves neither the patient nor the clinician. Competing fiscal and fiduciary responsibilities can divide the loyalty owed to patients. In Case 2, a financial decision by the practice group dictates which patients will be seen by the practice.

Ethical guidelines and some legal precedents question whether failure to pay for services constitutes a sufficient reason for termination. According to the AMA's Council on Ethical and Judicial Affairs, "the patient's failure to pay a bill does not end the relationship, as the relationship is based on a fiduciary, rather than a financial, responsibility."[10] Legally, "[c]ourts are split on whether a patient's inability to pay or lack of insurance justifies a physician's termination of the physician/patient relationship, especially when the patient continues to require medical attention."[11]

Because many practices do not accept medical assistance, if a patient's insurance changes to public insurance, the patient may suddenly be unable to find a physician. When a patient's insurance has been dropped by a practice, physicians are obligated to help patients make other arrangements for care, which may include helping them to contact their insurer or payer to find other physicians in the same specialty. It may be more difficult to find adequate alternative care to manage a complicated medical issue with a new physician.

Physicians have traditionally provided some patients with charity care, and medical associations historically support this practice. The AMA "has long recognized an ethic [*sic*] obligation of physicians to assume some individual responsibility for making health care available to the needy."[12] The AMA Council on Ethical and Judicial Affairs document, "Caring for the Poor," concludes that every "physician has an obligation to share in providing care to the indigent."[12]

5. **Does patient noncompliance change a physician's obligations to a patient? How so? Does providing care to a noncompliant patient increase exposure to malpractice liability?**

Patients themselves have obligations in the physician–patient relationship, and the quality of care for a patient who routinely misses appointments can suffer. For many conditions, it becomes impossible for a physician to provide safe and effective care without routine follow-up. Many medications have potentially toxic side effects and must be monitored. When standards of medical practice cannot be adhered to consistently, the physician may appear to be providing medical care that fails to meet minimal standards of care. Even if a patient is informed of the risks and potential side effects of a given treatment, failure to keep future appointments may compromise care to such a degree that the physician may seek to terminate the relationship.

A physician can reiterate why monitoring is crucial for a patient's condition and why adequate follow-up is mandatory. Physician and patient may contract for a period of time in which these problems will be addressed, with the understanding that the relationship will be terminated if attendance does not improve. All such conversations and agreements should be clearly documented in the patient's chart.

As long as the physician and the physician's staff are making good-faith efforts to ensure the patient's compliance and are documenting those efforts, it is unlikely that risk of malpractice liability is elevated in caring for noncompliant patients. Moreover, terminating a relationship with a noncompliant patient without first attempting to improve compliance, to provide sufficient explanation or notice of the termination, or to assist in finding another physician *would* probably increase the risk of malpractice liability—and certainly the potential risk would be greater than that associated with trying to provide care for the patient.

6. **If caring for a patient makes a physician uncomfortable for any reason (e.g., patient use of racist or sexist language, sexually explicit comments), is the physician still obligated to provide care? Under what circumstances can a physician terminate a relationship because of personal distress?**

Many physicians find that the physician–patient relationship offers great personal satisfaction. However, any relationship can suffer from miscommunication, an inability to bridge cultural gaps, or a breakdown in useful interaction despite the best efforts of those involved. When the physician–patient relationship breaks down, the loyalty that a physician owes the patient cannot be discontinued abruptly. Unexpected or sudden termination of the physician–patient relationship leaves the patient without needed resources and constitutes abandonment.

Case 3 illustrates a situation in which inappropriate attempts by the patient to become socially intimate with the physician may be grounds for terminating the physician–patient relationship. The role of boundaries in establishing safe interaction can be summarized as follows:

> Boundaries in the patient–physician relationship prevent exploitation of either of the 2 parties by allowing the 2 parties to set appropriate limits during the interaction…. Mutually understood boundaries provide protection for the patients in the relationship by allowing certain limits on physical space and contact and emotional involvement. Physicians also may have a number of psychological vulnerabilities. Caring for patients may foster strong emotions in physicians; boundaries protect the physician from overextending in this regard.[13]

Some patients may not appreciate these boundaries and may ask their physicians personal questions, offer repeated gifts and compliments, or attempt to engage in a relationship outside the clinic. In these situations, the physician should carefully point out to the patient the behavior that transgressed boundaries and explain why that behavior warrants concern. If the patient asks unwanted and intrusive personal questions, the physician can make it clear to the patient that such questions are inappropriate. Reiteration of commitment to the physician–patient relationship in its context and to the patient's specific medical care should be emphasized. Sensitivity is warranted to the emotional pain or loss of face that the patient might experience.

7. **Consider alternative methods of dealing with the "difficult" patient. What steps might allow a physician to negotiate a more effective relationship with a "difficult" patient?**

Case 4 explores a difficult physician–patient relationship in which trust and some degree of ease between physician and patient never develop. A patient may present with anger for various reasons, including poor interactions with healthcare professionals in the past, difficulty navigating the healthcare bureaucracy, or mistrust of the healthcare system and its agents. These difficulties may predate the establishment of the physician–patient relationship and cause difficulty from the initial contact. The patient may seem suspicious of the physician's advice and motivation, while the physician becomes wary and frustrated with the patient, perhaps feeling that patient expectations can never be met adequately. The difficult physician–patient interaction can become more tenuous as misunderstandings and poor communication lead to defensive behavior and assumptions about each other's motives.

Difficult relationships with patients stem from a variety of causes. One study found that "patients perceived as difficult are more likely to have a depressive or anxiety disorder, poorer functional status, unmet expectations, reduced satisfaction, and greater use of health care services."[14] "Difficult" patient behavior may reflect greater need and psychological distress and poor coping skills. Patients should be given the opportunity to express the reasons for their dissatisfaction. Similarly, although it may be difficult to do, physicians should examine their own behavior, consider how it contributes to the relationship, and consider changes that may help to resolve the conflict. In situations in which it appears that patients' anger is in response to their circumstances, rather than in response to identifiable actions on the part of the physician or staff, it is often helpful not to respond to their angered utterances and instead focus on listening to their needs while attempting to maintain compassion. When patients behave aggressively with verbal abuse, physicians must resist the impulse to respond in kind, or act in a way that would escalate the encounter, short of putting themselves or others in danger.

GOAL SETTING, DECISION MAKING, AND IMPLEMENTATION

8. **If you decide to maintain a strained relationship with a patient, how can you establish clear boundaries and common goals to work toward a more effective therapeutic relationship?**

Patients may need guidance to understand the limits of the professional relationship and to help identify inappropriate behavior and establish acceptable behavior, especially when neurologic impairment, such as impaired judgment or disinhibition, contributes. If appropriate, written descriptions of acceptable and unacceptable behavior, including a description of the consequences of unacceptable behavior, can be provided, and caregivers can be involved to remind patients of appropriate interactions. If a patient makes repeated phone calls and demands more time and attention than the physician or office staff can provide, physicians can establish ground rules (e.g., specific limits on the number or duration of phone calls per week) and explore other ways to meet the patient's needs. Only after efforts at restoring the relationship or redefining limits fail should termination of the physician–patient relationship be considered.

9. **What threshold or degree of disruptive conduct by a patient is sufficient to make terminating the relationship with that patient ethically permissible?**

Although patients' needs and best interests should be given considerable deference, abusive patient behavior cannot go unchecked. One threshold for taking action is when disruptive patient behavior begins to interfere with the care or comfort of other patients. Patient advocates, practice managers, or other neutral parties may help to establish better communication, clear expectations for behaviors, and consequences if those expectations cannot be met. Because a patient may require time to change conduct, a reasonable trial period during which the patient receives constructive and appropriate feedback is often indicated. Terminating the relationship at the first violation of the agreement, for example, might appear retaliatory.

Bernat, 55–6, Ch. 3

Despite best efforts, some difficult patient behaviors may warrant termination of the relationship.[15] Patients who threaten harm may require the physician to consult legal advisors and utilize security personnel to protect staff and other patients. In the extreme case in which threats are made or dangerous behaviors enacted, the physician's duty to protect others from harm may warrant immediate termination of the relationship.

10. What steps should be taken by a physician who has decided to terminate a physician–patient relationship to ensure that all ethical and legal obligations to the patient have been met?

Regardless of the reasons for terminating the relationship, physicians should review state laws or regulations (e.g., from the state licensing board) and published guidelines by state or national medical societies such as the AMA and AAN. The AMA Code of Medical Ethics (8.115) states:

> Physicians have an obligation to support continuity of care for their patients. While physicians have the option of withdrawing from a case, they cannot do so without giving notice to the patient, the relatives, or responsible friends sufficiently long in advance of withdrawal to permit another medical attendant to be secured.[16]

The AAN has similar guidelines:

> Once the relationship has begun, the neurologist must provide care until care is complete, the patient ends the relationship, or the neurologist returns the patient to the care of the referring physician. If the neurologist justifiably desires to end the relationship, and if continued neurologic care is appropriate, he/she should assist in arranging care by another neurologist.[8]

The events leading to the decision to terminate the relationship should have been clearly documented in the patient's chart at the time of each occurrence, including missed appointments, reasons given for cancellation, incidents of verbal abuse, specific patient language and staff response, time of the events, and participants or witnesses to the behavior. Conversations with the patient to establish boundaries should also be recorded, with specific expectations and consequences for future transgressions clearly enumerated.

Although an in-person conversation explaining the reasons for termination is preferable as an initial step, the notification should also occur in writing.[10] The letter should include a brief explanation—in impartial language that is free of a judgmental or accusatory tone—of the reason for termination. The length of time that needed services will continue to be available should be clearly presented. The duration may vary, depending on the condition being treated and availability of clinicians competent to treat the condition. In areas with healthcare shortages and long waiting lists for appointments, a longer timeframe for termination may be appropriate to ensure that patients can secure care from another provider. The letter to the patient should be sent by certified mail with return receipt to document that the patient has received notification. Sample letters are available from medical societies or in published literature for reference.[17]

Bernat, 55–6, Ch. 3

The ethical duty not to abandon the patient remains, regardless of legal constraints and professional guidance.[15] Physicians should facilitate the transfer of care to another healthcare professional with both thoroughness and timeliness. Arguably, physicians should provide names and locations of recommended physicians; however, patients can also be directed to public resources or patient advocacy groups with links to physicians or centers with appropriate expertise. Privacy regulations (HIPAA) permit the physician to send records to another physician, even without a signed waiver for the purpose of medical care. The physician should also offer to communicate directly with the new caregiver regarding the patient's medical history and treatments, if this would reasonably facilitate patient care.

Once the patient is referred to another physician, copies of records are transmitted. A potential stumbling block beyond the control of the referring physician is the waiting time involved for new patient appointments with the new physician, a period during which the patient may not have access to care, except via the ED. If continued care cannot be established and the relationship must be terminated, state laws and medical society recommendations should be examined to ensure that regulatory requirements are met, as these vary according to healthcare plan and location. Regardless of legislative constraints, the ethical burden of the physician as the patient's fiduciary remains, prohibiting termination in a manner that would constitute abandonment.

KEY POINTS

- Unexpected or sudden termination of the physician–patient relationship is both ethically and legally problematic.
- Failure to pay for services should not be considered an indication for immediate termination of the relationship.

- Establishing clear boundaries within the physician–patient relationship requires clear and open communication and is necessary to prevent inappropriate interactions.
- In most cases, the physician should attempt to find suitable replacement care before termination of care is complete.
- The reasons for termination of care should be well documented in the patient's chart and clearly conveyed via letter.

KEY WORDS

Fiduciary relationship—relationship that is founded on trust in which physicians are held to a high standard of conduct to use their authority for patients' best interests.

Abandonment—a legal term that refers to the termination of the physician–patient relationship without reasonable effort to arrange for continued care.

REFERENCES

1. Baker RB, Caplan AL, Emanuel LL, et al., eds. *The American Medical Ethics Revolution: How the AMA's Code of Ethics Has Transformed Physicians' Relationships to Patients, Professionals, and Society.* Baltimore, MD: The Johns Hopkins University Press, 1999:117.
2. American Medical Association. Code of Medical Ethics. Principles of Medical Ethics. Available at www.ama-assn.org/ama/pub/physician-resources/medical-ethics/code-medical-ethics/principles-medical-ethics.shtml. Accessed March 29, 2012.
3. Spencer E. Professional Ethics. In: Fletcher J, Boyle R, eds. *Introduction to Clinical Ethics, 2nd ed.* Hagerstown, MD: University Publishing Group, 1997:289.
4. Beauchamp T, Childress J. *Principles of Biomedical Ethics, 5th ed.* New York: Oxford University Press, 2001:312.
5. Bernat, 51–2, Ch. 3.
6. American Medical Association. Code of Medical Ethics. Opinion 10.015, The Patient–Physician Relationship. Available at www.ama-assn.org/ama/pub/physician-resources/medical-ethics/code-medical-ethics/opinion10015.page. Accessed March 29, 2012.
7. American Medical Association. Code of Medical Ethics. Opinion 10.05, Potential Patients. Available at www.ama-assn.org/ama/pub/physician-resources/medical-ethics/code-medical-ethics/opinion1005.page. Accessed March 29, 2012.
8. American Academy of Neurology. Code of Professional Conduct. Section 1.3, Beginning and Ending the Relationship. [*PECN* appendix document A and available at www.aan.com/view/PECN]
9. DeWitt T, Roberts K. Teaching residents about patient and practice termination in community-based continuity settings. Arch Pediatr Adolesc Med 1995; 149:1367–70.
10. American Medical Association. Patient–Physician Relationship Topics. Ending the Patient–Physician Relationship. Available at www.ama-assn.org/ama/pub/category/4609.html. Accessed March 16, 2012.
11. Katz L, Paul MB. When a physician may refuse to treat a patient. Physician's News Digest, February 2002. Available at www.saul.com/media/article/1048_pdf_527.pdf. Accessed March 16, 2012.
12. American Medical Association. Council on Ethical and Judicial Affairs. CEJA C – I-92, Caring for the poor. Available at www.ama-assn.org/ama1/pub/upload/mm/code-medical-ethics/9065a.pdf. Accessed March 16, 2012.
13. Farber N, Novack D, Obrien MK. Love, boundaries, and the patient–physician relationship. Arch Intern Med 1997; 157(20):2291–4.

14. Jackson J, Kroenke K. Difficult patient encounters in the ambulatory clinic. Arch Intern Med 1999; 159(10):1069–75.
15. Bernat, 55–6, Ch. 3.
16. American Medical Association. Opinion 8.115, Termination of the Physician–Patient Relationship. Available at www.ama-assn.org/ama/pub/physician-resources/medical-ethics/code-medical-ethics/opinion8115.page?. Accessed March 16, 2012.
17. Willis D, Zerr A. Terminating a patient: Is it time to part ways? Fam Pract Manag 2005; 12(8):34–8.

SUGGESTIONS FOR FURTHER READING

Huss WH, Coleman M. *Start Your Own Medical Practice: A Guide to All the Things They Don't Teach You in Medical School about Starting Your Own Practice*. Naperville, IL: Sphinx Publishing, 2006:156.
Miller RD. *Problems in Health Care Law*. Sadbury, MA: Jones & Bartlett Publishers, 2006:442.

9 THE IMPAIRED PHYSICIAN

William Brannon, Jr., MD, FAAN

LEARNING OBJECTIVES

Upon completion of this chapter, participants will be able to:

1. Describe how to recognize behaviors that suggest that a physician is impaired.
2. Discuss the ethical rationale and the role of self-regulation in professionalism as it applies to reporting impaired colleagues.
3. Describe the types of programs that are available to assist impaired physicians and the success rate for treating impaired physicians.

LEARNING RESOURCES

Key chapters in Bernat's third edition—1, 2, 3

Key relevant AAN documents available at www.aan.com/view/PECN

A   B   C

CLINICAL VIGNETTES

CASE 1

Dr. Livingston is a 72-year-old general surgeon who has practiced in the community for more than 30 years; he is well liked and is a role model for young physicians. His colleagues recently noted that during surgery he was slower and occasionally seemed "mixed up" for otherwise routine procedures. At the instruction of one of his partners, and unknown to Dr. Livingston, the office staff started directing simpler cases to him and more complex cases to the other surgeons. He saw an established patient for a lump in her supraclavicular fossa in the same area where 5 years ago he had removed a mass that proved to be a benign lymph node. Without further evaluation, he surgically removed the mass, which again was benign. During the surgical procedure, which he performed alone, the staff noted that Dr. Livingston was tentative and slow. Postoperatively, the patient was found to have injury to the spinal accessory and supraspinatus nerves. With encouragement from his department chair, Dr. Livingston was sent to a neurologist for evaluation of possible cognitive impairment. His Mini-Mental State Exam score was 25, with errors in short-term recall and construction. Subjectively, his answers to many questions in the history were vague or evasive, and he and his wife minimized his problems as "senior moments," including the time that he became lost while driving in a familiar neighborhood. The neurologist suspected dementia and recommended more detailed neuropsychologic testing, which Dr. Livingston refused, claiming that he was safe to operate and that "that stupid memory testing can't determine whether I'm capable of operating."

CASE 2

Dr. Parker, a 36-year-old neurologist, joined a practice of 3 other neurologists—one senior member considering retirement and 2 who had been part of the practice for 6 years and had been granted partnership status. For the first half year of Dr. Parker's tenure, he developed a reputation of having an excellent work ethic and was well liked by his patients and his peers. He seemed to thrive on work and was willing to take call for his senior partner on frequent occasions. After 3 months in this practice, Dr. Parker developed a lingering respiratory illness associated with a chronic cough. His primary care physician prescribed a cough preparation that did not effectively control his symptom. He found a sample of a cough preparation containing hydrocodone that did effectively control his cough and restored his energy. After 4 weeks, he was symptom-free. After 6 months in the practice, Dr. Parker experienced the untimely death of a fellow resident who had been his close mentor during training. He became depressed and began to self-medicate with an antidepressant but found no benefit, and he began to use increased amounts of beverage alcohol. A few weeks later, family discord developed and evolved during ensuing months to divorce after he had refused marriage counseling and told his wife that he did not want to continue the marriage. His practice contract came up for renewal after he had been in the practice for 18 months. Disagreement with the provisions of the document and discord that had been brewing with the other members of the group for some time resulted in Dr. Parker's leaving the practice and accepting a position as a hospitalist–neurologist in a town some distance away.

In his new position, Dr. Parker quickly became known for his erratic temper, particularly with the nursing staff, and his seeming indifference to physicians who had referred patients for his care in hospital. In addition, he failed to make rounds at appropriate times, wrote inappropriate orders such as "TLC q2h at bedside." This behavior became of such concern that the nursing staff presented the problem to Dr. Parker's associate neurologist in the hospitalist practice. He was reluctant to become involved in someone else's problem, as he was also busy and did not want to "rock the boat" lest he lose a fellow worker and see his job requirements increase. The nursing staff referred the matter to the nurse manager, who spoke to Dr. Parker. Dr. Parker was indifferent to that discussion, and his behavior continued. When he failed to arrive at the start of his shift in the hospital and a crisis occurred on the floor, the nurse manager was informed and referred the matter to the hospital chief of staff. After his review, he referred the matter to the committee for impaired physicians, and an investigation was begun.

QUESTIONS FOR GROUP DISCUSSION

GETTING STARTED

1. Have you personally encountered a physician who you thought was impaired in the practice of medicine? If so, how did you feel about the situation? Did you consider ethical implications of the impairment that you observed? How should you respond to such an issue?

ASSESSMENT

2. What are similarities and differences in the cases? Are the physicians impaired? If so, what findings suggest impairment in each instance?
3. Discuss the ethical and professional issues related to cognitive impairment or dementia in physicians.
4. What are the signs of impairment by drug or alcohol use in practicing physicians?

MORAL DIAGNOSIS

5. What are the ethical and professional obligations of the neurologist in Case 1 who suspects that the practicing surgeon has dementia? Similarly, what are the ethical and professional obligations of the neurologist in Case 2 who was approached by the nurse manager about a colleague who she suspects may be impaired?
6. What are the obligations of the neurologists in each of the cases to the physicians who are suspected of impairment?
7. Discuss whether concerns for the safety of patients or concerns for the privacy of the physicians should prevail in each case.

GOAL SETTING, DECISION MAKING, AND IMPLEMENTATION

8. What current policies or procedures are relevant to reporting impaired colleagues?
9. What resources are available to assist physicians who are impaired by substance abuse? What is the success rate in treating physicians who are impaired by substance abuse?

That investigation led to the conclusion that Dr. Parker was impaired by addiction to hydrocodone in particular, was a user of any opiate he could obtain, and was an alcoholic.

COMMENTARY ON DISSCUSSION QUESTIONS

1. Have you personally encountered a physician who you thought was impaired in the practice of medicine? If so, how did you feel about the situation? Did you consider ethical implications of the impairment that you observed? How should you respond to such an issue?

An impaired physician is one who, by virtue of a physical or mental illness or control by substance or alcohol abuse, is unable to fulfill personal and professional responsibilities. The chance is that most physicians during their careers will encounter a colleague, a teacher, or an attending who is impaired. Although the exact incidence of impaired physicians is not known, estimates state that between 10% and 15% of all healthcare professionals will at some time during their careers misuse drugs, approximately 6% to 8% of physicians have substance use disorders, and up to 14% having an alcohol use disorder. It is believed that the overall prevalence of substance use and alcoholism among physicians is approximately the same as in the general public.[1] Other references place the number at around 10% to 15% at risk during some time in their careers.[2]

A 2005 study of physician willingness to report impaired colleagues found that 22% had reported an impaired colleague to a physicians' health program. Fewer than half of the respondents were aware of any guidelines for reporting an impaired colleague. Most respondents believed that the protection of society trumped the protection of individual's rights when it came to impaired physicians, and most reported that they would be more likely to report a colleague impaired because of substance abuse than they would to report one impaired because of cognitive decline or psychological impairment.[3] Another study sampled 3,500 physicians and reported that 64% of the sample completely agreed that all instances of significantly impaired or incompetent colleagues should be reported to their professional society, hospital or clinic, or other relevant authority. Women physicians, US medical school graduates, and those who practiced in hospitals, clinics, or academic centers were significantly more likely to agree that impaired colleagues should always be reported. Those in practice between 10 and 19 years, those in practice for more than 30 years, and those practicing in solo or 2-person groups were less likely to agree that an impaired colleague should always be reported. Barriers to reporting impaired colleagues who were discovered include the thought that someone else was taking care of the problem, belief that nothing would happen as the result of the report, fear of retribution, belief that it was not their responsibility, belief that punishment would be excessive, lack of knowledge on how to report, and belief that it could happen to them.[4]

Wynia pointed out that the word *professional* derives from the Latin and means to "speak forth" or to "declare aloud and publically."[5] He emphasized that the time honored idea of medical professionalism, which holds that medical practitioners are best suited to establish standards and values in the practice of medicine, is now directly challenged in that role. For example, as reported by DesRoches, 17% of physicians surveyed reported that in the 3 previous years they had come into contact with impaired colleagues, yet one-third of them had taken no action.[4] He noted that one-third of physicians in that report were not completely certain of their obligation to take action and one-third reported that they were unprepared to take action.

Until now, the obligation of physicians to report impaired colleagues may have been considered a supererogatory act (an act of goodness that is "above and beyond the call of duty" and thus represents a moral ideal[6]). With regulatory agencies assuming more of a role in the practice of medicine justified by the concern for patient safety, the supererogatory concept is replaced by direct ethical and legal obligations for physicians to become proactive in concern for impaired colleagues.

In a lengthy report from the Hastings Center, Morreim discusses the need for physicians to police themselves and the barriers to doing so, such as not having standards and facts to form a basis for judgment, the fear that the physician who reports a colleague may himself become a target for retribution, and uncertainty about whether or not the issue to be reported actually reflects a level of impairment.[7] Morreim reports that most states have statutes that require physicians to report impaired or otherwise questionably qualified colleagues. Further, the states provide additional considerations that bolster reporting requirements; namely, the duty to warn and the doctrine of fraudulent concealment, which holds that a physician who knows that he or another physician has caused patient injury, whether or not through negligence, should disclose that fact. Not to do so may constitute fraud, within the doctrine of fraudulent concealment, even if the failure to report is passive, as in simply keeping silent. That duty applies only to those actually treating patients and not to those bystanders who may have only heard about an issue of incompetence or negligence.[7]

Another issue is that of *qui tam*, or "one who sues on behalf of the king as well as himself." Qui tam arose in an effort by the US federal government, in a 1986 revision of the False Claims Act, to encourage citizens to help prosecute by reporting those who would defraud the government. Those reporters gain a share of the proceeds collected against the physician who may be convicted of such fraud.[7] Ethical issues continue to be paramount in practice in respect to duties regarding incompetent colleagues. Medical ethics as defined by the AMA require that, "a physician shall uphold the standards of professionalism, be honest in all professional interactions, and strive to report physicians deficient in character or competence, or engaging in fraud or deception, to appropriate entities"[8] and "a physician shall recognize a responsibility to participate in activities contributing to the improvement of the community and the betterment of public health."[9] In similar terms, Section 6.6 of the AAN Code of Professional Conduct requires that members assist in the identification and resolution of issues concerning impaired colleagues.[10]

Of particular interest, Bernat points out that neurologists encounter ethical issues in daily practice, and he discusses the principal ethical theories, stressing the concepts and rules to be learned.[11] He expands on the concepts that form the moral foundation of the physician–patient relationship[12] and stresses that physicians have a nonmaleficence–based ethical duty to colleagues and patients to help in identifying and assisting impaired physicians in their recovery, if such is possible.[13]

Bernat, 3–23, Ch. 1
Bernat, 24–48, Ch. 2
Bernat, 62–3, Ch. 4

ASSESSMENT

2. What are similarities and differences in the cases? Are the physicians impaired? If so, what findings suggest impairment in each instance?

In Case 1, the surgeon does have signs of early cognitive impairment that his colleagues noted and for which his office compensated, in itself a demonstration that the surgeon is impaired. In the case, preoperative evaluation of a patient was not adequately performed even though she previously had an enlarged lymph node in the same area. In addition to these factors, Dr. Parker resisted any further evaluation, which reflected a significant change in his behavior, and resistance to evaluation is the first sign to look for in a colleague who has mild cognitive impairment or is developing clear signs of dementia. In these early stages, the cognitively impaired physician is very good at hiding subtle deficiencies and will gloss over what seems to be a minor error in practice or signs of impaired cognitive function, such as a slight memory deficit or perhaps a mild word-finding difficulty, with a glib but plausible explanation. Other factors that may be important clues to the mental status of a practicing physician would include the stability of family relationships; business practices, particularly decisions on such issues as managing retirement funds; mistakes in writing prescriptions; delay or forgetfulness in keeping up with medical records; or errors in making notes. Changes in personality, such as withdrawing from participation in activities where others may view behavior, irritability in relationships with colleagues and hospital personnel, and failure to keep appointed rounds or to attend conferences, may all be clues to early cognitive impairment.

Cognitive changes are a normal part of aging and, in and of themselves, do not constitute evidence of mild cognitive impairment or dementia, the incidence of which increases considerably with age, which is perhaps a significant reason physicians shy away from becoming involved in reporting potentially cognitively impaired colleagues. Lobo-Prabbu et al. noted that the physician population in the United States is graying, with slightly more than 35% of physicians past age 55 as of 2006.[14] Barriers to identifying potentially cognitively impaired physicians may include:

1. Older physicians may have a lighter caseload and therefore less opportunity for peer review.
2. Younger physicians may feel uncomfortable voicing concerns about older colleagues out of respect or because the older physician may have been a mentor.
3. Hospital administrators may be reluctant to ask for a review of the privileges of older respected physicians who may have helped them keep their jobs.
4. Medical staff bylaws may not address special needs in credentialing the aging physician.

5. Subtle cognitive changes are difficult to identify.
6. Peers may be enablers by assisting their older colleagues and helping to hide their mental status changes.[14]

Although proactive measures to identify physicians with cognitive impairment and to establish guidelines for what to do when they are identified have received limited focus, some discussion has addressed potential changes that may be helpful, such as annual physical and mental status examinations for physicians over age 65 years who continue to practice.[14] Particularly important is the issue of identifying and treating potentially reversible cognitive impairments, as opposed to presuming the dementia is permanent and untreatable and encouraging or forcing the retirement of physicians who are demented. Approximately 20% of patients who appear to have dementia at first pass may have a treatable illness, depression among the most likely. Treatment could enable some physicians to return to active practice. Thus, it is even more important to strive for early recognition and diagnosis of those impaired by cognitive disturbance.

Case 2 illustrates a physician who is impaired by substance abuse that was likely triggered by a lingering respiratory illness, perhaps leading to depression and frustration because of his not feeling well and not being able to balance his active schedule. Hydrocodone not only helped his cough, but also may have induced a false sense of wellness. The next blow came from a personal emotional crisis from which the physician found no effective relief in self-treatment. Then followed the other issues of a dysfunctional family, overwork, and the necessity to earn a large income to support his habit, his family, and himself. None of his colleagues recognized his distress until things deteriorated to the point of his becoming a dangerous physician, forcing action to identify his deficiencies, which led to rehabilitation attempts and effective treatment. Wallace and colleagues point out the many stressors that affect physicians, including inordinately heavy workloads, with an increase in work superimposed; 50–60-hour workweeks when not on call; work shifts longer than 24 hours; and work in emotionally charged atmospheres that are associated with suffering, failures, fear, and death.[15] Physicians may also contend with difficult situations with patients, families, and hospital staff. The constant demand for rapid cognitive assessment while processing large data sets may have a negative effect on work quality. These factors may significantly contribute to a physician seeking some substance for relief and thus becoming an abuser. Combine this scenario with the fact that many physicians have no personal physician to turn to, and it becomes no surprise that physicians become impaired.

3. **Discuss the ethical and professional issues related to cognitive impairment or dementia in physicians.**

Ethically, we as physicians are bound to place the best interests of patients and their protection above all else in our practice. Included in that mandate is the obligation to be aware of the practice issues of those colleagues with whom we daily interact, whether by patient referrals, requests for consultations, or direct observation. As noted above, the identification of and willingness to seek assistance for the potentially cognitively impaired physician is inherently difficult and has many barriers.

In assisting a senior physician to recognize his age-related limitations, one may enlist the assistance of his junior associates or confidants who have worked with him in the operating room or in other venues to offer a private critique. One may seek assistance by inquiring into policies and resources of a hospital staff or state medical society and following those recommendations. Another option is to speak confidentially to a trusted colleague who would look into the issue and advise an appropriate course of action. It is better not to approach the impaired physician directly with what might be perceived as an accusation. Doing so may lead to further denial and entrench a defensive attitude toward the colleague trying to help.

4. What are the signs of impairment by drug or alcohol use in practicing physicians?

When a colleague comes to work reeking of alcohol, unable to navigate effectively, and not in a mindset conducive to good patient care, it is a "no-brainer" to recognize impairment. Generally though, most physicians are effectively able to hide their drug- or alcohol-induced impairment, sometimes for a long period. This author is aware of one physician who kept 2 cases of mouthwash in his office under the guise of combating bad breath. In fact, one case of bottles had its mouthwash replaced by Scotch whiskey, and the other case was mouthwash to hide the odor of the Scotch. Some years passed before the impairment became obvious after several errors occurred while he performed surgery. Behaviors indicating the possibility of substance abuse range from nearly normal to those of a disruptive person. Analyzing health and practice in a group of general surgeons in Wisconsin, Harms et al. noted that 10% of the group of 114 practicing surgeons drank alcohol daily, 25% of the group encountered physicians who were covering call while impaired by alcohol, and 7% of the study group were alcoholic.[16]

In addition to the usual signs of intoxication, more subtle signs may be detected, such as personality changes, including irritability, rigidity, and increasingly variable and inconsistent behaviors and interpersonal relationships. Those issues may be difficult to assess initially, as physicians in general are known for peculiarities in behavior and such issues may be thought simply a part of that latitude in eccentricity. Depression and substance abuse may mimic one another, making the distinction difficult. Nevertheless, a decline in productivity, making clinical rounds at odd times, excessive fatigue, sleep disturbances, deficient record keeping, and social withdrawal are red flags that suggest a more careful appraisal of a physician.[17]

Swiggert and colleagues have reported a spectrum of behaviors that range from aggressive through passive-aggressive to passive behaviors that are in themselves potentially disruptive. In the aggressive group are inappropriate anger or threats, yelling and publicly demeaning colleagues and team members, intimidating behaviors, using foul or vulgar language, throwing things, outbursts of anger, violence, and physical abuse. Passive-aggressive behaviors include hostile notes or emails, derogatory or belittling comments about the institution or groups, sexual harassment, and persistent complaining and blaming. More passive issues include chronic tardiness, failure to return telephone calls, inadequate or inappropriate chart notes, avoidance of responsibilities for meeting attendance, etc., refusal to participate in activities as expected, and inadequate or no preparation for duties.[18]

MORAL DIAGNOSIS

5. **What are the ethical and professional obligations of the neurologist in Case 1 who suspects that the practicing surgeon has dementia? Similarly, what are the ethical and professional obligations of the neurologist in Case 2 who was approached by the nurse manager about a colleague who she suspects may be impaired?**

Bernat, 62–3, Ch. 4

Confronting this kind of issue is difficult. Bernat points out that among the ethical obligations physicians have to colleagues and to the community are "to teach, to recognize, and rehabilitate impaired physicians."[13] The AAN in Section 6.1 of its Code of Professional Conduct requires that "the neurologist should cooperate and communicate with other healthcare professionals, including other physicians, nurses, and therapists, in order to provide the best care possible to patients"[19] and, in Section 6.3, that "a neurologist should not knowingly ignore a colleague's incompetence or professional misconduct, thus jeopardizing the safety of the colleague's present and future patients.[20] Violations of the AAN Code of Conduct may be a basis for disciplinary action against members of the AAN.[21]

The Joint Commission has mandated that each healthcare organization have in place bylaws or procedures for addressing issues of impairment among the medical staff. In MS.11.01.01, relating to a medical staff, elements of performance require that patient protection be paramount and that provisions for identification, diagnosis, and rehabilitation, rather than discipline of impaired physicians, be established.[22]

6. **What are the obligations of the neurologists in each of the cases to the physicians who are suspected of impairment?**

Medicine is a learned profession. In being so considered, practitioners have the privilege of self-regulation, wherein the members of the profession are allowed the autonomy and authority to determine the requirements for education and practice. Implicit then is the obligation—moral, ethical, and practical—to ensure that appropriate standards of excellence in education and practice are maintained so that the best interests of the patient are ensured. That obligation, by virtue of the traditions of medicine, accrues to each member of the profession—student and practicing physician alike. Morreim very elegantly discusses the barriers to reporting impaired colleagues, among them: inviting scrutiny of oneself (retribution is well known against whistleblowers, and no one wants that label), encountering possible allegations of attempting to stifle competition, and fear of lawsuits.[7]

A major problem is convincing physicians to fulfill their obligation by making known the faults of practicing physicians when those faults involve cognitive or skills decline because of age or because of incompetencies that result from inadequate continuing education or training. This obligation is mandated by the AAN and AMA.[8]

7. **Discuss whether concerns for the safety of patients or concerns for the privacy of the physicians should prevail in each case.**

Professional self-regulation is a foundation of the privilege that physicians have to provide the healthcare of an individual. Physicians have an obligation to report impaired colleagues. In accepting their role as healthcare professionals, they also must forfeit claim to some privacies and be willing to accept a level of scrutiny in their practices and, to some extent, in their private lives. Depending on the setting, a physician who is aware that another physician is impaired should inform the department chief, hospital chief of staff, or an appropriate committee of the state medical society or state licensing board. The Joint Commission, which has a prime mandate for patient safety, has mandated that each organization deal with impaired physicians through the medical staff, which has a responsibility to establish mechanisms and criteria for reviewing physician credentials and for establishing means to terminate an impaired physician's membership in the medical staff.[23]

GOAL SETTING, DECISION MAKING, AND IMPLEMENTATION

8. **What current policies or procedures are relevant to reporting impaired colleagues?**

Virtually all institutions where medicine is practiced have procedures and policy manuals available through the offices of the medical staff, the chief of staff, medical education, and various department chiefs of service. Additionally, each local and state medical society has in place a mechanism for assisting in the recognition, evaluation, rehabilitation, and disposition of impaired physicians. These programs are usually designed with the cooperation of the state medical licensing authority to rehabilitate or discipline an affected individual. Leape and Fromson have proposed that the current ad hoc approach to physician performance be replaced by a routine, formal, proactive system of monitoring that would use validated measures to focus on behavioral and clinical performance. Three required components would be objectiveness, fairness, and responsiveness.[24] Effecting this approach requires the cooperation of private practices, hospitals, and both state and local medical societies.

9. **What resources are available to assist physicians who are impaired by substance abuse? What is the success rate in treating physicians who are impaired by substance abuse?**

Resources available to assist in rehabilitating physicians who are incompetent because of illness or addiction include local hospitals, medical societies, and state medical associations. Some state medical associations, through a risk-management approach, seek to make physicians aware of the impairment issues as they begin practice. These are valuable resources for physicians as they mature in their practice.

Medical schools have student health services and advocacy to assist students who are in trouble from any cause. For practicing physicians, every jurisdiction has an available physicians health program to assist the physician who is facing impairment caused by substance abuse. These programs provide confidentiality, mandate formal treatment, and have a long-term monitoring effort. Merio and Greene reviewed physician views regarding the physicians health program in one state and noted that 78.4% of participants reported satisfaction with the program, whereas 15.4% expressed dissatisfaction.[25] The results of the treatment program were found to be better than similar programs for the general public. Ways in which the program was said to be helpful included maintaining sobriety, helping to provide job security, assisting in restoration of healthy relationships, and improving spiritual foundation. Respondents felt that the program was not as helpful with managing legal and malpractice issues. Only 4.7% of participants found the program entirely unhelpful.[25]

Holtman studied the disciplinary careers of drug-impaired physicians and found that of medical practice licenses revoked during an 11-year period, approximately 13% were restored.[26] Physicians disciplined for drug and alcohol abuse were more likely to have their licenses restored than those whose licenses were revoked for other reasons. Physicians whose licenses were revoked for substance abuse were also more likely to have a repeat disciplinary event.[26]

In addition to the ethical and potentially legal issues involved in reporting and dealing with impaired physicians,

> We need a better understanding of the types of stress involved in medical training and practice and the nature of the dangerous dysphoria it can produce. We must be willing to teach and talk openly about the disease of addiction. ... The measure of the health of our profession is not only how well we care for our patients, but also how well we take care of ourselves.[27]

KEY POINTS

■ An impaired physician is one who, by virtue of a physical or mental illness or control by substance or alcohol abuse, is unable to fulfill personal and professional responsibilities.

■ Estimates suggest that between 10% and 15% of all healthcare professionals will at some time during their careers misuse drugs, approximately 6% to 8% of physicians have substance use disorders, and up to 14% have an alcohol use disorder.

■ Patient protection is paramount, and physicians have an ethical obligation to report impaired colleagues.

■ Most states have statutes that require physicians to report impaired or incompetent colleagues.

■ Virtually all institutions where medicine is practiced have procedure and policy manuals with guidance on reporting impaired and incompetent colleagues.

■ Local and state medical societies and medical boards have mechanisms for assisting in the recognition, evaluation, rehabilitation, and discipline of impaired physicians.

■ The spectrum of questionable behaviors that should not be ignored include personality changes, irritability, rigidity, and increasingly variable and inconsistent behaviors and interpersonal relationships; decline in productivity; making clinical rounds at odd times; excessive fatigue; sleep disturbances; deficient record keeping; social withdrawal; disruptive conduct; inadequate or inappropriate chart notes; refusal to participate in activities as expected; and inadequate or no preparation for duties.

KEY WORDS

Impaired practitioner—one whose ability to practice medicine with reasonable skill and safety is impaired because of a physical, neurologic, psychiatric, or emotional illness, including deterioration through the aging process, loss of motor skill, or excessive use or abuse of drugs, including alcohol.

Incompetent practitioner—one who is unable to provide sound medical care (diagnostic and treatment services) because of deficient training, experience, qualifications, clinical skills, knowledge, or judgment.

Qui tam—abbreviation of the Latin phrase *qui tam pro domino rege quam pro se ipso in hac parte sequitur* ("who as much for [our] lord the king as for himself in this action pursues"). This concept allows a private individual who assists a prosecution to receive all or part of any imposed penalties. It is current in the United States under the False Claims Act (31 USC § 3729 et seq.), which allows a private individual with knowledge of past or present fraud committed against the federal government to bring suit on the government's behalf.

REFERENCES

1. Baldisseeri MR. Impaired healthcare professional. Crit Care Med 2007; 35(2) (Suppl):S106–16.
2. Berg KH, Seppala MD, Schipper AM. Chemical dependency and the physician. Mayo Clin Proc 2009; 84(7):625–31.
3. Farber NJ, Gilibert SG, Aboff BM, et al. Physicians' willingness to report impaired colleagues. Soc Sci Med 2005; 61:1772–5.
4. DesRoches CM, Rao SR, Fromson JA, et al. Physicians' perceptions, preparedness for reporting and experiences related to impaired and incompetent colleagues. JAMA 2010; 304(2):187–93.
5. Wynia MK. The role of professionalism and self-regulation in detecting impaired or incompetent physicians. JAMA 2010; 304(2):210–1.
6. Bernat, 12, Ch. 1.
7. Morreim EH. Am I my brother's warden? Responding to the unethical or incompetent colleague. Hastings Cent Rep 1993; 23(3).
8. American Medical Association. Code of Medical Ethics. Principles of Medical Ethics. Section II. Available at www.ama-assn.org/ama/pub/physician-resources/medical-ethics/code-medical-ethics/principles-medical-ethics.page. Accessed March 26, 2012.
9. American Medical Association. Code of Medical Ethics. Principles of Medical Ethics. Section VII. Available at www.ama-assn.org/ama/pub/physician-resources/medical-ethics/code-medical-ethics/principles-medical-ethics.page. Accessed March 26, 2012.
10. American Academy of Neurology. Code of Professional Conduct. Section 6.6, The Impaired Physician. [*PECN* appendix document A and available at www.aan.com/view/PECN]
11. Bernat, 3–23, Ch. 1.
12. Bernat, 24–48, Ch. 2.
13. Bernat, 62–3, Ch. 4.
14. Lobo-Prabbu SM, Molinari VA, Hamilton JD, et al. The aging physician with cognitive impairment: Approaches to oversight, prevention, and remediation. Am J Geriatr Psychiatry 2009; 17(6):445–54.
15. Wallace JE, Lemaire JB, Ghali WA. Physician wellness: A missing quality indicator. Lancet 2009; 374:1714–21.
16. Harms BA, Heise CP, Gould JC, et al. A 25-year institution analysis of health, practice, and fate of general surgeons. Ann Surg 2005; 242:520–9.
17. Boisaubin EV, Levine R. Identifying and assisting the impaired physician. Am J Med Sci 2001; 232:31–6.
18. Swiggart WH, Dewey CM, Hickson GB, et al. A plan for identification, treatment, and remediation of disruptive behaviors in physicians. Front Health Serv Manage 2009; 25(4):3–11.
19. American Academy of Neurology. Code of Professional Conduct. Section 6.1, Cooperation with Health Care Professionals. [*PECN* appendix document A and available at www.aan.com/view/PECN]
20. American Academy of Neurology. Code of Professional Conduct. Section 6.3, Criticism of a Colleague. [*PECN* appendix document A and available at www.aan.com/view/PECN]
21. Hutchins JC, Sagsveen MG, Larriviere D. Upholding professionalism: The disciplinary process of the American Academy of Neurology. Neurology 2010; 75:2198–2203.
22. The Joint Commission. Requirement MS.11.01.01. Available at www.massmed.org/Content/NavigationMenu6/JCAHORequirement/JCAHO_Requirement_M.htm. Accessed March 26, 2012.
23. Youssi MD. JCAHO standards help address disruptive physician behavior. Physician Exec 2002; 28(6):12–3.
24. Leape LL, Fromson J. Problem doctors: Is there a system-level solution. Ann Int Med 2006; 144:107–15.

25. Merio LJ, Greene WM. Physician views regarding substance use–related participation in a state physician health program. Am J Addict 2010; 19:529–33.
26. Holtman M. Disciplinary careers of drug-impaired physicians. Soc Sci Med 2007; 64:543–53.
27. Verghese A. Perspective: Physicians and addiction. N Engl J Med 2002; 346(20):1510–1.

SUGGESTIONS FOR FURTHER READING

Hendrie HC, Clair DK, Brittain HM, et al. A study of anxiety/depressive symptoms of medical students, house officers, and their spouses/partners. J Nerv Ment Dis 1990; 178(3):204–7.

Hughes PH, Conrad SE, Baldwin D, Jr., et al. Resident physician substance abuse in the United States. JAMA 1991; 265(16):2069–73.

Johnson TM. Physician impairment: Social origins of a medical concern. Med Anthropol Quart 1988; 2:17–33.

Jones JW, McCullough LB, Richman BW. Who should protect the public against bad doctors? J Vasc Surg 2005; 41(5):907–10.

Rosenthal MM. *The Incompetent Doctor: Behind Closed Doors.* Berkshire, UK: Open University Press, 1995.

Valliant GE, Sobowale NC, McArthur C. Some psychological vulnerabilities of physicians. N Engl J Med 1972; 287(8):372–5.

Verghese A. *The Tennis Partner.* New York: Harper Collins Press, 1998.

This is the story of one of Dr. Verghese's students who, addicted to cocaine, went through rehabilitation but ultimately committed suicide. A moving story that deserves the attention of all students of medicine.

Walzer RS. Impaired physicians: An overview and update of the legal issues. J Leg Med 1990; 11(2):131–98.

Williams WC. Old Doc Rivers. In: Williams WC. *The Doctor Stories*. New York: New Directions Publishing Corp., 1984.

This story portrays the tension between a physician's dedication to his patients and his inability to recognize and respond to his own health problems.

10

SEXUAL MISCONDUCT BY PHYSICIANS

Thomas Pellegrino, MD

LEARNING OBJECTIVES

Upon completion of this chapter, participants will be able to:

1. Define the terms *boundary violation*, *sexual impropriety*, and *sexual violation*.
2. Identify boundary violations and sexual misconduct between physicians, their patients, and persons under their supervision.
3. Cite ethical and professional statements that prohibit sexual contact between physicians and patients.
4. Describe an appropriate response when one suspects that a colleague is involved in sexual impropriety or a sexual violation.
5. Identify resources for evaluating and assisting physicians who are concerned about their ability to respect appropriate boundaries in the physician–patient relationship.

LEARNING RESOURCES

Key chapters in Bernat's third edition—3

Key relevant AAN documents available at www.aan.com/view/PECN

A

CLINICAL VIGNETTES

CASE 1

Dr. Edwards is 42 years old and single, having divorced 4 years ago. One of his patients is Charlotte Johnson, an unmarried 38-year-old woman with multiple sclerosis (MS). She has mild weakness of her left leg but is otherwise asymptomatic. Despite doing well with treatment, she is very anxious and frequently schedules appointments to seek reassurance about her course and prognosis. At one appointment, she tells Dr. Edwards how she appreciates his care and concern and invites him to her home for dinner to express her appreciation. Dr. Edwards is concerned that it would be inappropriate to accept her invitation, but he is reluctant to risk insulting her by refusing.

CASE 2

Dr. Stockwin is a 50-year-old male neurologist in solo practice. One of his patients, Frank Adamson, has severe MS. He is paraplegic, confined to a wheelchair, and has erectile dysfunction. Over the years, Dr. Stockwin has come to know Mr. Adamson's wife quite well. He finds her attractive but has always maintained a professional demeanor. On several occasions, Mrs. Adamson has confessed frustration about her husband's erectile dysfunction, and Dr. Stockwin has suggested counseling and urology consultation. Mrs. Edwards begins seeking frequent private conversations with Dr. Stockwin, during which she gives him small gifts. One evening while Dr. Stockwin is finishing his charts, Mrs. Adamson appears at the door, distraught and tearful. Although the office is closed, Dr. Stockwin lets her come in. The situation gets out of control, and she and Dr. Stockwin have sexual intercourse. They begin a regular sexual relationship.

CASE 3

Dr. Warren is a 60-year-old female neurologist who has been a widow for 5 years. One evening at a cocktail party she encounters a man whom she soon learns was the husband of a patient of hers who died 3 years ago. Mr. Robertson re-introduces himself and expresses gratitude for Dr. Warren's medical care and compassion during his wife's illness. He tells her that he has been very lonely since his wife's death. Dr. Warren confesses her own loneliness since the death of her husband. They begin seeing each other regularly and soon develop a sexually intimate relationship.

CASE 4

A new associate in a group of neurologists, while passing one of the exam rooms one day, hears Dr. Winchester, one of the senior partners in the practice, commenting to his patient about her "very sexy" underwear.

CASE 5

Dr. Jones is a gay male neurologist. His practice hires a male medical assistant whom Dr. Jones finds quite attractive; he senses that the attraction is mutual. One afternoon, the new medical assistant asks Dr. Jones if he would prefer that he stay after office hours to help clean up around the office.

QUESTIONS FOR GROUP DISCUSSION

GETTING STARTED

1. Have you ever encountered or observed inappropriate sexual behavior or relationships between a physician and a patient, a patient's family member, or an employee? What was your reaction?

ASSESSMENT

2. Are there issues of power or conflict in the interactions of the key actors in these cases that need to be addressed?

(continued)

3. What actions are considered sexual misconduct?
4. Do the cases have relevant contextual factors that either amplify or mitigate the potential sexual misconduct?
5. What are the needs of the patients, family members, or physicians involved? What are their preferences, and do these either amplify or mitigate the potential sexual misconduct?

MORAL DIAGNOSIS
6. What ethical standards and guidelines exist?

GOAL SETTING, DECISION MAKING, AND IMPLEMENTATION
7. What interventions would meet the needs of the patients in these cases and resolve moral problems?
8. If a physician becomes aware of sexual misconduct by another physician, what actions are required?

EVALUATION
9. Can you identify educational interventions that might help to prevent or resolve the moral problems posed by similar cases?

COMMENTARY ON DISCUSSION QUESTIONS

For group discussions on this sensitive topic, please be careful not to reveal the names or identifying characteristics of actual persons.

GETTING STARTED

1. **Have you ever encountered or observed inappropriate sexual behavior or relationships between a physician and a patient, a patient's family member, or an employee? What was your reaction?**

Sexual relationships between physicians and their patients have been forbidden since very ancient times.[1-3] One of the earliest proscriptions is in the Hippocratic oath (c. 500 BCE):

> Into as houses as I shall enter, I will go for the benefit of the ill, while being far from all voluntary and destructive injustice, especially from sexual acts both upon women's bodies and upon men's both of the free and of the slaves.[1]

Sexual acts were seen as an especially egregious example of "voluntary and destructive injustices,"[1] described as hubris (or hybris), a "self indulgent exploitation of one's power in order to dominate or dishonor." In other words, sexual acts between physicians and patients were (and are) considered inherently abusive, in that physicians use their special powers and privileges for their own sexual gratification rather than for the benefit of the patient.

Few reliable data are available concerning the prevalence of physician sexual misconduct. Research suggests that between 3% and 10% of US physicians have been involved in "sexual boundary violations."[4]

A review of 375 disciplinary actions by the Medical Board of California over an 18-month period found that 10% were for inappropriate sexual contact with patients.[4] The true extent of the problem is unknown because, as with many forms of sexual abuse or exploitation, instances of physician sexual misconduct may be under-reported.

Sexual misconduct is a form of boundary violation. Boundaries are the "parameters that describe the limits of a fiduciary relationship in which one person (a patient) entrusts his or her welfare to another (a physician)" and generally entail professional distance and respect.[5] "Boundary violations differ from 'boundary crossings', which are harmless deviations from traditional clinical practice, behavior, or demeanor."[6] Boundary crossings involve neither harm nor exploitation of the patient and include such activities as socializing with a patient at a charity event. Boundary violations, on the other hand, are typically harmful and exploit the patients' needs. Boundary violations can be erotic in nature, as well as financial, dependency, or authority based.[6]

ASSESSMENT

2. **Are there issues of power or conflict in the interactions of the key actors in these cases that need to be addressed?**

The physician–patient relationship is inherently unequal in many respects. Patients typically lack the knowledge and skills to diagnose and treat their own illnesses; they grant physicians the privilege of hearing their symptoms and sometimes their most closely held personal information, or of touching their bodies for appropriate purposes (e.g., physical examination), with the expectation of physicians' trustworthiness to act in their patients' best interests (fiduciary role). Sexual relationships between physicians and patients exploit the patients' vulnerability and trust by leveraging the physicians' privilege and authority primarily for the physicians' gratification rather than the patients' interests. Accordingly, such relationships are considered inherently unethical. The guidelines of the Federation of State Medical Boards of the United States stress that both sexual impropriety and sexual violation (see below) "exploit the physician–patient relationship, violate the public trust, and are often known to cause harm, both mentally and physically, to the patient."[7]

Sexual relationships between physicians and students or residents, or between physicians and their subordinates are also based on the inequalities of power and position. In each case, an unequal relationship is exploited for the benefit of the physician.

3. **What actions are considered sexual misconduct?**

In 1996, the Federation of State Medical Boards of the United States defined unacceptable behaviors, classifying them as either "sexual impropriety" or "sexual violation."[7] Either type of sexual misconduct is unethical and may be the basis for disciplinary action by a state medical board.

Sexual impropriety comprises behavior, gestures, or expressions that are seductive, sexually suggestive, disrespectful of patient privacy, or sexually demeaning to a patient, that may include, but are not limited to:

    a. Neglecting to employ disrobing or draping practices that respect the patient's privacy, or deliberately watching a patient dress or undress.

    b. Subjecting a patient to an intimate examination in the presence of medical students or other parties without the patient's informed consent or in the event that such consent has been withdrawn.

    c. Examining or touching genital mucosal areas without the use of gloves.

    d. Inappropriate comments about or to the patient, including but not limited to sexual comments about the patient's body or underclothing, sexualized or sexually demeaning comments to a patient, criticism of the patient's sexual orientation, comments about potential sexual performance during an examination.

    e. Using the physician–patient relationship to solicit a date or romantic relationship.

    f. Initiating a conversation regarding the physician's sexual problems, preferences, or fantasies.

    g. Performing an intimate examination or consultation without clinical justification.

    h. Performing an intimate examination or consultation without explaining to the patient the need for such examination or consultation, even when the examination or consultation is pertinent to the issue of sexual function or dysfunction.

    i. Requesting details of sexual history or sexual likes or dislikes when not clinically indicated for the type of examination or consultation.[7]

Sexual violation includes physical sexual contact between a physician and patient, whether or not initiated by the patient, or engaging in any conduct with a patient that is sexual or may be reasonably interpreted as sexual, including but not limited to sexual intercourse with oral, anal, or genital contact; inappropriate touching; or masturbation.[7]

4. Do the cases have relevant contextual factors that either amplify or mitigate the potential sexual misconduct?

In Case 1, Dr. Edwards has not yet initiated an inappropriate relationship with Ms. Johnson, but to accept her invitation would be outside normal professional boundaries. Given Dr. Edwards' own vulnerability (his recent divorce), the prospects for an inappropriate relationship are great. At the very least, to accept such an invitation would give the appearance of impropriety. Even if they did not engage in intimacy or sexual contact on this occasion, acceptance of the first invitation would make refusal of any future invitations much more difficult.

In Case 2, Dr. Stockwin's misconduct is with the patient's spouse rather than with the patient, but the sexual relationship has arisen from his relationship with the patient. The patient's vulnerability is being exploited for the sake of Dr. Stockwin's gratification. Even though their first sexual encounter appeared to be "spontaneous," Dr. Stockwin missed the early signs when Mrs. Adamson began bringing him gifts and discussing personal problems unrelated to her husband's MS.

In Case 3, unlike Case 1, Mr. Robertson is neither a patient nor a former patient of the physician, and unlike Case 2, the attraction between Dr. Warren and Mr. Robertson appears to be outside the context of the previous physicians–patient relationship between Dr. Warren and Mr. Robertson's spouse. Although Dr. Warren and Mr. Robertson first met during Mrs. Robertson's illness, they have not seen each other in the 3 years since she died.

The physician conduct in Case 4 is sexual impropriety and clearly outside the boundaries of the professional relationship. Even if offered in jest or if intended as an "ice breaker," Dr. Winchester's reference to the patient's "sexy underwear" is inappropriate. When does a compliment about a patient's appearance cross the line? For example, is there a difference between saying "that's a pretty sweater," "that sweater looks good on you," and "that sweater makes you look hot"?

Case 5 does not involve a patient or family member but illustrates another boundary issue for physicians who are employers or who are themselves employed. Sexual harassment in the workplace is defined by the US Equal Employment Opportunity Commission as:

> unwelcome sexual advances, requests for sexual favors, and other verbal or physical conduct of a sexual nature...when submission to or rejection of this conduct explicitly or implicitly affects an individual's employment, unreasonably interferes with an individual's work performance, or creates an intimidating, hostile or offensive work environment.[8]

5. **What are the needs of the patients, family members, or physicians involved? What are their preferences, and do these either amplify or mitigate the potential sexual misconduct?**

In Case 1, the patient's emotional concerns about her MS are appropriately met by Dr. Edwards, but her more frequent visits and her invitation to Dr. Edwards for dinner at her home may represent the emotional mechanism of transference, which is important to recognize, as it has the potential to escalate. Although a patient may feel attracted to a physician who is attentive, kind, and caring, doctors have a responsibility to provide competent care without exploitation of such vulnerability.

In Case 2, the patient is either unaware of his wife's feelings for Dr. Stockwin or unable to prevent her from acting on her feelings because of the impairment of his MS. His wife appears to have unmet emotional needs that are being expressed toward Dr. Stockwin by the mechanism of transference. Physicians' feelings toward patients via the mechanism of countertransference are often normal but can escalate and contribute to sexual impropriety or misconduct.[6]

Case 3 occurs 3 years after Dr. Warren was in a physician–patient relationship with Mr. Robertson's wife. Both Mr. Robertson and Dr. Warren have expressed their loneliness following the (separate) deaths of their spouses. Whether their subsequent relationship constitutes sexual misconduct is a matter of debate. The AMA's Council on Ethical and Judicial Affairs has advised that sexual relationships with former patients (and, by extension, their families) are unethical if the physician "exploits trust, knowledge, emotions, or influence derived from the previous professional relationship."[9]

Case 4, as presented, does not reveal the patient's experience. The needs and motivation of the physician in commenting on the patient's underwear, or in leaving the exam room door open so that the comment could be overheard, are unclear.

In Case 5, no patient exists; however, the physician appears to be acting on a sense of "mutual attraction" to the medical assistant. The analysis of this case is not dependent on the sexual orientation or gender of the physician and employee.

MORAL DIAGNOSIS

6. What ethical standards and guidelines exist?

Sexual acts between physicians and patients have been forbidden explicitly or implicitly by both ancient and modern codes of professional conduct.[2,3,9–13] Sexual contact between physicians and patients is unethical and unprofessional.

- The AAN Code of Professional Conduct specifically states, "The neurologist must not abuse or exploit the patient psychologically, sexually, physically, or financially."[12]
- The AMA Council on Ethical and Judicial Affairs Opinion 8.14 states, "Sexual contact that occurs concurrent with the patient–physician relationship constitutes sexual misconduct."[9]
- The US Federation of State Medical Boards declares, "Physician sexual misconduct exploits the physician–patient relationship, is a violation of the public trust, and is often known to cause harm, both mentally and physically, to the patient."[7]
- In the UK, the General Medical Council's guidance "Good Medical Practice," states "You must not use your professional position to establish or pursue a sexual or improper emotional relationship with a patient or someone close to them."[13]

GOAL SETTING, DECISION MAKING, AND IMPLEMENTATION

7. What interventions would meet the needs of the patients in these cases and resolve moral problems?

In Case 1, Dr. Edwards should politely refuse his patient's invitation. To avoid any concerns about hurting the patient's feelings, an explanation can be offered that he has a longstanding policy of not accepting such invitations from any patient. Dr. Edwards may also wish to consult with a respected colleague or undertake education regarding physician–patient boundaries to prevent future occurrences.

In Case 2, Dr. Stockwin's sexual relationship with a patient's wife is clearly an unethical sexual violation. The patient's well-being is neglected and may be undermined. The damage is done and cannot be reversed. If discovered, Dr. Stockwin is at risk for disciplinary action by the state medical board. This case also highlights the risks involved when physicians agree to meetings after hours, when no staff or other chaperones are present. Even if nothing untoward had occurred, Dr. Stockwin would have been highly vulnerable to a later accusation of inappropriate conduct.

In Case 3, it is unclear whether the relationship between Dr. Warren and Mr. Robertson constitutes sexual misconduct. She should consult a respected colleague or seek advice from a center with experience in identifying and treating physician misconduct.

In Case 4, the physician who overhears Dr. Winchester's comment about a patient's underwear is junior and new to the practice and, therefore, might fear retaliation on reporting the overheard comments. As a first step, the junior physician can seek guidance from a colleague outside the practice, without identifying Dr. Winchester. Alternatively, the junior physician could seek advice from the physician who is the head of the practice.

8. If a physician becomes aware of sexual misconduct by another physician, what actions are required?

The AAN Code of Professional Conduct (Section 6.6)[12] and many other professional codes widely agree that physicians have a professional responsibility to report impaired, incompetent, or unethical colleagues to appropriate authorities.[9–11,14] This responsibility is derived from the professional prerogatives that society confers on physicians and from the responsibility shared by all physicians to promote the health and well-being of patients and of society. In most cases of known or suspected sexual misconduct, the offending physician should be reported to the state medical board. The board will undertake a confidential investigation to determine if any action is warranted.[7] The decision to report a physician for suspected sexual misconduct can be a difficult and wrenching choice, considering the potential grave consequences to the accused physician and given that the reported physician may be

Bernat, 62, Ch. 3

a friend, colleague, or a superior in the workplace.[15] However, to fail to report sexual misconduct is to condone it and to enable the behavior with its attendant harm to patients and to the profession.

The potential consequences of sexual misconduct may be catastrophic for involved physicians and their families, colleagues, and patients. For example:

■ Physicians accused of sexual misconduct are subject to investigation and potential sanctions by the state medical board. Investigation may involve detailed interviews with patients, colleagues, office staff, family members, or others. Formal psychiatric or psychologic evaluation may be required. If a physician is found guilty of sexual misconduct, sanctions may include restriction, suspension, or revocation of a medical license. Mandatory treatment or continuing medical education, as well as continuing supervision and monitoring, may be required if any return to clinical practice is allowed. Hospital staff privileges, insurance plan participation, and prescribing privileges may be modified, suspended, or revoked. Any restriction of clinical privileges and any sanctions by the state medical board will be reported to the National Practitioner Data Bank and, depending on state law, may become public knowledge.[16]

■ Depending on the nature of the offense, physicians involved in sexual misconduct may be subject to civil litigation brought by victims or their families, practice partners, or others. In addition, criminal prosecution may occur. It should be noted that professional malpractice insurance or other personal liability insurance might provide no coverage in the event of voluntary or criminal wrongdoing. Financial loss, incarceration, or both may result.

■ Potential consequences for the physician's family relationships, personal reputation, and community standing are likely to be severe.

■ Sexual misconduct may result in severe emotional or other injury to patients. To the extent that the physician's judgment is clouded by his personal involvement with a patient, medical harm may occur as well.

EVALUATION

9. **Can you identify educational interventions that might help to prevent or resolve the moral problems posed by similar cases?**

Steps that might reduce the prevalence of sexual misconduct and perhaps reduce the risk of misunderstandings include:

■ Devoting more attention to this subject in education programming for medical students and residents. Several publications have recommended more detailed discussion of physician responsibilities and appropriate respect for sexual and professional boundaries and behaviors.[17,18]

- Clear and specific practice guidelines may help to protect patients and physicians. Wide variation exists among physician practices, e.g., regarding the need for chaperones for physical examinations and procedures. The need for a chaperone may depend on characteristics of the patient, the physician, the type of examination, and the reason for the examination.[19]
- Physicians should be encouraged to explain to patients what they are doing and why. No patient should have to wonder why her breasts or genitalia are being examined, or why he needs a testicular examination or rectal examination. Explicit permission from the patient should be obtained before medical students, office staff, or other physicians are permitted to be present during an interview or physical examination.
- The Center for Professional Health at Vanderbilt University Medical Center offers an online course entitled "Hazardous Affairs"[20] about professional boundaries and sexual misconduct. Physicians concerned about their ability to recognize and avoid potential sexual misconduct may find this course very helpful. The center also offers an intensive course for evaluation and treatment of physicians involved in sexual misconduct. Physicians may enroll themselves for this course, or their attendance may be mandated by state medical boards or other disciplinary authorities.[20]

KEY POINTS

- The nature of physicians' professional activities poses a potentially significant risk that physicians may engage in inappropriate social or sexual relationships with their patients or with others under their supervision.
- Such inappropriate social or sexual relationships may result in grave harm to patients and may have catastrophic consequences for physicians' professional careers.
- Prompt intervention by colleagues and urgent referral for expert professional help may prevent or mitigate harm to patients and may help to salvage a physician's career.
- Numerous professional and ethical codes are virtually unanimous in prohibiting sexual relationships between physicians and their patients.

KEY WORDS

Boundary crossings — harmless deviations from traditional clinical practice, behavior, or demeanor. Compare to *boundary violations.*

Boundary violations — harmful (or potentially harmful) behaviors that are outside the normal limits (boundaries) of the physician–patient relationship. Compare to *boundary crossings*.

Counter-transference — the inappropriate and sometimes unrecognized direction or redirection of a physician's feelings toward a patient, often, but not always, of an erotic or sexual nature.

Sexual impropriety —inappropriate sexual attitudes, language, or other activity that does not include actual physical contact between the perpetrator and the victim.

Sexual misconduct —behavior that includes physical sexual contact between the perpetrator and the victim.

Transference —the direction or redirection of a patient's feelings toward a physician or other healthcare professional, often, but not always, of an erotic or sexual nature.

REFERENCES

1. Miles S. *The Hippocratic Oath and the Ethics of Medicine.* New York: Oxford University Press, 2004.
2. The Oath of Asaph and Yohanan (6th c.?). In: *Sefer haRefuot, The Book of Medicines.* Available at www.med.umn.edu/phrh/oaths/hebrew/home.html. Accessed March 16, 2012.
3. Sun Ssu-maio (581–673) from "A Thousand Golden Remedies." Available at www.med.umn.edu/phrh/oaths/chinese-ssu-miao/home.html. Accessed March 16, 2012.
4. Swiggart W, Starr K, Finlayson R, et al. Sexual boundaries and physicians: Overview and educational approach to the problem. Sexual Addiction and Compulsivity 2002; 9(2–3):139–48.
5. Gabbard GO, Nadelson C. Professional boundaries in the physician–patient relationship. JAMA 1995; 273:1445–9.
6. Norris DM, Gutheil TG, Strasburger LH. This couldn't happen to me: Boundary problems and sexual misconduct in the psychotherapy relationship. Psychiatr Serv 2003; 54:517–22.
7. Federation of State Medical Boards. Addressing sexual boundaries: Guidelines for state medical boards. Dallas: FSMB, 2006. Available at www.fsmb.org/pdf/GRPOL_Sexual Boundaries.pdf. Accessed March 16, 2012.
8. The US Equal Employment Opportunity Commission. Facts about sexual harassment. Available at www.eeoc.gov/facts/fs-sex.html. Accessed March 16, 2012.
9. American Medical Association. Code of Medical Ethics. Opinion 8.14. Sexual misconduct in the practice of medicine. Available at www.ama-assn.org/ama/pub/physician-resources/medical-ethics/code-medical-ethics/opinion814.page?. Accessed March 28, 2012.
10. American College of Physicians. *Ethics Manual, 5th ed.* Ann Intern Med 2005; 142:560–82.
11. American College of Obstetricians and Gynecologists. Sexual Misconduct: ACOG committee opinion. Obstetr Gynecol 2007; 110 (2, pt.1):441–4.
12. AAN Professional Code of Conduct. Section 4.1 Respect for the Patient. [*PECN* appendix document A and available at www.aan.com/view/PECN]
13. General Medical Council. Good Medical Practice. Available at www.gmc-uk.org/guidance/good_medical_practice.asp. Accessed March 16, 2012.
14. Bernat, 62, Ch. 3.
15. Raniga S, Hider P, Spriggs D, et al. Attitudes of hospital medical practitioners to the mandatory reporting of professional misconduct. N Z Med J 2005; 118:U1781.
16. National Practitioner Data Bank. NPDB Guidebook. Available at www.npdb-hipdb.hrsa.gov/resources/NPDBGuidebook.pdf. Accessed March 16, 2012.
17. Kao AC, Parsi KP. Content analyses of oaths administered in US medical schools in 2000. Acad Med 2004; 79:882–7.
18. White GE. Medical students' learning needs about setting and maintaining social and sexual boundaries: A report. Med Educ 2003; 11:1017–9.
19. Gawande A. Naked. N Engl J Med 2005; 353:645–8.

20. The Center for Professional Health at Vanderbilt University Medical Center offers a variety of courses, seminars, and other resources for physicians. Available at www.mc.vanderbilt.edu/root/vumc.php?site=cph. Accessed March 16, 2012.

SUGGESTIONS FOR FURTHER READING

Galletly CA. Crossing professional boundaries in medicine: The slippery slope to patient sexual exploitation. Med J Aust 2004; 181:380–3.

Spickard A, Swiggart WH, Manley G, et al. A continuing education course for physicians who cross sexual boundaries. Sexual Addiction and Compulsivity 2002; 9:33–42.

INFORMED CONSENT AND REFUSAL

11

Thomas Cochrane, MD, MBA

LEARNING OBJECTIVES

Upon completion of this chapter, participants will be able to:

1. Describe the ethical foundation for the process of informed consent.
2. List the three necessary conditions for voluntary informed consent.
3. Identify circumstances in which the process of informed consent requires special attention.
4. Incorporate the process of informed consent into clinical practice.

LEARNING RESOURCES

Key chapters in Bernat's third edition—2, 8

Key relevant AAN documents available at www.aan.com/view/PECN

A   G   H

CLINICAL VIGNETTES

For each of the following cases, consider whether the informed consent of the patient is required. If it is, determine whether it can be obtained and the process for obtaining it.

CASE 1

Dr. Antezana, a healthy 46-year-old right-handed dentist, presents 1 hour after the acute onset of dysarthria, dense left hemiplegia (face, arm, and leg), and left-sided sensory loss. CT angiography reveals a proximal occlusion of the right middle cerebral artery. Either IV tPA or intra-arterial thrombolysis is likely to benefit him. He does not have anosognosia or other cognitive deficits and indicates that he fully understands the information presented to him and the recommendation for therapy, but he refuses thrombolytic therapy.

CASE 2

Mr. Green, a 52-year-old Jehovah's Witness, had a closed-head injury after being struck by a car 36 hours ago. Although he is currently stuporous, his neurologic prognosis is potentially very good. However, as a result of his trauma, he has severe upper gastrointestinal bleeding. The hematocrit has fallen from 35% to 22%, and endoscopic procedures have failed to stop the bleeding. He is at risk for shock, impaired cerebral oxygen delivery, and irreversible brain injury. Mr. Green's wife says that he is a firm believer in his church's teachings against accepting blood products and that he would steadfastly refuse transfusions, even if he would die as a result.

CASE 3

Mr. Heinz developed severe drug-induced hemolytic anemia during antibiotic treatment for pneumonia. His cardiac status is fragile, and he is likely to die unless he receives a blood transfusion. However, he refuses transfusion, despite extensive discussions over a period of several days. His refusal is not based on religious convictions but stems from a personal concern about "contamination." He says, "I desperately want to live, but I can't bear the thought of a contaminated blood product going into my body." Careful psychiatric evaluation reveals no evidence of an obsessive concern about contamination in general, nor does it reveal an indication of other psychiatric illness.

CASE 4

The attending in the SICU requests consultation regarding Ms. Charles, a 32-year-old previously healthy woman who fell from a ladder 3 days ago and sustained a high cervical-spine fracture. She is now quadriplegic with an extremely poor prognosis for recovery of movement. She did not have any head trauma and was conscious when found. She is now intubated because of ventilatory failure and is sedated because of discomfort with the endotracheal tube. Her husband, parents, and brother are all adamantly opposed to spinal stabilization surgery and request that LST be withdrawn. They describe Ms. Charles as an extremely active, athletic person and state that after actor Christopher Reeve became quadriplegic, she was emphatic that she would "never want to live like that." The family requests that ventilator support be withdrawn *without* waking her up. They want to spare her the distress of learning about her condition, as they know with certainty that she would decide against life support if she were not sedated.

CASE 5

Dr. Eklund is the principal investigator in a study of an experimental drug for the treatment of ALS. He is frustrated because enrollment in the study has been much slower than expected, threatening to delay or prevent approval of a therapy that could help many patients. Dr. Eklund is discussing the study with Ms. Reder, an ALS patient whom Dr. Eklund has known for some time. The study drug has a good safety profile thus far but carries a low risk (<1:10,000) of a lethal allergic reaction. Dr. Eklund happens to know that Ms. Reder's close friend died of an allergic reaction to a medication and that Ms. Reder herself has refused treatments in which anaphylaxis or other severe allergic reactions were described.

QUESTIONS FOR GROUP DISCUSSION

GETTING STARTED

1. Have you ever felt that the requirement for informed consent was a hindrance to "good medical care"?

ASSESSMENT

2. In Case 1, is Dr. Antezana's refusal of thrombolytic therapy informed? Why or why not?
3. If Dr. Antezana's stroke rendered him unable to discuss treatment options or express a preference, could he be treated with thrombolytics based on the emergency circumstances?
4. In Case 2, should Mr. Green's refusal of blood products, as explained by his wife, be honored? What if Mr. Green were conscious and possessed decisional capacity?
5. Imagine that Mrs. Green is accompanied by a church representative who is present with her permission during treatment discussions. The representative points out the biblical passages that are the basis for refusal of blood. Mrs. Green defers and refuses the transfusion and any further discussion of it. What concerns does this raise?
6. Does Mr. Heinz in Case 3 have capacity to refuse blood products? Is his decision rational? Must a person's refusal of recommended therapy be rational or based on accepted medical reasoning in order to be valid?
7. Does Ms. Charles in Case 4 have decision-making capacity? What are potential responses to the family's request that her ventilator be stopped without attempting to wake her up?
8. If Ms. Charles were awakened, refused spinal stabilization surgery, and asked to be sedated again and then extubated, should her wishes be honored?
9. Can Dr. Eklund in Case 5 omit presenting to Ms. Reder the remote risk of a lethal allergic reaction to the investigational drug? Could he change the standard presentation of this risk for her in order to emphasize its rarity?

MORAL DIAGNOSIS

10. In each of these cases, which ethical principles are in conflict?

GOAL SETTING, DECISION MAKING, AND IMPLEMENTATION

11. Could the treatment refusals of Dr. Antezana, Mr. Heinz, or Ms. Charles ethically be overridden? Describe the process that could be used to override each of their refusals. If it were possible to treat Dr. Antezana or Mr. Heinz without their knowledge, would it be ethically defensible?
12. What are possible responses to the scenario in which Mrs. Green is accompanied by the church representative (#5 above)?
13. Is it ethically permissible to conceal from Mr. Heinz the *actual* risks of a "contaminated" transfusion in an effort to persuade him to consent?

COMMENTARY ON DISCUSSION QUESTIONS

GETTING STARTED

1. Have you ever felt that the requirement for informed consent was a hindrance to "good medical care"?

Most care provided by clinicians is associated with benefit that outweighs risk. Occasionally, such as phlebotomy for routine blood tests, the risk is so minimal and the benefit so obvious that a formal consent discussion is unnecessary. As the potential risks or harms of a treatment increase, so does the requirement for clinicians to discuss them in the process of informed consent. However, even for complex, high-risk interventions (e.g., intra-arterial thrombolytic therapy for stroke), the information that would satisfy requirements for informed consent should arise in conversations between healthcare providers and patients or their surrogates in any case. The informed-consent process, even when required to be formally documented, does not over-burden medical care.

The requirement for informed consent might seem to be a hindrance because of the time necessary to conduct the conversation with the patient or family, especially when a patient questions or refuses an intervention that the physician has recommended and believes is necessary. However, the ethical and legal purpose of obtaining consent is to allow a competent patient to either agree or disagree with a clinician regarding the course of his or her treatment. The informed-consent process protects the patient's autonomy, and physicians should honor an informed, competent patient's choice, even if a poor clinical outcome would be the expected result.

ASSESSMENT

2. In Case 1, is Dr. Antezana's refusal of thrombolytic therapy informed? Why or why not?

Most frameworks for informed consent contain some version of the following 3 criteria:

1. The patient has been provided adequate *information* in understandable language and terminology about the risks and benefits of the proposed intervention and the alternatives to make a decision.
2. The patient is capable of understanding and evaluating the information (i.e., has *decisional capacity*).
3. The patient's consent is given *free of coercion.*[1]

Dr. Antezana has been given all of the relevant information, there is no reason to doubt his capacity for understanding it, and there is no evidence of coercion. Thus, his refusal is informed.

Decisional capacity, a term used within medicine and ethics, is determined by physician evaluation of the patient. *Competence*, the legal term used by the courts in ruling on a patient's ability to make decisions, is often based on a physician's assessment of the patient's decisional capacity. In this chapter, *competence* and *decisional capacity* will be used interchangeably.

3. **If Dr. Antezana's stroke rendered him unable to discuss treatment options or express a preference, could he be treated with thrombolytics based on the emergency circumstances?**

When treating a patient who lacks decisional capacity during a medical emergency, physicians invoke the doctrine of implied or presumed consent, which states that in an emergency situation in which it would be clearly harmful to the patient to delay a treatment that is beneficial and considered to be a standard of care in order to obtain consent, physicians may proceed without consent on the assumption that the patient would have provided consent if he were able.[2] The doctrine of implied consent cannot be invoked if a surrogate is available, if the treatment can be safely delayed, or if there is no emergency. In 1999, the Ethics and Humanities Subcommittee of the AAN concluded that this doctrine could be applied to the use of IV tPA if it is considered the standard of care.[3] The AAN and the American Heart Association now consider IV tPA the standard of care for ischemic stroke in some regions.[4,5] As a result, the Ethics, Law and Humanities Committee of the AAN recently updated its position to state that "if the patient lacks capacity and no proxy decision maker can be found after a reasonable effort, then the physician may administer the medication based on the principle of implied consent for emergency treatment."[6] Invoking the doctrine of implied consent does not eliminate the physician's responsibility to discuss tPA administration with the patient's surrogate, if available, in person or by telephone.[7] Because intra-arterial thrombolysis carries more risk, is an invasive procedure, and is not yet considered a standard of care, it would not satisfy the criteria for implied consent for emergency treatment.

Bernat, 25, Ch. 2

4. **In Case 2, should Mr. Green's refusal of blood products, as explained by his wife, be honored? What if Mr. Green were conscious and possessed decisional capacity?**

The fact that Mr. Green's refusal is made by his surrogate makes no difference, assuming that she is accurately representing his preferences. Honoring an informed refusal made on the basis of deeply held and stable values—whether religious or secular—is a demonstration of respect for individual choice. In the case of refusal of blood products by an adult member of the Jehovah's Witness faith, established ethical reasoning and legal precedent exist for respecting patients' refusal. However, the directive to honor patients' refusal does not eliminate the requirement for physicians to meet their obligations in the informed-consent process, including discussion of the risks, benefits, and alternatives to transfusion. One should not assume that Mr. Green or any patient, on the basis of religion, race, ethnicity, or other group membership, will make a particular decision. To do so is to overlook the patient's right for self-determination. To simultaneously respect the patient's beliefs and to provide the options necessary for informed consent can seem contradictory. If Mr. Green were conscious, a physician could say words similar to, "I wish to respect your beliefs, and at the same time I want to be certain that you're aware of all the treatment options available to you. May I explain them to you?" In fact, a similar statement should be made to his wife when she is acting as his surrogate.

5. **Imagine that Mrs. Green is accompanied by a church representative who is present with her permission during treatment discussions. The representative points out the biblical passages that are the basis for refusal of blood. Mrs. Green defers and refuses the transfusion and any further discussion of it. What concerns does this raise?**

Just as physicians might be concerned that Mrs. Green is being "coerced" by the church representative, the church representative may also be worried that Mrs. Green is being coerced by the physicians. Coercion exists whenever "powerful negative incentives" are employed by one party to influence the decision of another.[1,8] In this case, coercion could arise from the implied threat of the disapproval of church members. Coercion just as easily could occur if the healthcare team exaggerates the risks of refusing transfusion. Bernat states that when a physician exaggerates or overemphasizes the risks (or benefits) of a treatment or an alternative in order to manipulate a patient's behavior, the physician is practicing subtle coercion through the use of deception.[2]

Bernat, 26, Ch. 2

Bernat, 25, Ch. 2

Persuasion, on the other hand, occurs when one person comes to believe in something through the merit of reasons advanced by another person.[9] Persuasion can be distinguished from coercion by the lack of an implied threat. Not only is persuasion by physicians permissible, many would consider it part of physicians' duties to their patients. When a physician considers one course of action clearly preferable to another, it would be irresponsible simply to accept a patient's refusal without first trying to ensure that the patient's decision is informed. Through attempts at persuasion, the physician can ensure that the patient understands the relevant medical facts and the risks and benefits associated with the alternatives. An attempt at persuasion can sometimes reveal the fact that a patient's decision is influenced by lack of understanding, exaggerated fears, prejudices, or confused thinking in the setting of an illness.

Clinicians should also remain sensitive to the influence of *framing effects* on patients' judgments. Clinicians can sometimes influence patient or surrogate decisions simply by changing the wording of a question or statement. As an example, one can influence decisions by describing a patient's prognosis in terms of probability of either survival or death. It is easy to perceive "a 1% chance of survival" as *different* from "a 99% chance of death." A patient may give one response if asked, "would you want us to do everything possible to save your life if your heart stopped beating?" and quite a different response after a full disclosure and discussion of the nature of the interventions that might be required and the likelihood of survival.

6. **Does Mr. Heinz in Case 3 have capacity to refuse blood products? Is his decision rational? Must a person's refusal of recommended therapy be rational or based on accepted medical reasoning in order to be valid?**

At least 3 responses are possible to this patient's refusal on the basis of his stated fear of the risks of transfusion: (a) his refusal could be accepted as an informed refusal, (b) it could be asserted that he *lacks capacity* with respect to this medical decision, or (c) it could be asserted that he has *capacity but is making an irrational choice*.

The criteria proposed by Bernard Lo can be used to analyze whether Mr. Heinz possesses decisional capacity:

- Does he appreciate that he has a choice?
- Does he appreciate the medical situation and prognosis as well as the risks, benefits, and consequences of available and recommended treatments?
- Is his decision stable over time and not impulsive?
- Is his decision consistent with his personal values and healthcare goals?[10]

Mr. Heinz appears to understand the situation and appreciates that he has a choice. The duration of his fear of contamination is unclear but is most likely longstanding. His statement that he fears "contamination" from the transfusion more than he fears harm or death that could result from refusing the transfusion is, in fact, a statement of his personal values and healthcare goals. Thus, he appears to have decisional capacity to refuse the transfusion.

Does the rationality or irrationality of the basis of his decision matter? According to Gert and Culver:

> to act irrationally is to act in a way that one knows, …or should know, will significantly increase the probability that oneself, or those one cares for, will suffer death, pain, disability, loss of freedom, or loss of pleasure; and one does not have an adequate *reason* for so acting.[11]

A *reason* is:

> a conscious, rational belief that one's action will help anyone, not merely oneself or those one cares about, avoid some… harms or gain some good, ability, freedom, or pleasure, and this belief is not seen to be inconsistent with one's other beliefs by almost everyone with similar knowledge and intelligence.[11]

Mr. Heinz's refusal could be considered irrational because it significantly increases the probability that he will die, and the risk of harm from contamination of a transfusion is negligible in comparison. However, a person may make a decision that appears to lack logic or reason on a superficial level but is consistent with a set of internal principles or values derived from the individual's life history.

Bernat,
29,
Ch. 2
The law, as Bernat observes, "generally does not permit physicians to overrule their competent patients' refusal of treatment merely on the basis of irrationality."[12] Although it may be tempting to label a patient as lacking capacity in order to justify overriding a patient's "irrational" decision, transfusing an adult against his wishes could be considered battery.

7. Does Ms. Charles in Case 4 have decision-making capacity? What are potential responses to the family's request that her ventilator be stopped without attempting to wake her up?

Because she is sedated, Ms. Charles does not have decision-making capacity. However, an important question is whether her capacity could be *restored* by withdrawing sedation. The family is asking the physician to discontinue LST of a patient whose capacity might be restorable. It is ethically impermissible to comply with the family's request. Respect for autonomy implies that if the patient can make a decision, then the patient should be given the opportunity to do so. If the patient's capacity can be restored, then the patient can either make the decision or, alternatively, choose to let surrogates make the decision.

8. If Ms. Charles were awakened, refused spinal stabilization surgery, and asked to be sedated again and then extubated, should her wishes be honored?

If these events were to transpire, it would appear that Ms. Charles has decision-making capacity and has made an informed refusal. However, 2 concerns exist regarding her capacity. First, at least initially, Ms. Charles's decision has not been shown to be stable over time and could be considered "impulsive," in the sense that the emotional shock of the injury may be unduly influencing her decision. Second, it is known that for patients with high spinal-cord injury or even locked-in syndrome, their self-assessments of quality of life can change over time, so that it could be argued that Ms. Charles cannot provide informed consent until she has more information about the actual (not imagined) quality of life with her disability and more precise estimates of her prognosis and rehabilitation options.[13] If it seems likely that a patient's preferences will change over a short period of time, one should be reluctant to act on a decision when that action has significant and irreversible consequences.

Case 4 demonstrates why one is not always ethically required to *immediately* honor a competent patient's medical decision, even if it appears to be rational and informed. The decision to withdraw LST, once acted upon, is irreversible. Conversely, a decision to *continue* LST can always be reconsidered, and it would seem acceptable for the healthcare team to insist that more time be allowed to pass before permitting withdrawal. A decision to override a competent patient's refusal of treatment should not be taken lightly.[14] Consultation with a hospital ethics committee and possibly with hospital legal counsel would be required. If Ms. Charles' refusal of LST remains consistent after she has recovered from the acute emotional shock of her trauma and after she has developed an informed sense of what life with her disabilities could be like, then her refusal of LST should be honored.

Bernat,
182,
Ch. 8

9. **Can Dr. Eklund in Case 5 omit presenting to Ms. Reder the remote risk of a lethal allergic reaction to the investigational drug? Could he change the standard presentation of this risk for her in order to emphasize its rarity?**

The standard in both research and clinical practice for disclosure of side effects is that clinicians must disclose any potentially serious adverse effects, even if they are extremely uncommon, and they must disclose any minor adverse effects if they are common. Thus, though it is rare, the risk of a lethal allergic reaction should be discussed with Ms. Reder. When enrolling patients in trials, researchers must adhere to the protocol for disclosure that was approved by the institutional review board. Dr. Eklund would not be permitted to conceal information that was required by the study protocol; additionally, as Ms. Reder's treating physician, he has a duty to discuss information that she would consider relevant.

One can argue that deceiving Ms. Reder in order to gain her consent to participate in the trial would serve the interests of future patients. However, this would amount to a decision to pursue the interests of future patients at the expense of the interests of the current patient, which would violate the physician's duty as a fiduciary of Ms. Reder.

MORAL DIAGNOSIS

10. **In each of these cases, describe which ethical principles are in conflict?**

Bernat,
9–13,
Ch. 1

Informed consent is a way of safeguarding patients' autonomy and self-determination. Respect for autonomy may sometimes seem to conflict with *beneficence*, the principle that physicians actively serve the best interests of their patients.[15] In Western medicine, the physician's obligation to honor a patient's autonomy typically supersedes the duty to the principle of beneficence. Patients with decision-making capacity are entitled to reject physician recommendations. Such decisions are often labeled "against medical advice," or AMA. When patients decline physician recommendations, it is important that they be treated in a way that leaves the door open for them to reconsider.

GOAL SETTING, DECISION MAKING, AND IMPLEMENTATION

11. **Could the treatment refusals of Dr. Antezana, Mr. Heinz, or Ms. Charles ethically be overridden? Describe the process that could be used to override each of their refusals. If it were possible to treat Dr. Antezana or Mr. Heinz without their knowledge, would it be ethically defensible?**

The decision to override the informed consent or refusal of a patient with capacity should rarely, if ever, be made. An ethics consultation is virtually mandatory in such circumstances. The purpose of consultation is not to request assistance in overriding the patient, but to determine whether such action is ethically justifiable. Gert and Culver have proposed strict criteria that could justify overriding a patient's treatment refusal:

a. The harms that the treatment will avoid or ameliorate must be very great (e.g., death or permanent disability).
b. The harms imposed by treatment must be comparatively much less.
c. The patient's desire not to be treated must be irrational, as defined by strict criteria.
d. Most rational persons would advocate that such treatment be forced in every similar instance.[11]

12. **What are possible responses to the scenario in which Mrs. Green is accompanied by the church representative (#5 above)?**

A reasonable initial approach might be to speak with Mrs. Green alone and assure her that the desire of the healthcare team is to respect her husband's wishes, regardless of whether they are consistent or inconsistent with church teaching. This approach avoids the appearance of arguing faith versus fact and demonstrates respect for the patient's faith and autonomy. It would not be appropriate to permit the church representative to guide the decision-making process without Mrs. Green's involvement. In general, such situations are opportunities to make use of an ethics consultation.

13. **Is it ethically permissible to conceal from Mr. Heinz in Case 3 the *actual* risks of a "contaminated" transfusion in an effort to persuade him to consent?**

Deception is virtually never ethically permissible in clinical care. Fortunately, it is probably rare that it is the most attractive option. In practice, most patients and surrogates accept a carefully considered, soundly justified treatment recommendation, even if several discussions are required. Indeed, in this case, discussing the actual risk of contamination from a blood transfusion may help Mr. Heinz to change his mind regarding the transfusion, although this would require more time and effort on the part of the clinician. The choice to deceive Mr. Heinz might seem "expedient" but would be a violation of trust and an act of disrespect.

KEY POINTS

- Informed consent, including informed refusal, is one of the most important ways to respect patient autonomy.
- Consent is considered informed when (a) the patient has been provided adequate information, (b) the patient is capable of understanding and evaluating the information, and (c) the consent is given free of coercion.
- Although a medical decision that appears irrational may be grounds for questioning a patient's competence (capacity to provide informed consent), a competent, informed adult should generally be permitted to make such a decision.
- A competent, informed refusal of LST should generally be honored but only after careful deliberation and assessment of the requirements of informed consent. Ethics consultation is highly recommended whenever competence is in question or when irreversible decisions with serious consequences are being contemplated.

KEY WORDS

Capacity—a medical term that refers to a clinical judgment concerning a patient's ability to make decisions.

Competence—a legal term used by the courts in ruling on a patient's ability to make decisions that is often based on a physician's assessment of the patient's decisional capacity. Patients are considered competent when they have the cognitive capacity to understand (a) their current condition, (b) the medical alternatives, and (c) the expected outcomes of each alternative.

Emergency, implied, or presumed consent—a patient who lacks decisional capacity can be presumed to consent to recommended therapies when (a) the therapy is urgent (important to preserve health) or time-sensitive (an emergency) and (b) a surrogate decision maker cannot be identified.

Informed consent—consent to (or refusal of) a medical intervention is considered informed and autonomous when the patient has adequate information, is capable of understanding and evaluating the information, and is not coerced.

REFERENCES

1. Faden R, Beauchamp T. *A History and Theory of Informed Consent*. New York: Oxford University Press, 1986.
2. Bernat, 25, Ch. 2.
3. American Academy of Neurology. Ethics and Humanities Committee. Consent issues in the management of cerebrovascular diseases. A position paper of the American Academy of Neurology. Neurology 1999; 53:9–11.
4. del Zoppo GJ, Saver JL, Jauch EC, et al., on behalf of the American Heart Association Stroke Council. Expansion of the time window for treatment of acute ischemic stroke with intravenous tissue plasminogen activator. A science advisory from the American Heart Association/American Stroke Association. Stroke 2009; 40:2945–8.
5. Adams, Jr. HP, del Zoppo GJ, Alberts MJ, et al. Guidelines for the early management of adults with ischemic stroke: A guideline from the American Heart Association/ American Stroke Association Stroke Council, Clinical Cardiology Council, Cardiovascular Radiology and Intervention Council, and the Atherosclerotic Peripheral Vascular Disease and Quality of Care Outcomes in Research Interdisciplinary Working Groups: The American Academy of Neurology affirms the value of this guideline as an educational tool for neurologists. Stroke 2007; 38:1655–711.
6. American Academy of Neurology. Ethics and Humanities Subcommittee. a joint committee of the AAN, ANA, and CNS. American Academy of Neurology policy on consent issues for the administration of IV tPA. April 11, 2011. [*PECN* document G available at www.aan.com/view/PECN]
7. White-Bateman S, Schumacher H, Sacco R, et al. Consent for intravenous thrombolysis in acute stroke: Review and future directions. Arch Neurol 2007; 64:785–92.
8. Bernat, 26, Ch. 2.
9. Beauchamp TL, Childress JF, eds. *Principles of Biomedical Ethics, 5th ed*. New York: Oxford University Press, 2001:95.
10. Lo B. Assessing decision-making capacity. Law Med Health Care 1990; 18:193–201.
11. Gert B, Culver C. The justification of paternalism. Ethics 1979; 89(2):199–210.
12. Bernat, 29, Ch. 2.
13. American Academy of Neurology. Report of the Ethics and Humanities Subcommittee of the American Academy of Neurology. Position statement: Certain aspects of the care and management of profoundly and irreversibly paralyzed patients with retained consciousness and cognition. Neurology 1993; 43(1):222–3. [*PECN* document H available at www.aan.com/view/PECN]
14. Bernat, 182, Ch. 8.
15. Bernat, 9–13, Ch. 1.

SUGGESTIONS FOR FURTHER READING

Ascension Health. Key ethical principles. Available at www.ascensionhealth.org/ethics/ public/key_principles/informed_consent. Accessed March 10, 2012.
Berg J, Appelbaum PS, Lidz CW, et al. *Informed Consent: Legal Theory and Clinical Practice*. New York: Oxford University Press, 2001.
Meisel A, Kuczewski M. Legal and ethical myths about informed consent. Arch Intern Med 1996; 156(22):2521–6.

12 ASSENT AND REFUSAL BY CHILDREN AND ADOLESCENTS

Patricia Evans, MD, FAAN, FAAP

LEARNING OBJECTIVES

Upon completion of this chapter, participants will be able to:

1. Understand the difference between assent and consent for children.
2. Describe the mature-minor doctrine.
3. Appropriately apply the term "emancipated minor."
4. Outline the process for determining whether a minor can provide consent for a medical procedure or must provide assent with parental consent.
5. Interpret and use ethical rationale for involving children in decision making regarding their illness and treatment.

LEARNING RESOURCES

Key chapters in Bernat's third edition—2, 8

Key relevant AAN documents available at www.aan.com/view/PECN

A

O

CLINICAL VIGNETTES

CASE 1

Christine is a 14-year-old girl who collapsed at an athletic event. CT of the brain revealed a large pontine mass. The neurosurgeons debulked the mass, which was a high-grade glioma. Later, the oncologist told Christine's parents that chemotherapy and radiation would be beneficial and possibly add decades to her life. Without it, she could die within a year. The oncologist wanted to discuss the treatments with Christine before starting, and her parents objected, stating that she did not need to be bothered with the details. At a recent visit, Christine spoke privately with the physician and a nurse and said that she knows that something is wrong, that she is afraid, and that she wishes she knew what the doctors and her parents were planning for her.

CASE 2

Benjamin is a 16-year-old, very bright but socially odd teenager whose medication until recently has helped to control his symptoms of Tourette syndrome. However, he now wishes to date and to be more "normal." He stopped taking all of his medications and, consequently, has more tics, including grunts and vocalizations. His family is distressed and insists that the neurologist "make him understand" how important it is that he stay on his medication.

CASE 3

Ashley is a 17-year-old who has had epilepsy for 5 years. She lives with her parents. The seizures are very difficult to control, despite attempts with a wide range of medications, which she has taken without any resistance. Ashley is the mother of a 4-month-old girl, who fortunately, has not exhibited any birth anomalies resulting from Ashley's need for antiepileptic therapy during pregnancy. Now that she has had the baby, Ashley's parents are interested in pursuing evaluation for epilepsy surgery; however, Ashley refuses, even though she admits that she understands that this may be the only option for her to achieve normal function and adequate seizure control.

QUESTIONS FOR GROUP DISCUSSION

GETTING STARTED

1. Have you ever encountered the circumstance in which an adolescent or mature child expresses a medical decision contrary to that of the parents? If so, how did you feel during that encounter?

ASSESSMENT

2. Compare and contrast the cases. What are the key contextual differences?
3. What is assent and how does it differ from consent?
4. What is the mature-minor doctrine? How would it apply in each of the cases?
5. Does the fact that Ashley has had a baby matter? What is an emancipated minor, and what decisions can an emancipated minor make without parental involvement?

GOAL SETTING, DECISION MAKING, AND IMPLEMENTATION

6. How could you persuade Christine's parents to involve her in discussions about her treatment? What could you do if they continued to refuse?
7. How could you resolve the dispute between Benjamin and his parents regarding treatment of his Tourette syndrome?

COMMENTARY ON DISCUSSION QUESTIONS

GETTING STARTED

1. **Have you ever encountered the circumstance in which an adolescent or mature child expresses a medical decision contrary to that of the parents? If so, how did you feel during that encounter?**

   Decision making that involves the healthcare of older children and adolescents should include, to the greatest extent feasible, the assent of the patient as well as the participation of the parents and the physician. Children cannot necessarily be considered rational and autonomous, but serious consideration should be given to their developing capacity to participate in decision making.[1] By recognizing the importance of assent, physicians empower children to the extent of their capacity.[2,3] Clearly, this is dependent upon the chronological age and the developmental age of the child. Even when a child's opinion or agreement should not be sought, involving the child in healthcare discussions may foster trust and a better physician–patient relationship.[1]

   Bernat, 34–6, Ch. 2

ASSESSMENT

2. **Compare and contrast the cases. What are the key contextual differences?**

   In each case, the patient, who is a child or adolescent, expresses a medical decision that is contrary to the parents' wishes. In Case 1, Christine's parents agree that she needs treatment of the brainstem glioma with radiation and chemotherapy but do not believe that Christine should be involved in any discussion of her treatments. Christine wishes more information. Although she is only 14 and thus incapable of providing consent for treatment, she is capable of providing assent. Nevertheless, because quality- and length-of-life issues are very much at stake, parents and child will need to come to terms on the critical need of care and consider carefully both the risk–benefit ratio of any procedure and how to best honor Christine's wishes and still decide the best course of action for her health.

   In Case 2, Benjamin is refusing medications for his Tourette syndrome. He may or may not have adequate insight as to the degree of impairment that his tics are causing him socially and emotionally. However, the tics are not in themselves directly harmful. His parents are appropriately concerned that the tics and noises that he makes will cause significant social problems. Therefore, the issues of assent, consent, and refusal are at stake.

   In Case 3, Ashley's epilepsy is difficult to control and, thus, is disruptive to her life and potentially dangerous to her. Despite having a baby, she is not an emancipated minor. She may or may not have the capacity to make decisions as a mature minor. Conversely, her frequent hospitalizations may make her exceptionally aware of the pros and cons of surgery. Ultimately, her parents are responsible for decision making. In deciding who should make the decision, care should be exercised to assess Ashley's emotional insight and her developmental capacity for decision making. She may now be considering her decision regarding surgery in the context of being a new mother.

3. What is assent and how does it differ from consent?

Bernat, 34–6, Ch. 2

Assent is the capacity to agree to a medical procedure or decision, and assent differs from consent in a number of important ways. Consent is a legal standard required of parents or emancipated minors to permit medical procedures, whereas assent is not legally required for medical care. However, the role of assent has become increasingly recognized as an important ethical process by which minors may participate in the medical decisions that directly impact them. Assent is not intended to replace the critical need for parental guidance, responsibility, and authority for the care of their children. One important aspect of development is for children to become aware of and responsible for their own health and decisions related to it.[1,2,4–7] Just as is the case with informed consent, obtaining assent is an interactive process in which decisions are made as a medical and family team effort.[1,7,8]

The Committee on Bioethics of the American Academy of Pediatrics states that assent should include at least the following elements:

a. Helping the patient to achieve a developmentally appropriate awareness of the nature of his or her condition.
b. Telling the patient what to expect with tests and treatments.
c. Making a clinical assessment of the patient's understanding of the situation and the factors influencing how the patient is responding (including whether inappropriate pressure is being placed on the patient to accept testing or therapy).
d. Soliciting an expression of the patient's willingness to accept the proposed care. Regarding this final point, we note that no one should solicit a patient's views without intending to weigh them seriously. In situations in which the patient will have to receive medical care despite his or her objection, the patient should be told that fact and should not be deceived.[1,9]

In some clinical situations, a persistent refusal to assent, or specifically dissent, may be ethically binding,[3] specifically in the context of research, when the intervention is investigational as opposed to a standard of care; when intervention is not essential to the child's welfare; or when intervention can be deferred without substantial risk.[1,10] Assent in research is a child's affirmative agreement to participate in the research. Absence of the child's objection to research participation cannot be considered assent; the child must say yes to participation.

Bernat,
34–6,
Ch. 2
Culture assigns authority for healthcare decision making to healthcare professionals and parents and, as result, reduces the role that children are allowed to play in their own healthcare.[2] Thus, those who care for children must provide for measures to solicit assent and to attend to possible abuses of power over children when ethical conflicts occur.

Bernat,
34–6,
Ch. 2
Doing so is particularly important regarding the initiation, withholding, or withdrawing of life-sustaining treatment.[2,5,9–15]

The range of options available when conflicts arise may include counseling, both for the immediate and the long term. On occasion, the need may arise to consult with the hospital ethics committee. Rarely will the need for legal intervention occur.[1,7,8]

4. What is the mature-minor doctrine? How would it apply in each of the cases?

The *mature-minor doctrine* provides for minors to give consent to medical procedures if they can show that they are mature enough to make decisions on their own. It is a relatively new legal concept, and as of 2002, it was adopted as a statute in only a few states, including Arkansas and Nevada.[16] In several other states, including Pennsylvania, Tennessee, Illinois, Maine, and Massachusetts, state high courts have adopted the doctrine as law.[17,18]

In the states where it exists, the mature-minor doctrine takes into account the age and situation of the minor to determine maturity, in addition to factors and conduct that can prove maturity. For instance, the Arkansas statute states, "any unemancipated minor of sufficient intelligence to understand and appreciate the consequences of the proposed surgical or medical treatment or procedures, for himself [may offer consent]."[16] The standard is typical of the requirements of the mature-minor doctrine.

The mature-minor doctrine has been consistently applied in cases in which the minor is 16 years or older, understands the medical procedure in question, and the procedure is not serious. Application of the doctrine in other circumstances is more questionable. Outside of reproductive rights, the US Supreme Court has never ruled on the doctrine's applicability to medical procedures.[4,16–18]

In each of the cases presented, a medical team can turn to the mature-minor doctrine for assistance in approaching the appropriate care of the teenagers. However, it is important to remember that the mature-minor doctrine is more helpful when the minor is seeking treatment that the parents do not wish the minor to have; it is far less helpful when a minor is refusing treatment, regardless of parental wishes.[1]

Regardless of the clinical situation, the mature-minor doctrine is not intended to be a substitute for finding ethical and developmentally appropriate ways for a child to understand his or her own healthcare concerns and, when possible, participate in some, most, or all of the necessary decision making. Therefore, Benjamin (Case 2) and Ashley

Bernat,
181–2,
Ch. 8

(Case 3) may both be mature enough to refuse medication; however, each child must be assessed individually, with attention given to the severity of the consequences if medication is refused.[1–3,10–13,15,17,19]

5. Does the fact that Ashley in Case 3 has had a baby matter? What is an emancipated minor, and what decisions can an emancipated minor make without parental involvement?

Emancipation of minors is a legal mechanism by which minors are freed from control by their parents or guardians, and the parents or guardians are freed from any and all responsibility toward the children. Until emancipation is granted by a court, minors are still subject to the rules of their parents or guardians. In most countries, adolescents below the legal age of majority (adulthood) may be emancipated in some manner: through marriage, attaining economic self-sufficiency, obtaining an educational degree or diploma, or participating in a form of military service. However, this does not typically include having a child.[17,18]

Adolescents, defined by the World Health Organization as those 10 to 19 years old, can give independent consent for reproductive health services if their capacities for understanding have sufficiently evolved. The international Convention on the Rights of the Child limits parental powers and duties by adolescents' "evolving capacities" for self-determination.[20] Emancipated minors' self-determination may also be recognized, for instance, on marriage or default of adults' guardianship.[9]

In the case of Ashley, who is refusing evaluation for surgery for her refractory epilepsy, several ethical issues are involved. First, one must be concerned that cumulative injury from her seizures may impair her decision-making capacity. Second, the impact on her capacity to continue to care for a minor child must be considered, regardless of whether she has epilepsy surgery. A neuropsychologic evaluation can help to assess her comprehension, her level of emotional operation, and her capacity to make an informed decision. One could persuasively argue that her firsthand experience with chronic illness and frequent hospitalizations would heighten her understanding of surgery and its risks. Indeed, her capacity to refuse may be far more informed than the average 17-year-old.[15,20–24] Finally, in only a few months, she will reach the age of majority and will be responsible for her own decisions.

GOAL SETTING, DECISION MAKING, AND IMPLEMENTATION

6. How could you persuade Christine's parents in Case 1 to involve her in discussions about her treatment? What could you do if they continued to refuse?

With such a sudden and devastating discovery that a child has a life-threatening condition that requires aggressive therapy, it is not surprising that family members would react with a wide range of emotions. Parents often think that they are protecting their children when they withhold information from them or exclude them from conversations about their own care.[25] Children understand much more than their parents assume; they need information and wish to be involved in their own care and in making decisions regarding it, even if they do not have final authority on the decisions. The Committee on Bioethics of the American Academy of Pediatrics states that "an incomplete ability to understand does not justify a lack of discussion with a child who desires involvement in his or her care and decision making."[25] Lastly, research suggests that a substantial proportion of parents who withheld information about dying from their children regretted their decision and suffered depression and anxiety.[25] Thus, efforts should be made to persuade Christine's parents to inform her of her diagnosis and involve her in her treatment decisions. If needed, a counselor versed in family dynamics can be helpful to mediate best ways to provide critically important information to a child who wants it. Additionally, such a counselor can provide excellent insight to the degree of emotional and intellectual development of the child and suggest very sensitive ways of sharing information that are developmentally appropriate for the child. Parents often benefit from separate counseling. Regardless, the medical team that can maintain a healthy regard for the emotional and developmental age of the patient will have a much better relationship with the patient and the parents.[7,15,19,23,24]

Bernat, 181–2, Ch. 8

7. **How could you resolve the dispute between Benjamin and his parents regarding treatment of his Tourette syndrome in Case 2?**

The principle of autonomy is well established in ethics and the law for adults, and were Benjamin above the age of majority, the case would have no ethical dilemma. His treatment refusal would be honored. However, because children are not cognitively or emotionally developed enough to make informed decisions, they are presumed in the law to lack competence (the legal equivalent of decision-making capacity). Their parents, therefore, are ethically and legally entitled to make decisions for them.[26] The law and ethics also presume that parents act in the best interests of their children; this does not mean that a child's wishes or concerns can or should be ignored when they differ from those of the parents. Several important factors should be considered in resolving the ethical dilemma of an adolescent's refusing treatment when his parents insist otherwise. These include a benefits–burdens analysis of treating or not treating, prognostic accuracy, and consideration of the child's decision-making capacity.[9,23,26,27]

In resolving the conflict between Benjamin and his parents, it is important to review several concerns. First, the nature of Tourette syndrome is such that adolescents may be prone to inattention to social cues and unaware of how their mannerisms and vocal tics may put off their peers.[27] Additionally, the goal of care for Tourette syndrome is not necessarily the elimination of tics, but a reduction to the degree that renders no social, physical, or emotional compromise.[26,27] Finally, tics spontaneously both resolve and worsen, but they certainly worsen in the context of stress or illness. Reviewing the current stresses and attempting to minimize or eliminate them may be sufficient.[26]

Two possible outcomes to this case would be ethically permissible. The first would be to monitor Benjamin's progress from a clinical standpoint and reassure his parents that little risk is involved in waiting and watching. Respecting Benjamin's choice may provide him the opportunity to assess the consequences of his decision; if his tics worsen and he is aware of it, he may then be more inclined to take his medication if the decision to resume treatment is his. A second option would be to resume therapy, provided Benjamin can be persuaded that the medication will be restarted at a low dose and monitored closely. However, if conflict still persists between Benjamin and his parents, psychological counseling to help coach insight and methods for conflict resolution for both the parents and the child can be helpful.

TOPICAL SYNOPSIS

It is critically important that healthcare providers understand the role of autonomy in adolescents to either refuse or assent to therapy. Assent is the capacity to agree to a medical procedure or decision. Although important for the ethical and humane care of children, it is not a legal standard of care. By contrast, consent is the legal standard to which parents are held in order to provide nonurgent medical care to their children. The mature-minor doctrine is helpful in identifying minors who may have emotional and developmental capacity to participate in healthcare decisions that have a direct impact on them, and like assent, it rarely has legal restraints. By contrast, a minor is considered emancipated when he or she is married, can demonstrate sufficient income on which to live, and is judged emancipated by a court of law. Additionally, mental-health care is permitted when a minor seeks mental-health care, treatment for sexually transmitted diseases, and either contraception or termination of pregnancy.

KEY POINTS

- Children and youth should be involved in discussions about their care whenever possible. Discussions should be tailored to the individual child's capacity for understanding. Parental support and participation are important.
- *Emancipated minor* is a status that is defined in the law; by contrast, the *mature minor* is a concept in law that encourages the involvement of mature minors to participate in their own care.

KEY WORDS

Assent—to agree, concur, or yield to a proposal, request, or suggestion. Minors may assent to a medical treatment or plan in the process of discussion with family and medical personnel.

Informed consent—process of authorization by a patient to medical interventions that was developed as a legal protection for patients to preserve their autonomy. The 3 critical elements of obtaining informed consent are that the medical professional gives adequate information to the patient in a way that the patient can understand, that the patient has capacity to consent or refuse, and that consent is given without coercion.

Emancipated minor—a child who has been granted the status of adulthood by a court order or other formality. A minor can earn emancipated status in 3 ways: (a) petitioning the court that he/she is financially independent, and the parents have no objections; (b) legally marrying, although state laws governing age of consent have precedence; (c) enlisting in the US Armed Forces; however, the military now has minimal education requirements. Note that a minor having a baby does not guarantee emancipation.

Mature minors—those who are not yet of majority age but are mature enough to participate in decision making relative to their own medical care. Minors may be recognized as competent based on a variety of factors, including age, maturity, intelligence, and the nature and risks of the proposed treatment. The mature-minor doctrine has been most consistently applied in cases in which the minor is near the age of majority, usually 15 years or older, and most importantly, displays the capacity to understand the nature and risks of treatment.

Refusal—the legal right for patients to decide to not have medical care, even life-sustaining care. As in consent, the same 3 elements are required: the medical provider must give adequate information to the patient in a way that the patient understands, refusal is given without coercion, and the patient is competent to either consent or refuse.

REFERENCES

1. Bartholome WG. Informed consent, parental permission, and assent in pediatric practice. Pediatrics 1995; 96(5 Pt 1):981–2.
2. Bernat, 34–6, Ch. 2.
3. King NMP, Cross AW. Children as decision makers: Guidelines for pediatricians. J Pediatr 1989; 115:10–6.
4. Oberman M. Minor rights and wrongs. J Law Med Ethics 1996; 24(2):127–39.
5. Capron AM. Right to refuse medical care. In: *Encyclopedia of Bioethics*. New York: The Free Press, 1978:1498–507.
6. Dickens BM. Adolescents and consent to treatment. Int J Gynecol Obstet 2005; 89(2):179–84.
7. Kuther TL. Medical decision-making and minors: Issues of consent and assent. Adolescence 2003; 38:343–58.
8. Diekema DS. Conducting ethical research in pediatrics: A brief historical overview and review of pediatric regulations. J Pediatr 2006; 149:S3–11.

9. Committee on Bioethics, American Academy of Pediatrics. Informed consent, parental permission, and assent in pediatric practice. Pediatrics 1995; 95:314–7.
10. Leikin SL. Minors' assent or dissent to medical treatment. J Pediatr 1983; 102:169–76.
11. Leikin S. Minors' assent, consent, or dissent to medical research. IRB 1993; 15:1–7.
12. Shield JPH, Baum JD. Children's consent to treatment: Listen to the children—they will have to live with the decision. Br Med J 1994; 308:1182–3.
13. Leikin S. A proposal concerning decisions to forgo life-sustaining treatment for young people. J Pediatr 1989; 115:17–22.
14. Rothman SM, Brenner P, Rouse F, et al. A community-based clinical selective in end-of-life care. J Palliat Med 1998; 1:257–64.
15. Scott E. Judgment and reasoning in adolescent decision making. Villanova Law Review 1992; 31:1607–69.
16. Arkansas State Code. A.C.A. § 20-9-602(7). Available at www.youthrights.net/index. php?title=Arkansas_Consent_Age_for_Medical_Procedures. Accessed July 24, 2012.
17. American Academy of Pediatrics Committee on Bioethics. Guidelines on forgoing life-sustaining medical treatment. Pediatrics 1994; 93:532–6.
18. Schlam L, Wood JP. Informed consent to the medical treatment of minors: Law and practice. Health Matrix: J Law Med 2000; 10(2):141–74.
19. Bernat, 181–2, Ch. 8.
20. Rights under the Convention on the Rights of the Child. Available at www.unicef.org/crc/index_30177.html. Accessed March 21, 2012.
21. Sundstrom D. Seizures and teens: maximizing health and safety. Except Parent 2007; 37:77–9.
22. Biglan A, Brennan P, Foster S, et al. *Helping Adolescents at Risk: Prevention of Multiple Problem Behaviors*. New York: Guilford Press, 2004.
23. Fletcher JC, Spencer EM, Lombardo PA. *Fletchers' Introduction to Clinical Ethics. 3rd ed.* Hagerstown, MD: Univ Pub Group, 2005.
24. *Diagnostic and statistical manual of mental disorders-text revision,4th ed.* Washington, DC: American Psychiatric Association, 2000.
25. Levetown M for the Committee on Bioethics of the American Academy of Pediatrics. Communicating with children and families: From everyday interactions to skill in conveying distressing information. Pediatrics 2008; 121:e1441–60.
26. Williams M. Ethical perspectives in neurology. In: *Movement Disorders: Continuum: Lifelong Learning in Neurology*. 2007; 13(1):154–7.
27. Schuerholz LJ, Baumgardner TL, Singer TL, et al. Neuropsychological status of children with Tourette's syndrome with and without attention deficit hyperactivity disorder. Neurology 1996; 46(4):958–65.

13 INTELLECTUAL DISABILITY

Michael Shevell, MDCM, FRCPC, FANA, FAAN

LEARNING OBJECTIVES

Upon completion of this chapter, participants will be able to:

1. Define intellectual disability according to present consensus criteria and delineate its attributes.
2. Identify those factors that render the intellectually disabled individual "never competent."
3. Identify the surrogate decision-making model that is most applicable for children or adults with intellectual disability.
4. Describe important ethical safeguards in research protocols involving subjects with intellectual disability.

LEARNING RESOURCES

Key chapters in Bernat's third edition—13, 16
Key relevant AAN documents available at www.aan.com/view/PECN

A

CLINICAL VIGNETTES

CASE 1

John was diagnosed with Fragile X syndrome by molecular studies of the FMR1 gene. Now 12 years old, he attends a special school and has not acquired basic reading and writing skills. His intelligence quotient (IQ) is in the high 50s, with better nonverbal than verbal skills. He has autistic traits that include repetitive behaviors, a desire for sameness, and an indifference to companionship. He has significant attentional difficulties for which he takes methylphenidate, and aggressive outbursts for which he takes risperidone. He lives with his parents and older sister. His mother's 50-year-old brother also has Fragile X syndrome and has lived in a group home since the death of his parents 5 years ago.

One day during recess at school, John impulsively raced across the street to retrieve a ball and was struck by a car. He was intubated and taken to the emergency department, where he remains comatose, and a head CT scan shows severe diffuse cerebral edema and an epidural hematoma. His parents refuse to provide consent for surgery to evacuate the hematoma or to insert an intracranial pressure monitor.

CASE 2

Samantha is a 35-year-old woman with Down syndrome (Trisomy 21). During her first year of life, she had surgery for duodenal atresia and a severe congenital heart malformation (endocardial cushion defect). She is an only child. She attended regular school but cannot read. Her IQ is in the mid 60s. She lives with her parents, who are both retired and in their early 70s. They are her legal guardians. She attends a local sheltered workshop, where she assembles headsets for use on airplanes.

Five years ago Samantha had hemolytic uremic syndrome and then developed chronic renal failure. She is on peritoneal dialysis 3 times per week. Her parents, who thought she was on a waiting list for kidney transplantation, asked why it was taking so long and were told by the nephrologist that she is not eligible for a kidney transplant because of her intellectual disability. They ask their neurologist if this is true.

CASE 3

Steven is a 7-year-old boy who had severe birth asphyxia. He has spastic tetraplegic cerebral palsy with athetosis and dystonia. He is wheelchair bound, nonverbal, and fed by others. He communicates laboriously using a Bliss board. His significant motor limitations preclude valid IQ testing.

Steven has frequent partial seizures with secondary generalization that are refractory to anticonvulsant medications, and he has had status epilepticus several times. He was evaluated for epilepsy surgery but is not a candidate. Steven's neurologist asks his parents to enroll him in a clinical trial of a novel anticonvulsant medication that has passed phase I and II human studies in adults. Both the parents and the neurologist will receive financial compensation for study participation from the sponsoring pharmaceutical company, with a bonus for completing the study. The primary outcome measure is seizure frequency over 6 months. The study requires monthly office visits and blood sampling.

QUESTIONS FOR GROUP DISCUSSION

GETTING STARTED

1. Do the patients in these cases meet criteria for the diagnosis of intellectual disability? Have you cared for patients with intellectual disability? Has a patient's intellectual disability affected the way that you provided care to the patient? How?

(continued)

CASE 1: JOHN

2. What factors may account for John's parents' refusal of surgery for the epidural hematoma?
3. Whose interests should be considered in making this decision? What ethical basis ought to be used to make the decision?
4. If the neurologist involved disagrees with the parents' decision, how should she proceed?

CASE 2: SAMANTHA

5. Is intellectual disability a sufficient reason to exclude Samantha from the organ-transplant list?
6. Should Samantha be asked her wishes? What weight should be assigned to them?
7. How can this situation be addressed?

CASE 3: STEVEN

8. Is it ethically permissible for Steven's parents to enroll him in the research study?
9. Is it ethically permissible for Steven's parents to be compensated for Steven's participation in the research study?
10. What safeguards protect persons with intellectual disability who participate in research?
11. What guidelines are available to help guide the informed-consent process for medical treatment and research in individuals with intellectual disability?

COMMENTARY ON DISCUSSION QUESTIONS

GETTING STARTED

1. **Do the patients in the cases meet criteria for the diagnosis of intellectual disability? Have you cared for patients with intellectual disability? Has a patient's intellectual disability affected the way that you provided care to the patient? How?**

Intellectual disability is a disability characterized by significant limitations both in intellectual functioning (reasoning, learning, problem solving) and in adaptive behavior, which covers a range of everyday social and practical skills.[1] Systems of support are necessary to maximize the individual's function and expected participation in family, educational, and societal settings. Onset occurs before the age of 18 years.

Most, if not all, neurologists will encounter patients with intellectual disability in their practices, especially as many of these patients live long lives.[2] The prevalence of intellectual disability is 2%–3% in the general population. Intellectual disability is more than an IQ score below an arbitrary cutoff; however, IQ scores are useful to stratify the severity of intellectual disability. The patients in the cases presented can be reliably diagnosed with intellectual disability.

CASE 1: JOHN

2. What factors may account for John's parents' refusal of surgery for the epidural hematoma?

Parents are intrinsically assumed to make decisions that are in their child's interests and are vested with the moral and legal authority to do so. As the primary caregivers, it is they who will invariably contend with the consequences of their choices. Thus, when parents refuse treatment for a child that the healthcare team believes would be beneficial, it is important to explore their understanding of the child's condition and prognosis and their understanding of the risks and benefits of treating or not treating the child. These understandings can often be discovered with open-ended questions. Perhaps John's parents' understanding is that his injuries are so severe that any intervention is futile. They might not want to subject him to additional harm or pain. They could be concerned that if he survives with severe neurologic deficits and care needs, their ability to care for him and to cope could be overwhelmed.

3. Whose interests should be considered in making this decision? What ethical basis ought to be used to make the decision?

Parents or guardians make medical decisions for children with intellectual disability. Because children with intellectual disability never have a capacity for autonomous decision making (a status known as "never-competent") and never possess the potential for developing autonomy,[3] the substituted-judgment model for decision making is not applicable, as this standard asks a surrogate to try to reproduce the decision that the patient would have made by applying the patient's values and preferences.[4] The "best interest" model, which balances the benefits of the patient's saved life against the burdens of that life, can be applied.[5–8] Parents are permitted to incorporate competing and conflicting interests into their decision, including consideration of the burdens of caring for the child and the effect of doing so on the rest of the family.[8] In this particular instance, the burden of Fragile X syndrome on John's life has not been excessive, and he has been capable of many normal activities. It is too early to predict the outcome of treating his traumatic brain injury and, thus, too early to conclude that the burdens of his saved life would be excessive. An argument can be made that his parents' refusal to consent to treatment is ethically impermissible at this time. The decision *not* to treat his brain injury is irreversible because he will die or suffer worse neurologic injury without treatment; however, the decision to initiate treatment is reversible. If it becomes clear after the initiation of treatment that the neurologic prognosis is poor, John's parents could ethically subsequently decide to limit or withdraw treatment. Thus, it is ethically preferable to initiate treatment of John's traumatic brain injury.

Bernat, 389–91, Ch. 16

Bernat, 88–9, Ch. 4

Bernat, 89–90, Ch. 4

Bernat, 318–9, Ch. 13

4. If the neurologist involved disagrees with the parents' decision, how should she proceed?

Treating physicians are not obliged to accept without question parental decisions that appear not to be in a child's best interests. The parents and physicians should discuss the parents' reasons for their decision, and the parents should be offered the opportunity to express their concerns. The neurologist should explain, in terms that the parents can understand, the range of outcomes with or without treatment. The neurologist can also describe the option of initiating treatment and later withdrawing it if the prognosis becomes grave, as the family may not be aware of this option. If necessary, a family meeting can be facilitated by an impartial mediator, such as an ethics consultant. If an impasse between the professional staff and the family continues and, considering that the treatment decision is an emergency, if the ethics consultation team concurs that it is ethically impermissible for the parents to decide *not* to treat John, then they may need to obtain advice from hospital legal counsel or possibly obtain a court order to treat the child.

CASE 2: SAMANTHA

5. Is intellectual disability a sufficient reason to exclude Samantha from the organ-transplant list?

Samantha has no apparent contraindication to renal transplantation other than her mild-to-moderate intellectual disability. Organs for transplantation are a scarce resource, and the Organ Procurement and Transplantation Network/United Network for Organ Sharing (OPTN/UNOS) has established objective criteria for ranking the eligibility and priority of patients on its waiting lists. Thus, tension exists between the ethical principle of justice, which supports giving Samantha a kidney,[9] and the principle of just allocation of scarce resources, which allocates organs on the basis of medical and psychosocial eligibility and the likelihood of perceived benefit.

Successful transplantation requires patient cooperation and adherence to a regimen of immunosuppression that typically involves multiple medications and frequent medical visits. Transplantation centers routinely conduct psychosocial evaluations of potential transplant recipients to determine if they will be capable of maintaining compliance with posttransplant care.[9] In 2007, the OPTN/UNOS board of directors, upon the recommendation of the OPTN/UNOS ethics committee, reaffirmed its position that "patients with disabilities should not be excluded from consideration for transplant *solely* by virtue of their disability" (emphasis added).[10] A survey of transplant centers in 2008 found that the use of neurodevelopmental delay in decisions regarding pediatric organ transplant listings was varied and inconsistent across programs and that no programs had formal processes for including the diagnosis of neurodevelopmental delay in the decision to list patients.[11] Further, 21% of programs reported that "severe delay" was an absolute contraindication to transplantation and 19% reported that "profound delay" was an absolute contraindication, whereas 40% indicated that neurodevelopmental delay (regardless of severity) was never an absolute contraindication.[11] Thus, children with intellectual disability are variably included or excluded from consideration of transplantation, depending on the policies of the local transplant program and the severity of the intellectual disability.

From ethical and transplant policy perspectives, it would not be appropriate to exclude Samantha from the transplant list solely because of her intellectual disability. Rather, she should be referred to a transplant center with expertise in evaluating and supporting patients with cognitive impairment, and a complete medical and psychosocial evaluation should be incorporated into the decision. The decision to include or exclude Samantha from the transplant list should be based on the conclusions of such an individualized objective and thorough evaluation.

6. Should Samantha be asked her wishes? What weight should be assigned to them?

Bernat,
389–91,
Ch. 16

Samantha's parents, who are her guardians, make medical decisions for her. She does not have decision-making capacity; yet, it is still appropriate to seek her assent or dissent regarding the evaluation for kidney transplantation[3] and, if she is found to be a candidate, for the transplantation surgical procedure. Assent is a person's affirmative agreement to undergo a recommended treatment or procedure. Assent, which is commonly used in pediatrics, stems from the principle of respect for persons. The treatment options should be explained at a developmentally appropriate level; however, if her developmental level is profoundly low (e.g., less than age 5 years), she may not be able to comprehend at all, and her parents should decide without asking her. It is potentially distressful to ask Samantha her opinion if her parents have already decided that she will be evaluated and treated if eligible.[12]

7. How can this situation be addressed?

Samantha's neurologist can advise her parents to take her to a transplantation center for evaluation of her eligibility for transplantation.

CASE 3: STEVEN

8. Is it ethically permissible for Steven's parents to enroll him in the research study?

The ethical and legal requirements for research involving children are more stringent than those for adults because children are considered vulnerable, as they cannot weigh the risks and benefits of participation on their own. Persons with intellectual disability are considered vulnerable for the same reasons. Specifically, the ethical and regulatory requirements are that the risks of research should be minimized for children. The concept of "minimal risk" is often applied and is defined as "where the probability and magnitude of harm or discomfort anticipated in the proposed research are not greater, in and of themselves, than those ordinarily encountered in daily life or during the performance of routine physical or psychological examinations or tests."[13] While blood drawing, as required by the protocol, would normally be considered in the minimal risk category, the monthly requirement is more frequent and therefore more burdensome than the risks or discomforts that Steven would encounter in normal care, and would not meet the current definition of minimal risk.[14] However, the research itself, on a new antiepileptic medication, has the potential to be directly beneficial to Steven and therefore may be allowed, as long as the risks are justified by the anticipated benefits and the risk–benefit relationship is at least as favorable to the child as the risk–benefit relationship of available alternative approaches (i.e., his existing epilepsy treatment).[15,16]

9. **Is it ethically permissible for Steven's parents to be compensated for Steven's participation in the research study?**

Clinical research involving children is necessary to evaluate the safety and efficacy of new medications in children, as the results of research on adults cannot be directly extrapolated to children. Compensation or other incentives to participate in research can help to achieve this goal; however, they must not be so excessive as to cause the child's parents to distort their decision making or to alter their perception of the risks of research.[17,18] Several types of payments exist, ranging from reimbursement for expenses, which is considered the least ethically problematic, to incentive payments, which may have the greatest potential to be an undue inducement to participate in research.[17] Payments for participation of children in research must be evaluated by the locally responsible IRB/REB in advance. Assuming a properly constituted IRB has reviewed the research protocol and its compensation, it is ethically permissible for Steven's parents to be so compensated.

10. **What safeguards protect persons with intellectual disability who participate in research?**

Multiple levels of safeguards exist, including:[19]

- The parent or guardian's custodial responsibility to provide care and avoid harm
- The investigator's professional integrity and code of ethics
- The sponsoring institution's IRB/REB committee's responsibility to review and monitor clinical research protocols

- The guidelines of the Office for Human Research Protections of the Department of Health and Human Services[20]
- The suggestions of the National Council for Bioethics in Human Research[21]
- The international standards articulated by the Council for International Organization of Medical Sciences (CIOMS)[22]

11. **What guidelines are available to help guide the informed-consent process for medical treatment and research in individuals with intellectual disability?**

Professional medical societies such as the AMA, the AAN, and the Child Neurology Society have adopted general standards on the ethical responsibilities of physicians that address respect for autonomy and the informed-consent process. The Office for Human Research Protections of the US Department of Health and Human Services offers guidance,[20] as does the FDA, including the Belmont report.[23] The NIH has a website specifically for children who want to learn about participating in research.[24]

KEY POINTS

- Healthcare professionals must be familiar with the ethical standards that govern those with intellectual disability in clinical practice and research.
- The "best interests" decision model should be applied to decision making in the context of intellectual disability.
- Access to care and research for those with intellectual disability must be balanced against protecting them from excessive risks.

KEY WORDS

Best-interests standard—a standard for surrogate decision making that asks how a reasonable person would balance the anticipated burdens borne as a result of a proposed course of treatment against the benefits that accrue from it.

Intellectual disability—a disability that originates before the age of 18 years, characterized by significant limitations in both intellectual functioning and adaptive behavior, which covers many everyday social and practical skills.

Never-competent—a status that applies to young children who, by virtue of their normal developmental age, cannot be considered to have capacity yet, or to older children or adults who, by virtue of intellectual disability, never acquire sufficient intellect to have capacity.

Parental decision making—decisions made by parents for children are based on the best-interests standard rather than on the substituted-judgment standard.

Substituted-judgment standard—a standard for surrogate decision making that involves making a judgment by "walking in a patient's shoes."

It requires the proxy to have a clear understanding of the patient's healthcare preferences, goals, and values, and the courage to apply and uphold them despite the proxy's own potential misgivings. The substituted-judgment standard cannot be used in making decisions for a patient with intellectual disability because of the impossibility of the patient having any history of previously expressed values.

ACKNOWLEDGMENTS

The author is grateful for the support of the Montreal Children's Hospital Foundation during the writing of the chapter manuscript. Alba Rinaldi provided secretarial assistance.

REFERENCES

1. American Association on Intellectual and Developmental Disabilities. Definition of intellectual disability. Available at www.aaidd.org/content_100.cfm?navID=21. Accessed March 11, 2012.
2. Shevell MI, Sherr E. Global developmental delay and mental retardation. In: Swaiman K, Ashwal S, Ferreiro D, eds. *Pediatric Neurology: Principles & Practice, 4th ed.* Philadelphia: Mosby Elsevier, 2006:799–820.
3. Bernat, 389–91, Ch. 16.
4. Bernat, 88–9, Ch. 4.
5. Bernat, 89–90, Ch. 4.
6. Bernat, 318–9, Ch. 13.
7. Bernat JL. Informed consent in pediatric neurology. Sem Pediatr Neurol 2002; 9:10–8.
8. Kopelman LM. The best-interests standard for incompetent or incapacitated persons of all ages. J Law Med Ethics 2007; 35:187–96.
9. Annunziato RA, Fisher MK, Jerson B, et al. Psychosocial assessment prior to pediatric transplantation: A review and summary of key considerations. Pediatr Transplantation 2010; 14(5):565–74.
10. Executive summary of the minutes OPTN/UNOS board of directors meeting. June 26, 2007. Available at http://optn.transplant.hrsa.gov/SharedContentDocuments/Executive_Summary_-_June_2007.pdf, Accessed March 22, 2012.
11. Richards CT, Crawley LM, Magnus D. Use of neurodevelopmental delay in pediatric solid organ transplant listing decisions: Inconsistencies in standards across major pediatric transplant centers. Pediatr Transplantation 2009; 13(7):843–50.
12. Shevell MI. Clinical ethics and developmental delay. Semin Pediatr Neurol 1998; 15:70–5.
13. Title 45 CFR 46.404. Research not involving greater than minimal risk. Available at www.hhs.gov/ohrp/humansubjects/guidance/45cfr46.html/. Accessed July 24, 2012.
14. Beauchamp TL, Childress JF. *Principles of Biomedical Ethics, 4th ed.* New York: Oxford University Press, 1994.
15. Title 45 CFR 46.405. Research involving greater than minimal risk but presenting the prospect of direct benefit to the individual subjects. Available at www.hhs.gov/ohrp/humansubjects/guidance/45cfr46.html/. Accessed July 24, 2012.
16. Wender EH. Assessment of risk to children. In: Grodin MA, Glantz LH, eds. *Children as Research Subjects. Science, Ethics, and Law*. New York: Oxford University Press, 1994:181–92.
17. Wendler D, Rackoff JE, Emanuel EJ. The ethics of paying for children's participation in research. J Pediatr 2002; 141:166–71.
18. Diekema DS. Conducting ethical research in pediatrics: A brief historical overview and review of pediatric regulations. J Pediatr 2006; 149:S3–11.

19. Shevell MI. Ethics of clinical research in children. Semin Pediatr Neurol 2002; 9:46–52.
20. Office for Human Research Protections. Available at www.hhs.gov/ohrp/. Accessed March 22, 2012.
21. National Council on Ethics in Human Research. Available at www.ncehr-cnerh.org/. Accessed March 22, 2012.
22. Council for International Organizations of Medical Sciences. Available at www.cioms.ch/. Accessed March 22, 2012.
23. The National Commission for the Protection of Human Subjects of Biomedical and Behavioral Research. The Belmont Report Ethical Principles and Guidelines for the Protection of Human Subjects of Research, April 18, 1979. Available at www.fda.gov/ohrms/dockets/ac/04/briefing/2004-4066b1_22_Belmont%20Report.pdf. Accessed March 22, 2012.
24. National Heart, Lung, and Blood Institute. Available at www.nhlbi.nih.gov/childrenandclinicalstudies/index.php. Accessed March 22, 2012.

14 DEMENTIA

Michael A. Williams, MD, FAAN

LEARNING OBJECTIVES

Upon completion of this chapter, participants will be able to:

1. Describe at least 2 ways in which dementia impairs decision-making capacity.
2. Identify ethical and legal procedures for representing the interests of incapacitated unbefriended patients when important, nonemergent medical decisions must be made.
3. Identify relevant policies at their institutions regarding informed consent and the authority of surrogates to make decisions on behalf of patients with impaired decisional capacity.

LEARNING RESOURCES

Key chapters in Bernat's third edition—2, 3, 4, 6, 15

Key relevant AAN documents available at www.aan.com/view/PECN

A   I   M   O

CLINICAL VIGNETTES

CASE 1

Sam, a 60-year-old man with an established diagnosis of frontotemporal dementia (FTD) with progressive nonfluent aphasia, is admitted to the orthopedic surgery service following a fall that resulted in a fractured hip. While he is in the hospital, liver enzymes are noted to be elevated and a CT scan shows a hepatic lesion. Sam's wife, Edna, who holds durable power of attorney for healthcare decisions for Sam, is advised of the test results and the need for a needle biopsy. Unaware of Sam's language impairment, the gastroenterology consulting team comes to see him while Edna is away. Because Sam is alert and interactive, they do not recognize his cognitive deficits, and with one of the residents witnessing, the fellow has Sam sign a consent form for the biopsy. When Edna arrives later in the day, the biopsy has already been performed. She immediately asks to speak with the physician who performed the biopsy without first speaking with her.

The attending physician who supervised the biopsy recognizes that he and his team erred in obtaining consent directly from Sam and apologizes to Edna. He promises to inform the hospital's committee for addressing medical errors so as to prevent any similar errors from occurring in the future.

CASE 2

Jan, a patient with moderate dementia, is found to have idiopathic normal-pressure hydrocephalus after she shows an unequivocal improvement in gait, bladder control, and awareness in response to CSF drainage by spinal catheter. The neurologist recommends shunt surgery, and Jan's family, who has seen the significant improvement, agree that the benefits of surgery outweigh the risks. However, by virtue of her dementia, Jan does not remember that she had gait impairment and incontinence, does not believe the diagnosis (anosognosia), and refuses to have surgery, saying, "I don't have any of the symptoms you're talking about." Her husband, family, and physician cannot convince her otherwise; yet, they are certain that shunt surgery is in her best interests. It could, they believe, improve the dementia and allow her to appreciate her own diagnosis. They question whether they can take Jan for surgery despite her apparent objection.

CASE 3

Edith is a 90-year-old woman with severe, end-stage Alzheimer dementia who resides in a nursing home. She is sent to the ED because of respiratory distress and is found to have pneumonia. It is obvious to everyone who evaluates her that she does not have decision-making capacity because she is nearly mute. The nursing home notes indicate that she has no family, no advance directive, and no guardian. A call to the staff indicates that she has had no visitors "for as long as anyone can remember." Because of falling oxygen saturation and tachycardia, she is intubated in the ED and is given IV fluids for rehydration. She is admitted to the ICU and responds sufficiently that she is safely extubated by the next morning. Although awake, she has no verbal communication except to say "no" or "stop" when the team tries to examine her. The nurses had restrained her hands overnight because she attempted to extubate herself at 3 am and pulled out the Foley catheter.

The chief resident, who is angry with the ED resident for intubating the patient and admitting her to an ICU bed that "could have been used for someone whose life is worth saving," writes a DNR order and tells the team on rounds that re-intubation would be futile and physicians are not required to provide futile treatment. However, the third-year medical student, who has recently completed the required second-year course in ethics, objects because the patient has no surrogate to make decisions on her behalf; the medical student believes that an ethics consultation is required. The chief resident scoffs at the suggestion and tells the student that the ethics taught in the lecture hall have no connection to the "real life" application of ethics in the hospital. The medical student responds that because hospital policy requires 2 physicians to verify that treatment is futile, the attending physician should be involved.

QUESTIONS FOR GROUP DISCUSSION

GETTING STARTED

1. Have you experienced ethical dilemmas in the care of patients with different types of dementia? How have these been handled?

ASSESSMENT

2. In each case, what are the patient's condition and prognosis? Is there any doubt or disagreement?
3. Do the patients in these cases have decision-making capacity?
4. Are the patients' preferences known? Is there any doubt or disagreement?
5. In the absence of an advance directive and a surrogate decision maker for an unbefriended patient, what procedures can or should be used for making healthcare decisions?
6. Do competing interests exist in any of the cases?
7. Do any issues of power or conflict in the interactions of the key actors in the cases need to be addressed?

MORAL DIAGNOSIS

8. Identify any relevant institutional policies that pertain to each case. Consider ethical standards and guidelines such as consensus statements by commissions or medical specialty societies.

GOAL SETTING, DECISION MAKING, AND IMPLEMENTATION

9. How can an ethics consultation be of benefit?

EVALUATION

10. What changes in institutional policy or educational interventions might help to prevent or resolve the moral problems posed by similar cases?

COMMENTARY ON DISCUSSION QUESTIONS

GETTING STARTED

1. **Have you experienced ethical dilemmas in the care of patients with different types of dementia? How have these been handled?**

The care of patients with dementia is common in neurology, and based on its epidemiologic data, the Alzheimer's Association estimates that by 2030, the number of people aged 65 and older with Alzheimer disease will reach 7.7 million—1½ times the estimated patient population in 2011 of 5.2 million.[1]

Although some evidence suggests that older patients are more likely than are younger patients to have advance directives,[2] it is still very common for patients with dementia not to have advance directives, for their surrogates to be appointed by virtue of state statute as opposed to the assignment of durable power of attorney for healthcare decisions, and for some patients with dementia to lack any family or friends to serve as their surrogate decision makers (i.e., they are unbefriended).[3] Other challenges in the care of patients with dementia include variants such as FTD and early-onset dementia, both disorders in which patients' clinical presentation does not match the expected presentation of an elderly person with obvious short-term memory problems, and consequently, the patients' impaired decision making may not be recognized in the course of casual conversation, especially by healthcare professionals who are not neurologists.

ASSESSMENT

2. In each case, what are the patient's condition and prognosis? Is there any doubt or disagreement?

In Case 1, Sam's diagnosis of FTD with progressive nonfluent aphasia is established, and his condition and prognosis are not at issue. Rather, the failure of the consulting team, and possibly the nursing staff on the orthopedic surgery ward, to recognize his lack of decision-making capacity has resulted in the performance of an elective procedure without valid consent.

Jan in Case 2 has been diagnosed with idiopathic normal-pressure hydrocephalus, and the prognosis with treatment is favorable based on her response to CSF drainage and published experience with shunt surgery.[4–7] The treating physicians and the family are in agreement; however, the patient herself does not recognize her neurologic deficits and thus sees no reason to have surgery.

In Case 3, although treatment with intubation, ventilation, and rehydration can stabilize Edith's medical condition, her dementia cannot be reversed. Furthermore, an 18-month longitudinal study of 323 nursing home residents with advanced dementia showed that 54.8% of residents died in the study period.[8] The probability of at least one episode of pneumonia was 41.1%, and the 6-month mortality rate of pneumonia was 46.7%. Therefore, the prognosis with end-stage dementia and aspiration pneumonia is poor. Although advanced dementia can be considered a terminal disease,[8] the issue of the futility of medical interventions will depend on whether the goals of care are to treat Edith's medical conditions to keep her alive, to alleviate or avoid the burdens of hospitalization and intensive care interventions, or to treat her dementia.

3. Do the patients in these cases have decision-making capacity?

Bernat, 362–3, Ch. 15

None of the patients in the cases presented has decision-making capacity,[9] but the cause is different in each case. Sam in Case 1 has FTD with progressive nonfluent aphasia, and although he can appear to interact much like a normal person, his ability to understand complex ideas (such as the content of the discussion for informed consent for his biopsy) and to communicate his wishes is impaired. For Jan in Case 2, the issue is anosognosia—the failure to recognize her own neurologic deficits. Although she can understand the explanation of her condition and the risks and benefits of shunt surgery, the anosognosia renders her incapable of appreciating both her circumstances and the likely consequences of either accepting or refusing the recommended shunt surgery. Thus, because of her lack of insight, her apparent refusal of shunt surgery is not informed and she does not have decision-making capacity.[10,11]

Bernat, 27–8, Ch. 2

In Case 3, Edith's lack of decision-making capacity with end-stage dementia is obvious and recognized by everyone involved in her care.

4. Are the patients' preferences known? Is there any doubt or disagreement?

Sam may have seemed to indicate agreement to the liver biopsy, but it is not clear whether the procedure was consistent with his wishes, as his aphasia may have prevented him from accurately expressing his wishes. Although it seems reasonable to presume that he would have wanted the biopsy (if he had capacity), such a presumption applies only in the circumstance of true emergencies and not for elective procedures. The best way to discern his preferences would have been for the gastroenterologists to contact his wife to discuss the proposed biopsy procedure and to inquire as to whether a biopsy would be consistent with his previously expressed preferences or goals of care.

Although Jan may appear to be expressing preferences not to have surgery, her capacity to have an informed preference is impaired by her anosognosia. Because decision-making capacity is not an all-or-none capacity, it is possible that Jan has the capacity to express preferences for lower-risk or less burdensome interventions, but she may not possess the capacity to express a preference for a beneficial surgery with limited and reasonable risks.[9]

Bernat, 362–3, Ch. 15
Bernat, 89–90, Ch. 4
Bernat, 318–19, Ch. 13

Edith's preferences are unknown and cannot be known because no family members or friends are available. Any decisions would have to be made according to the best-interests standard.[12,13]

5. In the absence of an advance directive and a surrogate decision maker for an unbefriended patient, what procedures can or should be used for making healthcare decisions?

Bernat, 9–11, Ch. 1

Consistent with the ethical principles of respect for persons and autonomy,[14] all patients with impaired decision-making capacity, even those who are unbefriended, deserve to have their interests represented when important medical decisions are made. Depending on the laws in the state where patients receive medical care, the most common mechanisms for identifying surrogates to represent the patients' interests are (a) requesting the ethics consultation team to determine whether the decision to write a DNR order is ethically permissible, (b) seeking a court-appointed guardian to approve the request for the DNR order, or (c) both.[15]

6. Do any competing interests exist in any of the cases?

In Sam's case (Case 1), no competing interests exist that relate to the intent to perform the biopsy; however, the hospital and its physicians now have an interest in acknowledging the error by the fellow and the resident in failing to recognize that Sam lacked decision-making capacity and that the medical record clearly indicated that his wife should make all decisions on his behalf. Performing an elective biopsy in the absence of valid informed consent can be considered battery.

In Jan's case (Case 2), the family members are interested in improving her health condition by persuading her to have the shunt surgery that she refuses, and they appear to have no competing interests.

In the case of Edith with advanced dementia (Case 3), the chief resident asserts that the interests of other patients in receiving ICU care should supersede Edith's interests. This is a specious argument based on the premise that physicians can arbitrarily take the interests of other unknown "potential" patients into consideration when deciding whether to admit a patient like Edith to the hospital or ICU. Although physicians should be mindful of the just allocation of scarce resources,[16] such decisions should not be made at the bedside, as a physician's first and primary duty is to the patient.[16,17] Scarce resources should be allocated according to hospital- or community-derived policies and procedures.[16] Even though Edith is in a state of advanced dementia, she has the same interests in access to appropriate healthcare and autonomy or to representation by a surrogate as all other patients. Bernat acknowledges the fiduciary duty that physicians have to "maintain the primacy of the patient's interests";[18] however, he also proposes that society's principal duty is to "provide chronic care, comfort care, and quality of life measures, but not further high-technology, life-prolonging measures for elderly patients who have exceeded their life expectancy."[19]

Bernat, 51, Ch. 3

Bernat, 362, Ch. 15

7. Do any issues of power or conflict in the interactions of the key actors in the cases need to be addressed?

Cases 1 and 2 have no obvious power conflicts. A power conflict *could* have existed in the case of invalid informed consent for Sam's biopsy, but the gastroenterology attending has mitigated the power differential by acknowledging the error to Sam's wife and apologizing for it. Even though the disclosure and apology are a highly appropriate best practice,[20] physicians should not expect that all apologies will result in forgiveness.[21]

In Case 3, a significant power differential between the chief resident and the third-year medical student exists. Such student–teacher power differentials are discussed cogently in Chapter 2 of this textbook. The medical student has correctly identified an ethical and legal dilemma and has shown significant courage in raising the issue on rounds and seeking to involve the attending physician despite the dismissive comments by the chief resident. The attending physician must be mindful to address the conflict and the ethical dilemma with the team in such a way that simultaneously respects the student's position and does not embarrass or intimidate the chief resident. The attending physician should take the opportunity privately to address the chief resident's behavior toward the medical student.

MORAL DIAGNOSIS

8. Identify any relevant institutional policies that pertain to each case. Consider ethical standards and guidelines such as consensus statements by commissions or medical specialty societies.

All hospitals have policies regarding informed consent and the authority of surrogates to make decisions on behalf of patients with impaired decisional capacity. Section 1.4 of the AAN Code of Professional Conduct and its guideline on ethical issues in the care of patients with dementia recommend for surrogate decision making for patients who lack capacity.[22,23] In most circumstances, healthcare professionals may reasonably assume that adults have decision-making capacity; however, in many situations, this assumption should be set aside. Neurologists who care for patients with dementia and cognitive impairment from other disorders, such as stroke or traumatic brain injury, are accustomed to assessing patients' capacity to participate in decisions. When the diagnosis is well established and a surrogate decision maker has been clearly identified, the onus is on physicians to be familiar with the patient's medical history and medical record. Although no ill intent was involved in the process of the biopsy for Sam in Case 1, the healthcare team's actions can be considered negligent, and they and the hospital are liable for the error.

Jan's circumstances in Case 2 are so infrequent that it is unlikely that a specific hospital policy would exist. However, an ethics consultation could be requested to determine, on the basis of justified paternalism,[24] whether the patient's family could take her to surgery against her apparent wishes. Alternately, the family could petition a court of law to have Jan declared incompetent (the legal determination of incapacity), have a member of her family appointed guardian, and allow the guardian to authorize the surgery. Doing so would be ethically and legally similar— though not identical—to parents making a decision for a child to have shunt surgery or shunt-revision surgery against her wishes.[25]

Short of these procedures, Jan's family has more latitude in persuasion than does the healthcare team, as healthcare professionals must take care not to coerce patients. In fact, this author has cared for a patient whose anosognosia initially led the patient to refuse shunt surgery. The family was eventually able to persuade the patient to have surgery, after which the patient's symptoms improved dramatically, as was hoped. When told about his symptoms and his initial refusal of surgery, the patient said that he had no recollection of his symptoms but that, knowing his own personality, he was not surprised that he refused surgery. He then thanked the physicians and family for persuading him to have the surgery.

Pertaining to Edith in Case 3, all hospitals have access to ethics consultants and attorneys who can advise regarding the patient's unbefriended status and the need for a guardian, and the law in most states addresses these matters.[15] The AAN guideline for the care of patients with dementia recognizes that for many patients with advanced dementia, palliative care may be more appropriate than further attempts at curative care.[15,23,26] This guideline also indicates that the use of restraints in patients with dementia may be ordered when the restraints contribute to the safety of the patient (as was the case when Edith was attempting to extubate herself) but not when their use is simply a convenience for the staff. Therefore, now that Edith is safely extubated, the need for restraints should be re-evaluated and the least invasive method should be used.[27]

Bernat, 369–73, Ch 15

Bernat, 368–9, Ch. 15

GOAL SETTING, DECISION MAKING, AND IMPLEMENTATION

9. How can ethics consultation be of benefit?

In Sam's case, although an ethics consultation may not be needed, the hospital's policies and procedures for responding to errors should be activated (see Chapter 5).

As mentioned above, an ethics consultation could be very helpful for Jan in Case 2 and would be an example of an ethics consultation performed for the resolution of an ethical dilemma, as opposed to a conflict between the family and the healthcare team. The decision to proceed with surgery on the basis of justified paternalism for a patient who "appears" to have decisional capacity can be quite difficult. Justified paternalism is the implementation either by family or physicians of medical decisions that override a patient's "apparent" preferences when (a) the patient lacks decision-making capacity, (b) the probability is high that the patient would be harmed if the patient's "apparent" decision were allowed and an intervention contrary to the patient's "apparent" preference were not allowed, and (c) the risk of the intervention chosen by the family or physicians is proportionally lower than the risk of the patient's choice.[24] This scenario usually occurs when a patient is capable of verbally or physically expressing a choice but, owing to neurologic impairment, is found to lack an appreciation of the consequences of the choice and thus lacks decision-making capacity. Evaluation of Jan's decisional capacity by an independent neurologist or psychiatrist would be helpful to the ethics consultants and the family. The decision to proceed with an intervention against a patient's "apparent wishes" on the basis of justified paternalism nearly always requires an ethics consultation. Additionally, even if a court of law would have to declare Jan incompetent, a judge is very likely to consider the recommendations of the ethics consultants in reaching a decision.

For Edith in Case 3, an ethics consultation, as suggested by the medical student, is highly recommended. The consultants can represent her interests in deliberation with the healthcare team. The ethics consultants cannot recommend that a DNR order *must* be written; they can only indicate whether Edith's current condition and prognosis make the decision by the healthcare team to write a DNR order ethically permissible. In some states, the ethics-consultation process alone may be sufficient to authorize a DNR order as ethically permissible; however, such orders generally apply only to the current hospital stay and not to future hospital stays. Therefore, it may be necessary for the hospital to petition a court of law for a guardian for the patient so that an enduring DNR order can be entered into the patient's medical record at the nursing home where she resides.

EVALUATION

10. What changes in institutional policy or educational interventions might help to prevent or resolve the moral problems posed by similar cases?

In Case 1, the hospital committee responsible for reviewing medical errors may wish to review the procedures for identifying patients who are known to lack decision-making capacity and whose surrogates are available for discussion and consent. The identification procedures should occur at the time of admission and should appear in the hospital chart (whether electronic or paper), and the procedures for a time out before any invasive intervention should include an assessment of whether the appropriate surrogate has provided consent.

In Case 2, the hospital may wish to review its procedures for ethics consultation and determination of decision-making capacity. Circumstances of justified paternalism may be so infrequent that a more general policy of seeking ethics consultation is preferable to a specific policy.

Lastly, Case 3 highlights the issue of review of hospital procedures for safeguarding the interests of unbefriended patients and for preventing unilateral decisions by physicians to declare treatment futile or to write DNR orders. Even when patients' family members or surrogates are present, the healthcare team has an obligation to discuss end-of-life care planning with them before DNR orders can be written.

KEY POINTS

■ All patients with impaired decision-making capacity, even those who are unbefriended, deserve to have their interests represented when important medical decisions are made.

■ Decision-making capacity is not an all-or-none capacity, and some patients may be able to express preferences for lower-risk or less burdensome interventions but may not possess the capacity to express a preference for a beneficial invasive intervention with limited and reasonable risks.

KEY WORDS

Anosognosia—unawareness of one's neurologic deficits as a result of the neurologic illness itself.

Decision-making capacity—the capacity of individuals to make decisions on their own behalf, while taking into consideration the potential benefits and burdens of the decision.

Justified paternalism—the implementation either by family or physicians of medical decisions that override a patient's "apparent" preferences when (a) the patient lacks decision-making capacity, (b) the probability is high that the patient would be harmed if the patient's "apparent" decision were allowed and an intervention contrary to the patients "apparent" preference were not allowed, and (c) the risk of the intervention chosen by the family or physicians is proportionally lower than the risk of the patient's choice. This scenario usually occurs when a patient is capable of verbally or physically expressing a choice but, owing to neurologic impairment, is found to lack an appreciation of the consequences of the choice and thus lacks decision-making capacity.

Unbefriended—term describing a patient who (a) lacks decision-making capacity, (b) lacks an advance directive, and (c) lacks family, friends, or other persons who are available and willing to make surrogate decisions on behalf of the patient.

REFERENCES

1. Alzheimer's Association. 2011 Alzheimer's Disease Facts and Figures. Alzheimers Dement 2011; 7(2):208–44.
2. Pollack KM, Morhaim D, Williams MA. The public's perspectives on advance directives: Implications for state legislative and regulatory policy. Health Policy 2010; 96:57–63.
3. Karp N, Wood E. Incapacitated and Alone: Health Care Decision-Making for the Unbefriended Elderly. Washington: American Bar Association Commission on Law and Aging, 2003.
4. Marmarou A, Bergsneider M, Klinge P, et al. The value of supplemental prognostic tests for the preoperative assessment of idiopathic normal-pressure hydrocephalus. Neurosurgery 2005; 57(3 Suppl):S17–28.
5. Relkin N, Marmarou A, Klinge P, et al. Diagnosing idiopathic normal-pressure hydrocephalus. Neurosurgery 2005; 57(3 Suppl):S4–16.
6. Tarnaris A, Williams MA. Idiopathic normal pressure hydrocephalus: Update and practical approach on diagnosis and management. Neurosurg Q 2011; 21:72–81.

7. Marmarou A, Young HF, Aygok GA, et al. Diagnosis and management of idiopathic normal-pressure hydrocephalus: A prospective study in 151 patients. J Neurosurg 2005; 102(6):987–97.

8. Mitchell SL, Teno JM, Kiely DK, et al. The clinical course of advanced dementia. N Engl J Med 2009; 361(16):1529–38.

9. Bernat, 362–3, Ch. 15.

10. Appelbaum PS. Assessment of patients' competence to consent to treatment. N Engl J Med 2007; 357:1834–40.

11. Bernat, 27–8, Ch. 2.

12. Bernat, 89–90, Ch. 4.

13. Bernat, 318–19, Ch. 13.

14. Bernat, 9–11, Ch. 1.

15. American Bar Association. Adult guardianship statutory table of authorities (6/11). Available at www.americanbar.org/content/dam/aba/uncategorized/2011/2011_aging_gship_stat_table_of_authorities_6_11.authcheckdam.pdf. Accessed April 3, 2012.

16. Andrews R, Cleaveland CR, Cutler C, et al. American College of Physicians Ethics Manual, 6th ed. Ann Intern Med 2012; 156:73–104.

17. American Academy of Neurology. Code of Professional Conduct. Section 1.2, Fiduciary and Contractual Basis. [*PECN* appendix document A available at www.aan.com/view/PECN]

18. Bernat, 51, Ch. 3.

19. Bernat, 362, Ch. 15.

20. Wojcieszak D, Saxton JW, Finkelstein MM. *Sorry Works! 2.0 Disclosure, Apology, and Relationships Prevent Medical Malpractice Claims*. Bloomington, IN: AuthorHouse, 2010.

21. Berlinger N, Wu AW. Subtracting insult from injury: Addressing cultural expectations in the disclosure of medical error. J Med Ethics 2005; 31:106–8.

22. American Academy of Neurology. Code of Professional Conduct. Section 1.4, Informed Consent. [*PECN* appendix document A and available at www.aan.com/view/PECN]

23. American Academy of Neurology Ethics and Humanities Subcommittee. Ethical issues in the management of the demented patient. Neurology 1996; 46:1180–3. [*PECN* document I available at www.aan.com/view/PECN]

24. Childress J. *Who Should Decide? Paternalism in Health Care*. New York: Oxford University Press, 1982:102–26, Ch. V. Justified paternalism.

25. Williams MA. Ethical considerations in hydrocephalus research that involves children and adults. In: *Hydrocephalus. Selected papers from the International Workshop in Crete, 2010.* Acta Neurochir Suppl 2012; 113:15–9.

26. Bernat, 369–73, Ch 15.

27. Bernat, 368–9, Ch. 15.

15 PRINCIPLED APPROACH TO NEUROLOGICALLY IMPAIRED DRIVERS

Matthew Rizzo, MD, FAAN • Katherine G. Shearer, MD

LEARNING OBJECTIVES

Upon completion of this chapter, participants will be able to:

1. Recognize ethical issues associated with assessment of fitness to drive in patients with cognitive impairment.
2. Describe how to apply objective methods for assessing driving abilities and appropriately advising patients, their families, and state licensing authorities.
3. Describe the legal and ethical considerations in evaluating and reporting patients with impaired driving abilities.

LEARNING RESOURCES

Key chapters in Bernat's third edition—3, 4

Key relevant AAN documents available at www.aan.com/view/PECN

A   I   J   K

CLINICAL VIGNETTES

CASE 1

A 70-year-old widow was arrested for driving 75 mph and crossing the center line to pass slower cars on a city street with a 35 mph speed limit. The police confiscated her license, her daughter drove her home, and she promised not to drive. Two weeks later she was arrested again for dangerous driving. She felt that the car ahead was waiting too long at an intersection, so she pushed it with her car directly into the path of traffic. In the presence of a policeman, she offered the car's driver $200 for damages and for not telling her daughter. Neurologic evaluation revealed the diagnosis of frontotemporal dementia. She is not allowed to drive, but she keeps trying. Her family asks the neurologist for advice.

CASE 2

A 45-year-old man presented with a nonconvulsive staring episode that led to the MRI that showed a frontal glioblastoma, which was treated with surgery followed by radiation therapy. He was treated with levetiracetam, and his postoperative EEG showed mild background slowing and no epileptiform activity. He recovered from surgery and, after 3 months, had mild residual motor dysfunction and cognitive impairment. He has had no further staring spells. His neurologist recommended that he not resume driving, but the patient disagreed and insisted on a formal driving assessment. A neuropsychologist found mild impairments of executive function and attention, and an occupational therapist found that, in a driving simulator, the patient could operate the controls and hold his speed and lane position as well as many other drivers could. Despite this objective evidence, the neurologist still recommends that the man should not drive. The patient and his family are upset.

QUESTIONS FOR GROUP DISCUSSION

GETTING STARTED
1. Have you ever evaluated a patient who you thought had impaired driving ability? What is challenging about addressing this problem?

ASSESSMENT
2. How can you determine if a driver is safe or unsafe? Are the drivers in the cases capable of decision making? Are they self-aware?
3. Is age or diagnosis alone a sufficient criterion for testing or restricting driving?

MORAL DIAGNOSIS
4. What is the ethical or legal justification for restricting a patient's driving?
5. Can "conspiring" with the family to hide the patient's keys be ethically justified?

GOAL SETTING, DECISION MAKING, AND IMPLEMENTATION
6. How do you advise patients regarding their fitness to drive?
7. What are the legal considerations in evaluating and deciding whether to restrict a potentially unsafe driver?
8. What should the neurologist tell the patient whose response is, "I will keep driving in spite of your recommendation"? What should the neurologist document in the chart?

COMMENTARY ON DISCUSSION QUESTIONS

GETTING STARTED

1. Have you ever evaluated a patient who you thought had impaired driving ability? What is challenging about addressing this problem?

Many neurologic disorders (e.g., dementia, brain tumor, movement disorders, stroke, demyelinating disorders, sleep disorders), psychiatric disorders, medical disorders, and medication side effects can impair one's ability to drive. Patients with these conditions should be asked about their driving and, if indicated, evaluated for their ability to safely operate a motor vehicle. A patient's ability to drive can be evaluated by many tests, including neuropsychological testing, driving simulation, on-road testing, and assessment of overall physical ability (balance, strength, coordination).[1] This issue can be challenging because it requires consideration of not only the patient's interests, but also those of the public, specifically the safety of other drivers and pedestrians. Patients often become upset when their driving privileges are restricted, as they view it as an imposition on their lives and freedom. Older adults in the US are susceptible to increased risk of depression and decreased quality of life when they stop driving.[2]

ASSESSMENT

2. How can you determine if a driver is safe or unsafe? Are the drivers in the cases capable of decision making? Are they self-aware?

Driving is one of the most complex tasks that patients undertake on a daily basis. The driver attends to stimuli (e.g., visual, auditory, vestibular, and somatosensory) and interprets the situation on the road; formulates a plan based on the sensory input, the driving situation, and previous experience; executes an action (e.g., applying the accelerator, brake, or steering controls); and monitors the outcome as a source of feedback for subsequent corrective actions. Errors can occur at any of these stages.

The risk of errors increases with deficits of attention, perception, response selection (which depends on memory and decision making), response implementation (executive functions), and awareness of cognitive and behavioral performance (metacognition). Age-related decline affects many neurologic functions that are necessary for safe driving, such as vision, hearing, cognition, and motor skills. The driver's emotional state, degree of wakefulness, psychomotor factors, and general mobility are also relevant.[3]

Many patients are unaware that their driving skills are impaired, leading to mismatch between their self-report of driving fitness and observed performance. Patient self-ratings of being a "safe" driver correlate poorly with on-road testing; self-ratings of being an "unsafe" driver correlate better.[4] Other factors that should concern physicians about impaired driving skills include moving violations, crashes, self-imposed restriction on driving distance, and avoidance of driving in heavy traffic, at night, or in bad weather.[4]

Drivers who lack awareness of their impaired cognition and behavior are at greater risk of having a car crash because they may not compensate for their unrecognized impairments. The driver in Case 1 with frontotemporal dementia is an example of such an unsafe driver who has a condition of cognitive failure known as *anosognosia* (from the Greek: *a*, without; *nosos*, disease; *gnosis*, knowledge). The patient in Case 2 has decisional capacity and is aware of his capabilities.

Physicians and caregivers often rely on intuition to restrict a patient's driving, but decisions made without adequate evaluation may unfairly deny some patients their driving privileges and mobility or, conversely, unwisely permit crash-prone patients to drive. Making appropriate and informed clinical recommendations about driving ability is crucial to the safety of the patient and everyone else on the road. The American Automobile Association has developed a CD-ROM, "Roadwise Review: A Tool to Help Seniors Drive Safely Longer," that assesses 8 abilities of the subject to predict driver safety: leg strength, general mobility, head/neck flexibility, high- and low-contrast visual acuity, working memory, visualization of missing information, visual search, and useful field of view.[5]

3. Is age or diagnosis alone a sufficient criterion for testing or restricting driving?

Licensed drivers aged 60 years and older have among the highest crash rates per mile of all age groups, approaching the rate of risky and much less experienced drivers under 25 years old.[6] Older drivers are more likely to be killed or injured in a car crash than are younger adults.[7,8,9] Drivers aged 80 years and older have higher crash death rates per mile driven than all but teenage drivers.[9] Thus, in the interests of their patients' safety, neurologists should screen elderly patients for skills and abilities that are relevant to driving safety and order further assessment as clinically indicated by the results of screening; however, restricting a patient from driving on the basis of age or diagnosis alone, without an appropriate evaluation, is not warranted.

Working-aged adults may be at increased risk for driving errors and crashes because of poor sleep attributable to onerous work schedules in our "24-hour society" or because of common sleep disorders such as obstructive sleep apnea syndrome.[10,11] The National Highway Traffic Safety Administration found that drivers most at risk to be sleepy are young people between the ages of 16 and 29, males, shift workers, and people with untreated sleep disorders. Driving while drowsy is both a legal and a moral issue.[12]

MORAL DIAGNOSIS

4. What is the ethical or legal justification for restricting a patient's driving?

Bernat, 9–11, Ch. 1

Bernat, 12–13, Ch. 1

Ethical decisions on driving fitness should respect the principles of autonomy[13] and beneficence[14] of a patient, recognizing that driving cessation is often a landmark of decline and collapse of a patient's life space. Driving is a privilege, not a right, and it offers the benefit of increasing mobility, social intercourse, and quality of life for persons of all ages. Aging and neurologic and medical disorders impair cognition and motor function, reducing driver performance and increasing the risk of errors that may lead to crash and injury.

Ethical decisions that restrict the autonomy of a driver require an understanding, based on the best available evidence, of the probability and magnitude of any harm that may occur with a particular driver with a particular set of problems driving in particular traffic settings.

With respect to driving restriction, we generally focus on injury risk, but restricted drivers face other risks—social, legal, economic, and psychologic. Older adults are at increased risk of depression and decreased quality of life when they stop driving; however, risks and benefits to individual drivers must be balanced against risks and benefits to others.[15]

Bernat, 13–14, Ch. 1

The principle of justice[16] requires us to treat people fairly and equitably and to design licensure policies so that burdens and benefits are shared equitably. With regard to issuing or restricting driver licenses, the question of the degree of tolerable driver risk is a public health and societal choice that is generally beyond the purview of a clinician. The department of motor vehicles (DMV) in most states has boards or committees that review patients' records and make the final determination regarding the degree of risk posed by a particular patient.[17]

Individuals have full autonomy when they have the capacity to understand and process information. An information-processing framework for evaluating driver capacity relies upon a "functional" evaluation of multiple domains (cognitive, motor, perceptual, psychiatric) that are important for safe driving. This framework can be applied to many disorders, including conditions that have not been studied with respect to driving, and to patients with multiple conditions and medications. Neurocognitive tests, driving simulation, and road tests provide complementary sources of evidence to evaluate driver safety, and no single test is sufficient to determine whether a patient should drive or not. With respect to beneficence and autonomy, better science will enable better ethical decisions.[18]

Bernat, 52, Ch. 3
Bernat, 65, Ch. 3

A driver who disagrees with the physician's advice to stop driving may seek a second opinion from another physician or a state DMV. Patient confidentiality should be respected to the fullest possible extent, but a physician may report an unfit driver to the DMV authorities in good faith or if compelled by state law.[19,20] Physicians must place patient rights, welfare, and safety above personal considerations, including fiduciary (even if reporting might be construed as "bad for business"). Drivers should be informed of physician concerns and of intent to report. Decisions on driver fitness should maximize autonomy and minimize harm. Justice dictates that costs and benefits of licensure should be shared among drivers and other members of society.

5. Can "conspiring" with the family to hide a patient's keys be ethically justified?

Neurologic and medical disorders increase the risk of driver errors that may lead to crashes. Drivers normally monitor their performance and internal state, and when feedback fails to match expectations, they normally detect the discrepancy and take corrective action. Drivers with cognitive impairments are less likely to realize their errors (impaired situation awareness) or self-impaired status (anosognosia) and are more likely to drive, unknowingly, while impaired. Anosognosia is not an all-or-none phenomenon, and subtle undiagnosed forms of it may hinder patients with a range of perceptual and cognitive impairments, such as those with sleep disorders, metabolic disorders, or medication effects, who are not aware of how sleepy or cognitively impaired they really are.

Bernat, 28, Ch. 2

Patients with Alzheimer disease or frontotemporal dementia, like the 70-year-old woman in Case 1, are especially prone to lack awareness of impairment[21] and may resist, even aggressively, the idea that they are no longer capable of driving safely. In these cases, the principle of beneficence would supercede autonomy. In fact, it can be argued that patients who lack awareness of their deficits are not autonomous because they cannot make informed decisions, and therefore, justified paternalism[22] with cooperation of their family may be ethically permissible. It would be more harmful to allow the patient to drive than not, considering the added risk to property passengers, pedestrians, and other drivers.[15,23] Because of incapacity and lack of awareness, the driver is no longer capable of deciding for himself or herself and requires assistance. It can be argued that families have a shared responsibility for driver safety.[24] When the patient is a danger to herself or others it is ethically justified to hide the keys; this is an act of beneficence and protection of a vulnerable person—not deception or conspiracy.

GOAL SETTING, DECISION MAKING, AND IMPLEMENTATION

6. How do you advise patients regarding their fitness to drive?

The impact of a medical condition on a patient's driving ability and safety depends on the natural history, severity, and treatment of disease. For example, a patient with a single seizure with a well-defined cause (e.g., an adverse response to IV lidocaine) may return to driving quickly (generally 3–6 months, depending on state laws). Patients with stroke may lose the ability to drive, but some may recover sufficiently to resume driving. Patients with Alzheimer or Parkinson disease may drive safely at first but, because of inevitable progression of their disease, later become unfit to drive. Interestingly, many at-risk older drivers have not been diagnosed with a neurologic disorder, and preclinical Alzheimer disease increases the relative risk of fatal crashes in older drivers.[25]

The AMA/National Highway Traffic Safety Administration,[26] American Academy of Ophthalmology,[27] American Association of Motor Vehicle Administrators,[28] and the Federal Motor Carrier Safety Administration have formulated guidelines for at-risk drivers with visual, cognitive, or medical impairments.[29]

In 2010, the AAN updated its algorithm for evaluating cognitively impaired drivers.[4,30] Clinical dementia rating (CDR) scale scores of 0.5 to 1.0 should prompt evaluation of driver risk factors, such as caregiver report of marginal or unsafe skills, history of citations, history of crashes, driving less than 60 miles per week, situation avoidance, aggression or impulsivity, score of less than 24 on the Mini-Mental State Examination (level C evidence), and other factors (alcohol, medications, sleep disorders, visual impairment, motor impairment).

Most patients with neurodegenerative disorders (such as the patient in Case 1) will eventually have to stop driving, and healthcare professionals should be prepared to discuss this prospect. Risk-mitigation strategies include encouraging family support for alternate transportation, professional driving evaluation, voluntary surrender of driving privileges, and DMV referral. With forewarning and preparation, patients can reduce their driving over time, preparing for eventual cessation. In contrast, patients with an episodic disorder (such as epilepsy) may have to stop driving until a subsequent evaluation shows that the underlying condition is sufficiently recovered and that performance and behavior have returned to safe levels, as determined by evidence-based criteria and state laws.

The patient in Case 2 showed the ability to control the speed and lane position in a driving simulator, but the problem is that the real-world validity of performance in a driving simulator may be difficult to prove,[31] and an unsafe driver may exhibit a reasonable performance under low-demand conditions and over limited time frames. The patient's neuropsychological impairments were relatively mild, and his request to return to driving appears to be reasonable given the results of his tests. The simulator results are unlikely to have been validated against real-world driving, but at least they suggest that the patient sufficiently recovered to be tested on the road to determine if he could safely return to driving. He is taking prophylactic anticonvulsant medication, and with only a single nonconvulsive staring spell, no evidence exists to support a diagnosis of epilepsy that would preclude driving.

Evidence is lacking regarding fitness for driving in the complicated patient in Case 2, but based on multiple risk factors and the high likelihood of neurocognitive decline, and because the patient may lack the awareness to self-restrict his driving when he declines, some neurologists may make the judgment that the risk of harm to the patient and other road occupants outweighs the benefit of mobility to the patient and may recommend that the patient not exercise the privilege to drive. Yet, best intentions assumed, it is not clear that ethical reasoning supports this judgment. In the absence of sufficient evidence of unfitness, the principles of beneficence and autonomy would militate against any recommendation that the patient cease driving because evidence is insufficient that either the patient or society would be safer if his driving were restricted. On the other hand, the patient's mobility, social interactions, work, and quality of life would all stand to suffer, and society would lose a potential worker who, as a result, would need additional social support; i.e., there is loss without benefit at several levels.

A more justifiable ethical tack that makes no unwarranted assumptions of driving fitness or risk and no unjustified restrictions of patient autonomy would be for the neurologist to advise the patient of concerns of driving safety and make arrangements to re-evaluate the driver in a follow-up appointment. The timing of such follow-up would depend on the nature and natural history of the condition (dementia, acute stroke, post-surgery, encephalopathy, obstructive sleep apnea, multiple sclerosis, etc.) in the driver under consideration. For example, in the case of CDR scale score of 0.5, the AAN recommends a 6-month follow-up. The recommendations and course of action for the patient's driving may become clearer over time; meanwhile, the patient's autonomy will not have been unduly restricted nor his quality of life unfairly diminished.

Many unsafe drivers resist driving restrictions, especially from concerns of losing their independence. These concerns can be mitigated by the patient planning alternative transportation options with the family or making use of community transport programs; doing so often improves patient compliance with driving restrictions. Patients who continue to resist giving up their licenses should be referred to the DMV for a driving evaluation and with legally binding administrative dispositions, such as enrollment in a driving education program, license restriction, or license revocation.

7. What are the legal considerations in evaluating and deciding whether to restrict a potentially unsafe driver?

In most states, reporting a potentially unsafe driver to the authorities is left to the physician's discretion. The AAN found that most states have "full legal immunity in place for physicians who observe all applicable laws in good faith"; however, this does not always shield the physician from civil litigation.[32] The AMA and National Highway Traffic Safety Administration suggest that physicians be required to report patients who pose a threat to themselves or others because of their driving or who are noncompliant with recommendations to cease driving.[26] Doctors who fail to advise sleepy patients about potential adverse consequences for driving may be liable for civil and criminal penalties.[6] The pitfall of following these suggestions is that the law does not protect the privacy and confidentiality of the physician reporters, who may then be subject to reprisals, including malpractice suits. Section 4.2 of the AAN Code of Professional Conduct states that physicians should respect the law.[33] Further, the law does provide precedent that physicians can be caused to divulge otherwise confidential patient information, especially where public health is a concern,[32,34] for instance, by subpoena of physician records. However, until all physicians are confident that their recommendations or actions are safeguarded, not all physicians will comply.[35] Evidence suggests that mandatory reporting is a policy on a collision course with itself[34] and may compromise the physician–patient relationship, leading patients to withhold pertinent medical information that may be needed for future care. Therefore, the AAN does not support mandatory reporting but supports optional reporting in good faith. Good faith (*bona fide* in Latin) reporting refers to sincere and honest disclosure of facts or opinions that might have importune results, such as license revocation. In these cases, the AAN and AMA would have state legislatures protect physicians who report impaired drivers to state licensing authorities from lawsuits based on breach of confidentiality.[25]

8. What should the neurologist tell the patient whose response is, "I will keep driving in spite of your recommendation"? What should the neurologist document in the chart?

If the clinical evidence raises questions of driver fitness, in line with evidence-based guidelines,[3] and the patient resists the advice to cease driving, a doctor may refer the person to the state DMV for a driving evaluation. Private driving tests are often not covered by insurance, and physicians do not want to coerce patients to take tests that they do not want or cannot afford, especially if insufficient evidence exists for the predictive validity of the tests. The driver is more likely to show up if license renewal depends on taking the test; state driving tests are included in the licensing fee. It is possible to make a convincing argument for driver cessation or testing based on family report, driving history, clinical evidence (including disease severity), and cognitive test scores.

Most patients respect the opinion of a thoughtful healthcare provider and would strive to avoid potential risks understood in terms of crashes and injuries to themselves, passengers, and family members. Alternate transportation planning is helpful, but sometimes the family has to hide the car keys in the interest of patient safety (as noted above). Physician concerns should be documented in the patient's chart, and if the provider has serious concerns (and evidence suggests that with patients whose CDR = 2, the provider should have concerns), the provider may report the patient to the state officials for legal disposition. If the report is competent and in good faith, the likelihood of reprisal is low. Most individuals are not purely selfish when it comes to the safety of others.[36]

KEY POINTS

■ Identification and evaluation of patients with unsafe driving skills secondary to their neurologic and medical conditions is an important responsibility of neurologists, as these patients are at an increased risk of injury or death from driving accidents. Therefore, neurologists must consider both the patients' interests and those of the public, which differs from the usual ethical analysis that is focused primarily on patients' interests.

- Restriction of driving is seen by patients as a restriction on their lives and liberty, and many are unwilling to part with their licenses.
- Evidence-based guidelines for evaluating driver safety exist to aid ethical decisions on driving fitness that respect principles of beneficence and maximize autonomy of patients.
- A dissenting driver may seek a second opinion from another physician or a state DMV.
- Patient confidentiality should be respected to the fullest possible extent, but a physician may report an unfit driver to the authorities in good faith or may be compelled by state law to do so.
- Physicians must place the patient's rights, welfare, and safety above all other personal interests, including fiduciary (even if reporting might be "bad for business").
- Drivers should be informed of physician concerns and of intent to report.
- Decisions on driver fitness should maximize autonomy and minimize harm.
- Justice dictates that costs and benefits of licensure should be shared among drivers and other members of society.

KEY WORDS

Anosognosia—unawareness of one's neurologic deficits as a result of the neurologic illness itself.

Justified paternalism—the implementation either by family or physicians of medical decisions that override a patient's "apparent" preferences when (a) the patient lacks decision-making capacity, (b) probability is high that the patient would be harmed if the patient's "apparent" decision were allowed and an intervention contrary to the patient's "apparent" preference were not allowed, and (c) the risk of the intervention chosen by the family or physicians is proportionally lower than the risk of the patient's choice. This situation usually occurs when a patient is capable of verbally or physically expressing a choice but, because of neurologic impairment, is found to lack an appreciation of the consequences of the choice and thus lacks decision-making capacity.

REFERENCES

1. Dawson JD, Anderson SW, Uc EY, et al. Predictors of driving safety in early Alzheimer's disease. Neurology 2009; 72:521–7.
2. DeCarlo DK, Scilley K, Wells J, et al. Driving habits and health-related quality of life in patients with age-related maculopathy. Optom Vis Sci 2003; 80:207–13.
3. Rizzo M, Sparks JD, McEvoy S, et al. Change blindness, aging and cognition. J Clin Exp Neuropsychol 2009; 31(2):245–56.
4. Iverson DJ, Gronseth GS, Reger MA, et al. Quality Standards Subcommittee of the AAN. Practice parameter update: Evaluation and management of driving risk in dementia. Neurology 2010; 74(16):1316–24. [*PECN* document J available at www.aan. com/view/PECN]
5. American Automobile Association. Roadwise Review: A Tool to Help Seniors Drive Safely Longer. Available at www.seniordriving.aaa.com/evaluate-your-driving-ability/interactive-driving-evaluation. Accessed July 25, 2012.

6. National Highway Traffic Safety Administration (NHTSA). Traffic safety facts 2007: Older population (Rep. No. DOT HS 810 992). Washington, DC: National Highway Traffic Safety Administration, 2008.
7. National Highway Traffic Safety Administration (NHTSA). Traffic safety facts 2005: Older population (Rep. No. DOT HS 810 622). Washington, DC: National Highway Traffic Safety Administration, 2006.
8. Centers for Disease Control and Prevention. Web-based injury statistics query and reporting system (WISQARS) [an interactive database system that provides customized reports of injury-related data]. Available at www.cdc.gov/injury/wisqars/index.html. Accessed March 27, 2012.
9. Insurance Institute for Highway Safety (IIHS). Fatality facts, 2006: Older people. Available at www.iihs.org/research/fatality_facts_2006/olderpeople.html. Accessed March 27, 2012.
10. Tregear SJ, Tiller M, Greenberg MI, et al. Sleep apnea and motor vehicle crashes— A systemic review and meta-analysis. National Occupational Injury Research Symposium, Pittsburg, PA, 2008.
11. National Sleep Foundation. Drowsy driving. Available at www.sleepfoundation.org/article/sleep-topics/drowsy-driving. Accessed March 27, 2012.
12. N.J.S.2C:11-5. Death by auto or vessel. www.njleg.state.nj.us/2002/Bills/A1500/1347_R2.HTM. Accessed March 27, 2012.
13. Bernat, 9–11, Ch. 1.
14. Bernat, 12–13, Ch. 1.
15. Gianola FJ. Public safety versus patient interest: Which to choose? JAAPA 2007; 20(2):49, 51.
16. Bernat, 13–14, Ch. 1.
17. Maryland Department of Transportation. Motor Vehicle Administration. Medical Advisory Board Referral. Available at www.mva.maryland.gov/About-MVA/INFO/26200/26200-03T.htm#Contact_info. Accessed March 27, 2012.
18. Rizzo M. A 70-year-old man trying to decide if he should continue driving. JAMA Clinical Crossroads 2011; 305:1018–26.
19. Bernat, 52, Ch. 3.
20. Bernat, 65, Ch. 3.
21. Bernat, 28, Ch. 2.
22. Childress J. Who Should Decide? Paternalism in Health Care. New York: Oxford University Press, 1982:102–26, Ch. V. Justified paternalism.
23. Snyder CH. Dementia and driving: Autonomy versus safety. J Am Acad Nurse Pract 2005; 17(10):393–402.
24. Rapoport MJ, Herrmann N, Molnar FJ, et al. Sharing the responsibility for assessing the risk of the driver with dementia. CMAJ 2007; 177(6):599–601.
25. Lundberg C, Hakamies-Blomqvist L, Almkvist O, et al. Impairments of some cognitive functions are common in crash-involved older drivers. Accid Anal Prev 1998; 30(3):371–7.
26. Carr D, Schwartberg J, Manning L, et al. Physician's Guide to Assessing and Counseling Older Drivers, 2nd ed. Washington, DC: NHTSA, 2010.
27. American Academy of Ophthalmology. Policy Statement: Vision Requirements for Driving. March 2006. Available at www.aao.org/about/policy/upload/AAODrivingPolicyWebcopy.pdf. Accessed March 27, 2012.
28. American Association of Motor Vehicle Administrators/National Highway Traffic Safety Administration. Driver fitness medical guidelines. Washington, DC: National Highway Traffic Safety Administration, 2009.
29. Tregear SJ, Rizzo M, Tiller M, et al. Diabetes and motor vehicle crashes: A systematic evidence-based review and meta-analysis. Proceedings of Driving Assessment 2007: The Fourth International Driving Symposium on Human Factors in Driving Assessment, Training, and Vehicle Design. Stevenson, WA. July 2007. Iowa City, IA: The University of Iowa, 2007:343–50.

30. Iverson DJ, Gronseth GS, Reger MA, et al. Practice parameter update: Evaluation and management of driving risk in dementia. Report of the Quality Standards Subcommittee of the AAN. Neurology 2010; 74(16); 1316–24. [*PECN* document K available at www.aan.com/view/PECN]
31. Fisher D, Rizzo M, Caird JK, et al., eds. *Handbook of Driving Simulation for Engineering, Medicine and Psychology*. Boca Raton, FL: CRC Press/Taylor & Francis Group, 2011.
32. Bacon D, Fisher RS, Morris JC, et al. American Academy of Neurology position statement on physician reporting of medical conditions that may affect driving competence. Neurology 2007; 68:1174–7.
33. American Academy of Neurology. Code of Professional Conduct. Section 4.2, Respect for Agencies and the Law. [*PECN* appendix document A and available at www.aan.com/view/PECN]
34. Appel J. Must physicians report impaired driving? Rethinking a duty on a collision course with itself. J Clin Ethics 2009; 20(2):136–40.
35. Drachman DA. Who may drive? Who may not? Who shall decide? Neurology 1988; 24(6):787–8.
36. Andersson H, Lindberg G. Benevolence and the value of road safety. Accid Anal Prev 2009; 41(2):286–93.

SUGGESTIONS FOR FURTHER READING

Bajaj JS, Saeian K, Hafeezullah M, et al. Patients with minimal hepatic encephalopathy have poor insight into their driving skills. Clin Gastroenterol Hepatol 2008; 6:1135–9.

Casuso J. Prominent firm files lawsuit in Farmers Market tragedy. The LookOut News. Available at www.surfsantamonica.com/ssm_site/the_lookout/news/News-2004/July-2004/07_14_04_Prominent_Firm_Files_Lawsuits_in_Farmers_Market_Tragedy.htm. Accessed March 28, 2012.

Dubinsky RM, Stein AC, Lyons K. Practice parameter: Risk of driving and Alzheimer's disease (an evidence-based review): Report of the Quality Standards Subcommittee of the American Academy of Neurology. Neurology 2000; 54(12):2205–11.

Foley D, Masaki K, White L, et al. Practice parameter: Risk of driving and Alzheimer's disease. Neurology 2001; 56(5):695.

Hoff CM. Review of Selected 2007 California Legislation: Vehicle: Putting Seniors in the Drivers' Seats: Improving California's Mature Drivers Program with Chapter 129. 38 McGeorge L. Rev. 321. c2007.

Rizzo M, Robinson S, Neale V. The brain in the wild: Tracking human behavior in natural and naturalistic settings. In: Parasuraman R, Rizzo M, ed., *Neuroergonomics: The brain at work*. New York: Oxford University Press, 2007:113–28.

16 REQUESTS FOR ENHANCED FUNCTION IN HEALTHY INDIVIDUALS

William P. Cheshire, Jr., MD, MA, FAAN

LEARNING OBJECTIVES

Upon completion of this chapter, participants will be able to:

1. Identify the distinction between therapy and enhancement.
2. Describe the ethical arguments for and against prescribing pharmacologic agents for the purpose of enhancing cognitive capacity beyond normal.
3. Incorporate into neurologic practice a method for responding appropriately and caringly to a patient's request for prescription for a drug to enhance cognitive function.

LEARNING RESOURCES

Key chapters in Bernat's third edition—20

Key relevant AAN documents available at www.aan.com/view/PECN

A   L

CLINICAL VIGNETTES

CASE 1

Sophia is a 25-year-old graduate student who has been treated for several years for multiple sclerosis (MS), with symptoms of paraparesis, visual impairment, and loss of coordination. Pursuing a career in patient advocacy, she is in the midst of writing her doctoral dissertation in healthcare policy and complains of mental fatigue and impairment in short-term memory. She cites two randomized, double-blind, placebo-controlled studies that demonstrate that donepezil improves cognition in MS[1,2] and requests a prescription.

CASE 2 (PART A)

Peter, a 20-year-old premed student, achieved a mediocre grade on his first organic chemistry exam. Many of his classmates, according to an article in the university newspaper, admitted to using diverted prescriptions for methylphenidate (Ritalin), dextroamphetamine/amphetamine (Adderall), and atomoxetine (Strattera) as "study aids" to improve alertness, mental focus, and "mental fitness." Peter, who hoped to gain admission to a top medical school, felt that he was falling behind the accelerating performance curve of his peers. To have a "fair chance" at academic success, he requested a prescription for something to help him study.

CASE 2 (PART B)

Ten years later, Peter has completed college, medical school, internship, and residency training in neurology and has signed on to a high-volume practice position so that he can pay his student loan debt. He enjoys seeing patients, but the hours are long, he is on call every other night, and fatigue has set in. Because he does not want to be a patient of a close colleague, he visits a neurologist in a nearby town to request a prescription for modafinil, as he believes that it will help him serve his patients better by sustaining his alertness and concentration, especially post-call. He is worried about making medical errors when fatigued and reasons that modafinil will help him avoid errors and the risk of malpractice liability.[3] He also requests prescriptions for anxiety, insomnia, and headaches.

CASE 3 (PART A)

As a 16-year-old high school student, Tracy was diagnosed with attention deficit hyperactivity disorder (ADHD). Her erratic academic performance, impulsivity, and inattentiveness improved on methylphenidate (5 mg bid), and she did well academically and socially. She was also a competitive gymnast whose parents encouraged her to aim for a gymnastic scholarship to college. On days that she did not take methylphenidate, she perceived that she was less able to focus on athletic performance or learn to perfect her form and technique. Tracy's father, an internist, asked a colleague to increase her prescription to an additional 5–10 mg of methylphenidate each afternoon for her gymnastic training. He wanted his daughter to make the most of her interests and perform to the best of her ability. Further, he contended that enhanced focus while practicing could reduce the risk of distraction and injury, as another gymnast had recently fallen and suffered a cervical spine injury.

CASE 3 (PART B)

Ten years later, Tracy is now a financial analyst for a highly competitive Wall Street firm. She follows global markets around the clock and carries her smartphone and laptop everywhere. She is on top of her game professionally, as are her competitors, and she strives to outpace them. She reasons that if she could improve her performance by another 10%, she could exceed her productivity targets more quickly, which would reduce her stress and enable her to spend more time with her family. Tracy recalls the performance edge that she felt when she took methylphenidate in school. While she no longer has any symptoms of ADHD, she wonders whether advances in neuropharmacology might help her to reach her aspirations. She has read financial reports that predict sizeable markets for cognitive-enhancing "smart drugs" now in development. She requests a prescription for the very latest "brain-boosting pill."

QUESTIONS FOR GROUP DISCUSSION

GETTING STARTED

1. Have you ever received a request from a patient for a prescription drug for the purpose of augmenting mental performance? How did you feel about the request? Did you consider the ethical implications?

ASSESSMENT

2. What laws and professional standards govern the prescribing of controlled substances for off-label indications? How do those standards apply to the cases under discussion?

3. What is the distinction between *medical therapy* and *enhancement of normal function through medical means*? Is a clear distinction between "restoring to wellness" and "making better than normal" always possible? What is meant by "normal"? What is meant by "better"?

4. What has traditionally been, and what should be, the professional role of the physician regarding therapy versus enhancement?

5. Compare and contrast the cases. What are the goals of cognitive enhancement in each case?

6. What factors motivate the desire for enhancement in each case? What might be some alternative ways of addressing those needs? Is every identified need "medical"?

MORAL DIAGNOSIS

7. In respect to patient autonomy, do adults with decision-making capacity have the ethical and legal right to refuse medical therapy? Does the principle of respect for autonomy entail the right to receive enhancing interventions of their choosing?

8. Might any forms of subtle coercion diminish the patient's autonomous decision in any of the cases?

GOAL SETTING, DECISION MAKING, AND IMPLEMENTATION

9. For each case, describe your reasons for concluding that writing the prescription is either appropriate or inappropriate. Also, describe what you would document in the chart and how you would educate and guide the patient to use the drug responsibly and safely.

EVALUATION

10. How might enhancement clinics affect the just distribution of medical resources?

11. Who should decide the boundaries of therapy and enhancement, and where ought the line that separates them be drawn?

COMMENTARY ON DISCUSSION QUESTIONS

GETTING STARTED

1. **Have you ever received a request from a patient for a prescription drug for the purpose of augmenting mental performance? How did you feel about the request? Did you consider the ethical implications?**

Requests from patients for prescriptions for neuroenhancement are increasing.[4] Although some physicians support the granting of these requests based on autonomy and the freedom to write off-label prescriptions, others are uncomfortable because of the uncertainties involved, such as the malpractice liability risk. Strong ethical arguments can be made both in favor of and against the prescription of neuroenhancement. However, at this writing, no consensus has been reached.

ASSESSMENT

2. **What laws and professional standards govern the prescribing of controlled substances for off-label indications? How do those standards apply to the cases under discussion?**

Prescription of medications for off-label use is both common and legal.[5] The US Food and Drug Administration regulates prescription drugs and prohibits the pharmaceutical industry from promoting drugs directly to consumers for unapproved uses, but it allows such off-label prescribing by physicians. Although off-label prescribing often lacks the scientific evidence that labeled indications have, such prescribing provides an opportunity for innovation and for the compassionate treatment of illnesses. Categorization by the US Drug Enforcement Administration of certain drugs as controlled substances represents a second line of legal restraint that applies to amphetamines.

Off-label prescribing occurs frequently in the treatment of chronic pain. Because patients with complaints of cognitive inadequacy gauge their symptoms subjectively, requests for neuroenhancing drugs may become more common. Neuropsychometric testing in these patients can be valuable in detecting the presence of a cognitive disorder or in quantifying the cognitive impact of depression, loss of sleep, or sedating medications. However, normal cognitive test results may not dissuade the patient who seeks to be better than normal from requesting an enhancing drug.

3. **What is the distinction between *medical therapy* and *enhancement of normal function through medical means*? Is a clear distinction between "restoring to wellness" and "making better than normal" always possible? What is meant by "normal"? What is meant by "better"?**

Cognitive enhancement refers to interventions that increase, amplify, or intensify mental capacities (e.g., alertness, vigilance, problem-solving ability, motor skills, or mood) in excess of normal levels for individuals or for humankind. Cognitive enhancement might be achieved through neuropharmacology or, potentially in the future, through electronic devices that influence cerebral function.[6]

The availability of drugs designed to improve mental function in patients with cognitive disorders has stimulated debate regarding whether and how such drugs should also be prescribed for cognitive enhancement in healthy people. This idea is hardly new. For centuries, people of many cultures have enjoyed caffeine,[7] the most widely used of psychoactive substances. Caffeine increases alertness, reduces fatigue, and improves performance on tasks that require vigilance.[8] However, the use of even a mild enhancer such as caffeine by a healthy person entails side effects, which may include anxiety, depression, palpitations, insomnia or rebound headaches, and at toxic doses, psychosis or suicide.[9,10]

The use of more potent stimulant drugs requires proportionately greater ethical caution, if not restraint, because of the associated potential adverse consequences. A clear example of such a stimulant is cocaine, which causes such addictive and socially destructive effects that its use beyond the medical indication of topical anesthesia is legally prohibited.[11]

The aims of cognitive enhancement are variously defined, and no single measure adequately defines intelligence. Cognitive performance encompasses many capacities, including but not limited to attention, vigilance, short- and long-term memory, implicit and explicit memory, integration of information, creativity, planning, modeling, judgment, restraint, and even the ability to forget. Each of these aspects of cognition has a neurochemical substrate that is potentially alterable through pharmacologic intervention. In recent years, elucidation of the molecular mechanisms that underlie such cognitive functions has laid the foundation for the development of more targeted approaches to cognitive neuropharmacology.[7,12,13]

Although it is important to distinguish the ethical categories of "therapy" and "enhancement," at times, they overlap or defy precise definition. The President's Council on Bioethics offered the following definition as a starting point:

> "Therapy" is the use of biotechnical power to treat individuals with known diseases, disabilities, or impairments, in attempt to restore them to a normal state of health and fitness. "Enhancement," by contrast, is the directed use of biotechnical power to alter, by direct intervention, not disease processes, but the "normal" workings of the human body and psyche, to augment or improve their native capacities and performances.[14]

Evaluation of which factors are relevant to distinctions of "normality" in regard to health and which attributes constitute "better" is the subject of ongoing philosophical and social debate. Central to this discussion are questions about the nature of optimal health and the purposes of intelligence. The AAN Ethics, Law and Humanities Committee, in its guidance on responding to requests from patients for neuroenhancement, took a pragmatic approach, stating:

> "Normal adult" patients in the context of neuroenhancement may be defined as patients who, after appropriate evaluation, neither 1) satisfy accepted criteria for medical or mental health disease, disorder, or injury (collectively described as medical or mental health condition), nor 2) satisfy accepted criteria to be considered at risk for a medical or mental health condition that can be prevented with appropriate measures.[4]

The ethical implications of cognitive enhancement intensify in parallel with the potency of the drugs used, as shown in this classification scheme with 4 categories of potency (fizzle, perk, jolt, and shock).[15]

The *fizzle* category includes proprietary substances and over-the-counter supplements that are marketed as cognitive enhancers despite a lack of evidence. Examples include ginkgo biloba and piracetam. The ethical concerns for fizzle drugs are truthfulness in advertising and the need for better education to deter exploitation of uninformed or vulnerable individuals.[15] The *perk* category comprises mild dietary stimulants such as caffeine. The ethical concerns are minimal. Coffee and tea consumed in moderation are safe, pleasant, and beneficial for most people. If taken in excess, caffeine can cause insomnia, anxiety, palpitations, and headaches.[15] The *jolt* category includes prescription drugs such as methylphenidate, modafinil, and amphetamine that exert a moderate stimulant effect. Each has clearly defined medical indications substantiated by clinical research studies.[15] The *shock* category covers hypothetical novel drugs that would have far greater potency or would radically alter the brain. Ampakines, which have enduring effects on the neurobiology of memory, are in this category.[15,16]

Aside from issues of medical safety, the jolt and shock categories raise profound ethical questions. The use of these drugs for enhancement purposes raises questions about which cognitive functions ought to be maximized, by what means, and for what intent. Further, widespread use of enhancing drugs might raise societal performance expectations to a level that could be burdensome to sustain, particularly by those who cannot or will not take enhancing drugs. Additionally, enhancement options could cultivate an attitude of dissatisfaction with one's natural abilities or impatience with the performance of others. Reliance on drugs to augment mental performance could undermine the virtues of discipline, study, personal effort, and perseverance, at least in regard to tasks that require short-term learning. The tainted history of the use of steroids and other drugs to enhance physical performance in athletes is instructive in the principle of fairness in competition.

4. **What has traditionally been, and what should be, the professional role of the physician regarding therapy versus enhancement?**

Except perhaps in the case of cosmetic surgery, the historical understanding of the proper role of the physician in society is restricted to the treatment and prevention of disease. Physician participation in cognitive enhancement represents a paradigm shift in the traditional role of physicians and the historical underpinnings of Western medicine, which, if it were to become routine medical practice, could result in the sick having to compete with the well for access to finite healthcare resources.[17]

5. **Compare and contrast the cases. What are the goals of cognitive enhancement in each case?**

Chatterjee has identified 3 general areas of neurologic enhancement: (a) improving normal motor skills and movement; (b) improving normal cognitive function, concentration, attention, and memory; and (c) improving normal mood and affect.[18] In Case 1, the rationale for prescribing donepezil is indisputably therapeutic, aiming to restore brain function that has been impaired by MS. Although donepezil is not labeled for the treatment of MS, a therapeutic rationale and limited evidence suggest that it may improve cognition in some patients with MS.[1,2] The alleviation of symptoms of disease falls squarely within the traditional healing purpose of medicine.

In Case 2 (Part A), although the student's aspirations are admirable, his means of achieving them are questionable. Peter, a premedical student, believes that his academic performance is slipping and that his peers have an advantage with the help of stimulants. In Case 2 (Part B), Peter's motivation has changed to what he *perceives* to be altruism. He rationalizes that if he enhances his cognitive performance, he would be able to serve his patients better or perhaps to serve more of them.

The most notable aspect of Case 3 (Part A) is that Tracy does not request a new prescription. She is already taking methylphenidate for ADHD. She only requests a dosage increment for the purpose of increasing the apparent effect on mental focus in her athletic performance. Here, the determination of whether methylphenidate is therapeutic or enhancing is blurry. In fact, it could be both therapeutic and enhancing. In Case 3 (Part B), her motivations remain competitive but are now oriented toward cognition and job performance. She seems to perceive her cognitive abilities as commodities to be maximized and leveraged for the sake of material gain.

6. **What factors motivate the desire for enhancement in each case? What might be some alternative ways of addressing those needs? Is every identified need "medical"?**

In Case 1, the neurologist knows the patient well and thus is better qualified to assess her motivations and propensity for use of the drug than if this were an initial visit. The longstanding physician–patient relationship can engender a sense of loyalty in both parties. In response, the neurologist might find it difficult to decline the patient's request if the indications were unclear. The neurologist is also likely to be swayed by the desire to assist Sophia in her choice to pursue a career despite her MS.

In Case 2 (Part A), what is the neurologic disease for which Peter seeks treatment? Assuming that his physician has evaluated him and excluded cognitive, metabolic, and psychiatric illness, what remains is a mismatch between Peter's academic expectations and his performance. However, it is not clear that academic disappointment should count as a neurologic illness. Case 2 (Part B) illustrates some of the potential long-term consequences of choosing activities beyond one's abilities, such as working long hours and facing fatigue. These problems are not unique to physicians. It might be tempting to resort to a wakefulness-promoting drug with the aim of overcoming fatigue and chronic sleep deprivation, but it is doubtful whether any habitual drug can be an adequate substitute for restorative sleep and other elements of a healthy lifestyle.[19]

It is important to consider in Case 3 (Part A) whether the goal of performance enhancement for gymnastic training is to satisfy Tracy or her father. Although her father is a strong advocate for medication, the risk would fall to Tracy. Bernat points out that the process of informed consent fails to relieve concerns about enhancing treatments that parents permit for their children.[20]

Bernat, 496–8, Ch. 20

MORAL DIAGNOSIS

7. **In respect to patient autonomy, do adults with decision-making capacity have the ethical and legal right to refuse medical therapy? Does the principle of respect for autonomy entail the right to receive enhancing interventions of their choosing?**

Bernat, 9–11, Ch. 1

Whereas neurologists are obligated to honor patients' autonomy,[21] the AAN Ethics, Law and Humanities Committee opines that neurologists have no obligation to write prescriptions for neuroenhancement simply because patients demand it, stating:

> Thus, neurologists who have reason to believe that neuroenhancement will result in more harm than benefit to a patient may ethically refuse to provide it on the basis of nonmaleficence. While such refusal may appear paternalistic, physicians have no ethical obligation to provide patients with treatments or medications simply because they want them. However, physicians are obligated to explain their refusal in terms that are understandable to patients without being demeaning or disrespectful.[4]

Bernat,
34–6,
Ch. 2

An important autonomy consideration in Case 3 (Part A) is that as an adolescent, Tracy should have a say in whether she wishes to take the higher dose for this indication, consistent with the principles of assent and dissent for children.[22,23]

8. Might any forms of subtle coercion diminish the patient's autonomous decision in any of the cases?

In Case 2 (Part A), Peter claims that his exclusion from the resource of stimulant medication places him at an unfair academic disadvantage. A student's decision to request a stimulant prescription is not a purely autonomous one. The power of academic pressure and, for that matter, peer pressure should not be underestimated.

GOAL SETTING, DECISION MAKING, AND IMPLEMENTATION

9. For each case, describe your reasons for concluding that writing the prescription is either appropriate or inappropriate. Also, describe what you would document in the chart and how you would educate and guide the patient to use the drug responsibly and safely.

Case 1 is comparatively straightforward. In the interest of diagnostic accuracy, the neurologist should perform a thorough mental status examination or, preferably, obtain neuropsychological testing, which will also establish a baseline by which the outcome can be measured. Considering that the evidence in support of donepezil to improve cognitive function in MS is preliminary, donepezil's use for this purpose is still investigational and would not likely be covered by the patient's health insurance. The neurologist is obliged to disclose the potential burden of out-of-pocket expense and to assist the patient in weighing the cost against the anticipated or measured benefit of the drug.

In Case 2 (Part A), Peter claims that his exclusion from the resource of stimulant medication places him at an unfair academic disadvantage alongside his medicated peers. Writing a prescription for an enhancing drug might be easier for the physician than it would be to take the time to advise Peter that failure on a single test in a single subject is unlikely to affect his chances of getting into medical school (despite his fears) and that, in the long term, use of the drug is not in his best interest. Helpful advice to Peter should first explore nonmedical strategies to improve his performance. Perhaps he could reorganize his schedule and priorities; e.g., study with others or seek guidance in how to study. Although one could argue that reliance on enhancing medication for academic success undermines the dignity of human achievement and steals from students like Peter the opportunity for a sense of personal accomplishment attained through willful commitment, discipline, and perseverance, Peter's near-term focus on his grades may not allow him to appreciate the relevance of these greater concerns to his particular circumstances.[7,13] The neurologist should also counsel Peter regarding the safety implications of stimulant drugs that have serious potential side effects such as cardiovascular or neuromuscular overstimulation.[24] The precautionary principle also applies because the long-term consequences of chronic stimulant use on the developing brain have been insufficiently studied.

In Case 2 (Part B), Peter's altruistic argument may be more compelling, but it does not dismiss safety concerns, and it depends on Peter's enhanced performance being sustainable and translated to improved quality of care. If studies were to show that physician use of stimulant medication post-call reduced the rate of medical errors, would physicians be obliged to take them?[25] Similar questions have been raised regarding the ethics of fatigue countermeasures in the military.[26]

In Case 3, the patient is a teenager. As Bernat suggests, more stringent protection is necessary when neuroenhancement drugs are considered for use in children (who are less capable of comprehending medical risks and providing informed consent) and when the drugs' long-term effects on the developing brain are not well known.[20]

Bernat, 496–8, Ch. 20

EVALUATION

10. How might enhancement clinics affect the just distribution of medical resources?

Suppose that you were to write for Peter a prescription for methylphenidate and the following month Peter scores a higher grade on his next organic chemistry exam. How would you then handle the same requests from 20 of Peter's classmates who appear in the neurology clinic waiting area requesting an appointment and a prescription? Although the "wisdom of the masses" in demanding these drugs has been questioned,[27] illicit use of stimulant drugs nonetheless is increasingly widespread on university campuses among students who acquire diverted prescriptions from those who are being treated for ADHD.[7] Suppose that stimulant use among undergraduate, graduate, or professional students were to gain in acceptance.[28] Over time, their routine use could elevate personal and societal expectations to a level where people left behind the accelerating-performance curve, either because of medical contraindications to taking stimulants or by choice, would eventually fall short.[7] Those with normal cognitive functioning might begin to feel inadequate or be perceived as inferior.

The development and marketing of brain-enhancing drugs raises questions about the just distribution of limited medical resources, i.e., the principle of distributive justice. Neurologists would be obliged to ensure that the practice of "cosmetic neurology"[18] does not impede the access of sick patients to neurologic care. If large numbers of healthy individuals were to consume medical resources for the purpose of cognitive enhancement, patients with acute and chronic neurologic disorders could compete with them for services.[17] The neurologist's primary moral obligation is to patients with neurologic illness.

11. Who should decide the boundaries of therapy and enhancement, and where ought the line that separates them be drawn?

The ethical approach to these questions differs depending on whether the context is the bedside or public health and policy. In patient care, the needs of the patient at a given moment take priority over the interests of other patients or society. When indications are unclear, the neurologist may choose to prescribe a drug to improve cognitive function with the beneficent intent to help the patient to feel or function better. In the interest of nonmaleficence, the prescribing decision should also take into account the potential harms of the drug, both medical and social.

Bedside decisions, although individualized, do not occur in isolation, but combine to form a pattern of practice with broader implications. Some of these implications include concerns about exacerbating social divisions such that those with financial means could have the option to become "enhanced" while others would remain "unenhanced." Further apprehensions concern subtle coercive influences that might arise in a society that looks to pharmaceutical solutions to satisfy social, academic, and professional performance expectations. Although such dilemmas are not easily resolved at the bedside, informed-consent discussions should encourage the patient to consider his or her motivations for requesting an enhancing drug as well as the range of potential consequences.

CONCLUSION

Pharmaceutical agents, as with any biotechnology, have appropriate, inappropriate, and uncertain applications for improving cognitive capacity. Reflection and discussion of these cases provides an opportunity to explore the ethical implications of cognitive enhancement. These questions are not easily resolved and will likely remain at the forefront of neurology for years to come.

KEY POINTS

- As yet, no ethical consensus has been established concerning prescription neuroenhancement. The ethical distinction between therapy, which historically has been the primary concern of medicine, and enhancement is not always clear and depends on how one defines normal health and what counts as better than normal.
- Arguments for prescribing pharmacologic agents to enhance cognitive capacity include (a) respecting the autonomy of the patient who requests a prescription and (b) beneficence, intending to improve the patient's cognitive function.
- Arguments against prescribing such drugs include (a) nonmaleficence, out of concern about potential medical and psychiatric risks and cost to patients, (b) distributive justice, if enhancement practice were to consume

finite medical resources, and (c) wise stewardship of pharmaceutical technology, which may not be the most appropriate solution to social problems.

■ Physicians are not obligated—simply because patients want them—to provide patients with medications that physicians believe will result in more harm than benefit. Physicians are ethically obligated to respond to requests for pharmacologic enhancements respectfully and caringly and to explain the recommendation in terms that patients can understand.

KEY WORDS

Enhancement—the directed use of medical technology to augment native capacities and performance beyond what is normal for individuals or humankind.

Neuroenhancement—pharmaceutic or other biotechnologic interventions (such as brain-electronic interfaces) that are designed to increase, amplify, or intensify cognitive capacities such as alertness, vigilance, memory, problem-solving ability, motor skills, or mood.

Therapy—the directed use of medical technology to treat patients who are ill or at risk of becoming ill in attempt to prevent disease or restore patients to a normal state of health.

REFERENCES

1. Christodoulou C, Melville P, Scherl WF, et al. Effects of donepezil on memory and cognition in multiple sclerosis. J Neurol Sci 2006; 245:127–36.
2. Krupp LB, Christodoulou C, Melville P, et al. Donepezil improved memory in multiple sclerosis in a randomized clinical trial. Neurology 2004; 63:1579–85.
3. Cox DJ, Humphrey JW, Merkel RL, et al. Controlled-release methylphenidate improves attention during on-road driving by adolescents with attention deficit/hyperactivity disorder. J Am Board Fam Pract 2004; 17:235–9.
4. Larriviere D, Williams MA, Rizzo M, et al. Responding to requests from adult patients for neuroenhancements: Guidance of the Ethics, Law and Humanities Committee. Neurology 2009; 73:1406–12. [*PECN* document L available at www. aan.com/view/PECN]
5. Radley DC, Finkelstein SN, Stafford RS. Off-label prescribing among office-based physicians. Arch Intern Med 2006; 166(9):1021–6.
6. Hamilton R, Messing S, Chatterjee A. Rethinking the thinking cap. Ethics of neural enhancement using noninvasive brain stimulation. Neurology 2011; 76:187–93.
7. Cheshire WP. Drugs for enhancing cognition and their ethical implications: A hot new cup of tea. Expert Rev Neurother 2006; 6:263–6.
8. Fisone G, Borgkvist A, Usiello A. Caffeine as a psychomotor stimulant: Mechanism of action. Cell Mol Life Sci 2004; 61(7–8):857–72.
9. Broderick P, Benjamin AB. Caffeine and psychiatric symptoms: A review. J Okla State Med Assoc 2004; 97:538–42.
10. Tanskanen A, Tuomilehto J, Vilnamäki H, et al. Heavy coffee drinking and the risk of suicide. Eur J Epidemiol 2000; 16:789–91.
11. Cheshire WP. Cognitive enhancements considered from 221-B Baker Street. AJOB Neuroscience 2012; 3(2):35–6.
12. Glannon W. Psychopharmacology and memory. J Med Ethics 2006; 32(2):74–8.

13. Hall SS. The quest for a smart pill. Sci Am 2003; 289(3):54–7,60–5.
14. Kass L. A Report of the President's Council on Bioethics. *Beyond Therapy: Biotechnology and the Pursuit of Happiness*. Washington, DC: Harper Perennial, 2003.
15. Cheshire WP. The matter of the brightened grey. Ethics Med 2007; 23:35–8.
16. Lynch G. Glutamate-based therapeutic approaches: Ampakines. Curr Opin Pharmacol 2006; 6:82–8.
17. Cheshire WP. Just enhancement. Ethics Med 2010; 26:7–10.
18. Chatterjee A. Cosmetic neurology: The controversy over enhancing movement, mentation, and mood. Neurology 2004; 63:968–74.
19. Ellenbogen JM. Ethical perspectives in neurology: Sleep disorders. Continuum: Lifelong Learning in Neurology 2007; 13(3):248–51.
20. Bernat, 496–8, Ch. 20.
21. Bernat, 9–11, Ch. 1.
22. American Academy of Pediatrics. Committee on Bioethics. Informed consent, parental permission, and assent in pediatric practice. Pediatrics 1995; 95:314–7.
23. Bernat, 34–6, Ch. 2.
24. Silva RR, Skimming JW, Muniz R. Cardiovascular safety of stimulant medications for pediatric attention-deficit hyperactivity disorder. Clin Pediatr 2010; 49:840–51.
25. Cheshire WP. The pharmacologically enhanced physician. Virtual Mentor, AMA J Ethics 2008; 10(9):594–8.
26. Russo MB. Recommendations for the ethical use of pharmacologic fatigue countermeasures in the U.S. military. Aviat Space Environ Med 2007; 78(5 Suppl): B119–27.
27. Larriviere D, Williams MA. Neuroenhancement: Wisdom of the masses or "false phronesis"? Clin Pharmacol Ther 2010; 88:459–61.
28. Greely H, Sahakian B, Harris J, et al. Towards responsible use of cognitive-enhancing drugs by the healthy. Nature 2008; 456:702–5.

17 NEONATE WITH A SEVERE NEUROLOGIC DISORDER

Russell D. Snyder, MD, FAAN

LEARNING OBJECTIVES

Upon completion of this chapter, participants will be able to:

1. Define and explain the following terms and concepts as they apply to the ethical situations involving newborns: futility, autonomy, quality of life, best interests, disability, surrogate decision making, healthcare team responsibilities, conflict resolution, and truth telling.
2. Formulate a position regarding the management of a small, sick newborn with low potential for meaningful recovery.
3. Discuss the difficulty inherent in decision making when (a) uncertainty exists, (b) conflict exists between the healthcare team and surrogates, and (c) the individual is below the age of reason, has never been competent, is suffering, or has an unfavorable long-term outlook.
4. Distinguish the best interests of the neonate from the best interests of the surrogate decision makers or the healthcare team.
5. Delineate the limitations of futility decisions.

LEARNING RESOURCES

Key chapters in Bernat's third edition—2, 3, 13

Key relevant AAN documents available at www.aan.com/view/PECN

A N

CLINICAL VIGNETTE

Neurologic consultation was requested for advice regarding prognosis and treatment of a 3-day-old infant. The pregnancy had been complicated by vaginal bleeding at 3 months' gestation. Onset of labor was spontaneous at 24 weeks' gestation, and vaginal delivery was accomplished 3 hours later. The neonate, a boy, weighed 590 grams, was floppy and pale, had minimal spontaneous movement of the extremities, had a heart rate of 40, and lacked spontaneous respirations. Apgar scores were 1 at 2 minutes and 3 at 5 minutes. A neonatologist was present at the delivery.

After intubation and resuscitation, umbilical cord pH was 6.95, heart rate was 90, blood pressure was 48/30, and temperature was 36.8° C. Occasional small, spontaneous, and symmetrical movements of the extremities were noted that seemed to be "twitchy." No urine was produced for the first 18 hours. On day 2, bowel sounds were absent. Brain ultrasound revealed blood in the left lateral ventricle and a 1 cm cystic cavity in the right parietal area without mass effect. Occasional myoclonic jerks occurred. The EEG showed burst suppression.

On day 3, the fontanelle was full. Ultrasound showed germinal matrix hemorrhage on the left and blood in both lateral ventricles, with the cyst still present. Spontaneous movements had ceased. Ventilator support was still required, and dopamine was needed to maintain blood pressure. Spells of bradycardia were noted.

The parents were advised about the severity of the situation and the likely possibility of a neurologic outcome with major handicapping deficits. Anticipating the baby's death within several days, the healthcare team (HCT) suggested continuation of the ventilator and IV fluids but advised against aggressive care, i.e., no support of blood pressure or heart rate and no antibiotics or anticonvulsants. The HCT assured the parents that comfort would be provided to the neonate and that the infant would not suffer. Even though the parents expressed understanding of the situation, they insisted that all measures be undertaken to continue the baby's life. They felt that the HCT was mistaken and that a favorable outcome would occur. They said, "We believe in miracles."

The neurologist was asked to evaluate the situation, meet with the parents, and make recommendations regarding clinical outcome and the appropriate management of the neonate.

QUESTIONS FOR GROUP DISCUSSION

ASSESSMENT
1. What is the patient's medical condition and prognosis?
2. What treatment options exist?
3. Who are the appropriate decision makers?
4. Can the preferences of the neonate be determined?
5. What are the preferences of the patient's family (the surrogate decision makers)?
6. What are the preferences of the HCT?
7. Are any interests in conflict?
8. Would a decision by the HCT not to resuscitate the neonate at birth have been an ethically or legally permissible decision?
9. Should any institutional, legal, or other factors be considered?

MORAL DIAGNOSIS
10. What are some of the ethical issues in the case?
11. What justifications can be given for the ethically preferred resolution of the case?

(continued)

12. Can analogous cases be found in the medical or legal literature or in clinical experience?
13. What are the relevant guidelines for clinicians regarding the problem(s)?

GOAL SETTING, DECISION MAKING, AND IMPLEMENTATION

14. How is a satisfactory resolution to the case to be accomplished?

COMMENTARY ON DISCUSSION QUESTIONS

ASSESSMENT

1. What is the patient's medical condition and prognosis?

The multiple medical problems at birth such as those of this newborn often begin a cascade of events that lead to brain hemorrhage, periventricular leukomalacia, ventriculomegaly, and a high likelihood of significant long-term neurodevelopmental problems.

This neonate's medical conditions include prematurity, very low birth weight, intraventricular hemorrhage, developmental or acquired brain anomaly, and probable hypoxic injury to the brain, bowel, heart, and kidneys. The almost certain hypoxic-ischemic cerebral injury, evidence of other brain pathology, and multisystem disease greatly increase the risk of a poor outcome and make full neurologic recovery unlikely. Should this infant survive, he can be anticipated to have major deficits.[1-3] However, all medical prognostication, especially in sick neonates, involves a degree of uncertainty.

2. What treatment options exist?

Treatment options include (a) provision of palliative care and discontinuation of ventilator support, which would result in the baby's death; (b) continuation of ventilator support but withdrawal of other life-sustaining treatment (LST), including IV fluids, antibiotics, or vasopressors; (c) continuation of the ventilator and IV fluids and withdrawal of other LST such as antibiotics and pressors; or (d) use of all medically indicated treatments available. The HCT showed a preference for option (c).

In the Netherlands, it has been proposed that with appropriate ethical and legal procedures, the option of euthanasia for certain small, sick newborns would be permissible (the Groningen Protocol)[4]; however, this option has been the topic of considerable debate and has not gained widespread acceptance.

3. Who are the appropriate decision makers?

Bernat, 320–3, Ch. 13 With a neonate, the parents are the legal decision makers.[5] Difficulty occurs when the parents' desires are not consistent with the recommendations of the HCT. The best interests of the neonate should be the foremost consideration, but they are sometimes difficult to determine (see Questions 4 and 7). An examination of the infant immediately after birth by an experienced neonatologist is helpful in establishing the degree of viability and the prognosis.

Conflict develops when the HCT's preferred management plan is contrary to any decision the parents may make.[6,7] To override the parents' decision, the HCT must demonstrate that the parents' decision is not in the best interests of the neonate. The threshold for disqualifying the parents as the ultimate decision makers for a neonate is very high.

4. Can the preferences of the neonate be determined?

As a neonate cannot formulate or express preferences and is not autonomous, the parents and the HCT must be relied upon. Infants also cannot express views about their quality of life and about their present or future existence, which places considerable burden on the parents and the HCT. It is reasonable to assume that neonates would not wish to suffer. However, it is difficult to determine if a small neonate is suffering. Response to stimulation, frequency of crying, response to attempts at solace, and feeding behavior provide possible indicators.

Palliative care becomes an additional option when considering the neonate's best interests.[8]

5. What are the preferences of the patient's family (the surrogate decision makers)?

The parents in this case have expressed their preference that the neonate's life be preserved. They appear to have expectations for the infant's outcome that differ from the HCT's prognosis. The HCT can often deal with this difference in perspective by displaying compassionate understanding, by involving the parents in care and decision making, and by showing patience toward the parents' views. The HCT can explain to the parents the goals of the care being provided. The team need not have as one of its goals the changing of the parents' attitude.

6. What are the preferences of the HCT?

In the expectation of imminent death, the HCT in this case desires to continue with the ventilator and IV fluids without support of blood pressure or heart rate. The HCT realizes that the neonate has only a very small chance for a full and meaningful neurologic recovery without significant long-term deficits and believes that continued aggressive treatment in an attempt to continue the neonate's life may be harmful, painful, and potentially serve only to prolong suffering in the face of an ultimately poor outcome.

7. Are any interests in conflict?

The parents' interests conflict with those of the HCT. The parents are interested in continued survival, and the HCT is interested in relief of suffering and prevention of a life with a severe neurologic handicap, sensory deficits, difficulty in communication, and possibly limited life expectancy.[9] The best interests of the neonate must become part of this discussion. A best-interests decision involves concern for quality of life and the ultimate personhood. In the case of a neonate, the best-interests decision should place a high value on the neonate's life but also recognize that circumstances surrounding the birth can create a life of suffering. Healthcare providers have no moral obligation to apply all available therapy in every situation.[10]

Bernat, 327–8, Ch. 13

Many neonatal units have specialists who are familiar with situations such as the one in the case presented and can provide help toward resolving disagreements by appropriate patience, understanding, and compassion. Mediation by a third party is often helpful in resolution, especially when the mediation is approached in a nonjudgmental way. A consultation with a bioethics committee could prove useful if the bioethics committee is readily available and experienced in dealing with neonatal problems. Clergy can be involved as appropriate to the situation. Even when an unfavorable long-term outcome is anticipated, the parental desires should be weighted heavily in determining the treatment approach.[11]

8. Would a decision by the HCT not to resuscitate the neonate at birth have been an ethically or legally permissible decision?

A decision not to resuscitate at birth would most likely have resulted in an early death. Some argue that such a decision would have been appropriate, considering the infant's gestational age, birth weight, and clinical condition.[12] If the possibility that the infant may not survive is known in advance, the option to forgo resuscitation should be discussed with parents before delivery to obtain their permission.[13] However, in an urgent situation, such as often occurs in obstetrics, time may not be available for reflection by either the HCT or the parents. In such a situation, resuscitation is the appropriate intervention.

The choice facing the HCT at the time of the birth of a neonate with a severe neurologic disorder is never clear cut. Typically, it is not solely for life or death. The choice usually involves possible survival of the neonate in a severely disabled condition, which has been an intractable ethical issue for neonatologists and obstetricians for years.[6] No clinical test or objective indicator can accurately predict the outcome of a small, sick newborn in an ambiguous and uncertain situation, even after examination of the infant at birth. Without specific surrogate decisions, provision of LST is usually the best course to follow.[14,15]

Bernat, 323–7, Ch. 13

9. Should any institutional, legal, or other factors be considered?

The so-called Baby Doe regulations, which are federal regulations that were promulgated in modified form in the United States in 1984, state that the withholding of medically indicated treatment may only be undertaken when the infant is irreversibly comatose, the treatment would merely prolong dying or would not be effective in correcting the infant's condition, or the treatment would be futile or inhumane.[16]

The Born Alive Infants Protection Act, passed by the US Congress in 2002 stipulates that a born-alive infant must be provided with a minimum of a medical screening examination.[17] Subsequent care is not specified. State courts have thus far opined that parental preference is essentially irrelevant in the face of an emergency involving the birth of a borderline viable infant with the urgent immediate care left to the discretion of the HCT without surrogate input.[6] Neonatal intensive care units approach these regulations in various ways. The spectrum of management runs from full maintenance, with attention directed to all treatable problems, to withdrawal or withholding of ventilator support, vasopressors, antibiotics, and nutrition. Regardless of the approach, there is often a lack of malpractice litigation.

MORAL DIAGNOSIS

10. What are some of the ethical issues in the case?

Surrogate decision makers

Parents are the surrogate decision makers for children, and the parents in this case have opted for preservation of the neonate's life. The difficulty is that the parents and the HCT are not in agreement regarding the best interests and the probable quality of life for the infant if he survives. Although not an issue for this neonate, situations occur in which the parents or even other family members disagree regarding the management of a small, sick newborn. Most states have regulations that govern the order of supremacy, or hierarchy, among decision makers for when such conflicts occur.

Physician, the HCT, and the hospital

Death or disability is likely to occur in the small, sick newborn in this case, even if treatment is maximized. Although neonatal care for very-low-birthweight infants is improving and outcomes can be anticipated to become more favorable, recent figures indicate that in the 501–750-gram group, 47% of infants will die as neonates and 32% of the survivors will have major permanent disability.[2] A small statistical chance for meaningful survival remains. If the clinical situation is hopeless, the treatment offers little or no long-term benefit and may potentially be harmful, and suffering is being prolonged, the physician's ethical responsibility to provide continued treatment could cease.

The cost of care should not be a factor in the immediate management decision. It is often tempting to argue on the basis of distributive justice that if care is provided to *this* neonate, another neonate with a more favorable prognosis would be deprived of care; however, one study showed that the amount of resources devoted to care for infants who do not survive is not excessive.[18] The real cost to the healthcare facility for a day of care for a neonate in a newborn ICU is not the same as the charge that the facility makes for that day.

However, future needs of this infant, should he survive, will add greatly to cost and include medical care, habilitation, and education. Most parents are not familiar with the complex care required by an extremely premature infant in the hospital and after discharge. Early involvement of the institution's social and financial services is appropriate.

The HCT has an ethical responsibility to be an advocate for neonates and their best interests. Likewise, the HCT has a responsibility to respect the wishes of the parents. Physicians are inclined to focus on the management of neonates' medical problems, while the parents are grieving the pregnancy, their potentially impaired parenthood, and the possible death of their child. Support and encouragement from the HCT is vital throughout this stage and must consider and give attention to both cultural and ethnic diversity.

Futility

Futile treatment is therapy that has no beneficial physiologic effect on the patient's medical condition and merely prolongs suffering. However, treatment that permits a life to continue, including such management as ventilator support and blood pressure support, could be considered a physiologic benefit. We do not know that the neonate in this case is suffering.

The neonate

The primary responsibility of the parents and the HCT is the best interests of the neonate and includes the provision of comfort and the prevention of suffering and harm. Both the parents and HCT have an implicit responsibility to achieve a reasonable quality of life for the neonate. However, difficulty is encountered in the determination of a reasonable quality of life for this neonate, a nonautonomous individual.

Care must be exercised in making assumptins about quality-of-life decisions that devalue individuals with disabilities. Older persons with disabilities are not necessarily unhappy about their situation and seldom wish that they could have died at an earlier time.[19] A handicapped individual who has never known a full quality of life may not object to a limited quality. Studies in adults have shown that physicians underestimate the quality of life of their elderly patients and that many adults appreciate even a limited quality of life. The Down syndrome population provides an example of handicapped individuals who often have a reasonable quality of life.

In 1983 the President's Commission for the Study of Ethical Problems in Medicine and Biomedical and Behavioral Research stated:

> Permanent handicaps justify a decision not to provide life-sustaining treatment only when they are so severe that continued existence would not be a net benefit to the infant.

Though inevitably somewhat subjective and imprecise in actual application, net benefit is absent only if the burdens imposed on the patient by the disability or its treatment would lead a competent decision maker to choose to forgo the treatment.[20]

11. What justifications can be given for the ethically preferred resolution of this case?

Covert withholding and withdrawal of treatment is to be avoided. Even if the outcome is uncertain, the parents' wishes become paramount considerations. Additional medical investigations that would help to determine prognosis with a high degree of accuracy are not currently available. Although individual cases vary and no 2 cases are identical, prognostications founded on evidence- or consensus-based guidelines and those based on experiences of experts at other institutions provide a critical scientific foundation for prognoses that can be modified based on the individual physician's experience with patients in similar circumstances.

Where possible, in similar cases in which the infant has low birth weight and poor prognosis, discussions with the parents about the prognosis can start before birth. Even in the situation of this neonate, the HCT should continue to meet with the parents, displaying empathy and understanding. The family must be kept fully informed regarding status and prognosis, and the HCT can provide information in small frequent segments. It is important that the HCT assume a nondirective approach. When more than one treatment modality is available, the HCT can present these options to the parents for their consideration. It is often advantageous for one member of the HCT to be designated as the principle spokesperson. Also, involvement of other groups outside the immediate HCT, such as the bioethics committee and social services, may be helpful to all concerned.

12. Can analogous cases be found in the medical or legal literature or in clinical experience?

A 2005 survey of Flemish physicians who provided care to infants who died reported that an estimated 57% of deaths were preceded by end-of-life decisions. In 21%, the decision was to withdraw treatment; in 13%, to withhold treatment; in 16%, to administer drugs to alleviate pain in doses that may have shortened life; and in 17%, to purposefully administer a lethal dose of a drug.[21]

The Texas State Supreme Court, in dealing with an extremely premature birth, commented on the extent of the parental right to refuse LST. The Court decided that informed decisions about resuscitating an extremely premature infant can be made only by actually examining the infant at birth.[22] The standard to be applied when examining the infant at birth was not clarified by the Texas decision, which provided no predictors of outcome. After the initial emergency assessment by the HCT to treat or not to treat (usually involving a decision around resuscitation), parental consent is legally required for treatment decisions.[6,22] This Texas decision also implied that life was always preferable to death for a neonate.

13. What are the relevant guidelines for clinicians regarding the problem(s)?

In 2002, the AAP advised neonatologists that the survival of infants born at between 22 and 25 weeks of gestation is problematic. It is considered appropriate not to initiate resuscitation for infants who are younger than 23 weeks' gestation or who weigh less than 400 grams, but the overall condition of the neonate at birth should be taken into consideration,[23] a position that is shared among guidelines from many countries.[24] The increasing rate of initially viable premature births, the publicity concerning "miracle babies," and improvements in neonatal care will increase societal pressure against such decisions.[25,26]

The AAP 2007 policy on noninitiation or withdrawal of intensive care for high-risk newborns emphasizes that "the effects of treatment decisions on the infant's outcome are not always predictable." This report stresses the need for extensive contact, great empathy, and continued discussion with the surrogates.[11]

GOAL SETTING, DECISION MAKING, AND IMPLEMENTATION

14. How is a satisfactory resolution of the case to be accomplished?

A variety of options may be ethically acceptable. Considerations include the following:

a. The principal clinical questions concern the appropriateness of maintenance of ventilator support, treatment of hypotension and bradycardia, and other interventions that may be indicated. The HCT cannot refuse to discuss management options with the parents if their introduction or continuation becomes clinically indicated, and the team has a duty to tell the truth regarding these management decisions.

b. Conversations with the parents plus compassionate and empathetic explanations may be all that is necessary. The parents and the HCT must realize that doing everything possible or doing nothing are not the only two options.[23] Some institutions have special bioethics committees for the neonatal ICU that are constituted because of the unusual nature of the issues surrounding the neonate and because of the need for experience in dealing with these problems. Such a committee, if available, could help to resolve questions of parental authority and ethically permissible management plans.

c. Although it may be tempting for the HCT to involve Child Protective Services agencies or to pursue other legal options when it appears that the parents are not acting in the best interests of the neonate, legal involvement is seldom useful. Rarely, if ever, do decisions by parents to continue treatment constitute neglect or abuse. Legal involvement by its very nature often increases rather than decreases conflict. Additionally, legal involvement in this case seems inappropriate because the case is likely to resolve of its own accord in several days or less.

Bernat provides useful guidelines for treatment decisions for seriously ill neonates:

- Maintain communication with parents at every stage and encourage their participation in all decisions.
- Establish the precise diagnosis.
- Establish the prognosis with and without treatment.
- Identify and explain available treatment options.
- Provide emotional support and counseling.
- Determine if parents are adequate decision makers.
- Recommend the level of appropriate treatment.
- Assess compliance with all government regulations.
- Provide optimal palliative care for the infant.
- Request a review by the hospital ethics committee if treatment will be limited to ensure that the infant's interests are protected.
- Refer the case to court for judicial review (only in exceptional circumstances).[10]

Bernat,
327–8,
Ch. 13

KEY POINTS

- Management of a small, sick newborn with low potential for meaningful recovery is fraught with ethical and medical challenges.
- Conflicts between the HCT and surrogate decision makers may arise and should be managed by the HCT displaying compassionate understanding, by involving the parents in care and decision making, and by showing patience toward the parents' views. The team need not have as one of its goals the changing of the parents' attitude. The best interests of the neonate should be the foremost consideration.
- The best interests are sometimes difficult to determine for a neonate who is unable to express his or her own best interests. An examination of the infant immediately after birth by an experienced neonatologist is helpful in establishing the degree of viability and the prognosis. In the case of a neonate, the best-interests decision should place a high value on the neonate's life but also recognize that circumstances surrounding the birth can create a life of suffering. Healthcare providers have no moral obligation to apply all available therapy in every situation.

KEY WORDS

Very low birth weight—usually considered to be 500 grams or less.

Baby Doe regulations—regulations that state that withholding medically indicated treatment can only be undertaken when the infant is irreversibly comatose, the treatment would merely prolong dying or would not be effective in correcting the infant's condition, or the treatment would be futile or inhumane.

REFERENCES

1. Shankaran S, Johnson Y, Langer JC, et al. Outcome of extremely-low-birth-weight infants at highest risk: Gestational age ≤24 weeks, birth weight ≤750 g, and 1-minute Apgar ≤3. Am J Ob Gyn 2004; 191:1084–91.
2. Vohr BR, Allen M. Extreme prematurity—the continuing dilemma. N Engl J Med 2005; 352:7–72.
3. Marlow DM, Wolke D, Bracewell MD, et al. Neurological and developmental disability at six years of age after extremely preterm birth. N Engl J Med 2005; 352:9–19.
4. Verhagen E, Sauer PJ. The Groningen protocol—Euthanasia in severely ill newborns. N Engl J Med 2005; 352:959–62.
5. Bernat, 320–3, Ch. 13.
6. Annas GJ. Extremely preterm birth and parental authority to refuse treatment—the case of Sidney Miller. N Engl J Med 2004; 351:2118–23.
7. Payot A, Gendron S, Lefebvre F, et al. Deciding to resuscitate extremely premature babies: How do parents and neonatologists engage in the decision? Soc Sci Med 2007; 64:1487–500.
8. Bhatia J. Palliative care in the fetus and newborn. J Perinatol 2006; 26(suppl 1):S24–6.
9. Sayeed SA. The marginally viable newborn: Legal challenges, conceptual inadequacies, and reasonableness. J Law Med Ethics 2006; 34(3):600–10.
10. Bernat, 327–8, Ch. 13.
11. American Academy of Pediatrics Committee on Fetus and Newborn, Bell EF. Noninitiation or withdrawal of intensive care for high-risk newborns. Pediatrics 2007; 119:401–3.
12. Wood NS, Marlow N, Costeloe K, et al. Neurologic and developmental disability after extremely preterm birth. N Engl J Med 2000; 343:378–84.
13. Batton DG and the Committee on Fetus and Newborn. Antenatal counseling regarding resuscitation at an extremely low gestational age. Pediatrics 2009 124:422–7.
14. Young EWD, Stevenson DK. Limiting treatment for extremely premature, low birth-weight infants (500 to 750 g). Am J Dis Child 1990; 144:549–52.
15. Bernat, 323–7, Ch. 13.
16. Child abuse and neglect prevention and treatment program—HHS. Final rule. Fed Regist 1985; 50:14878–92.
17. Public Law 107–207, 116 Stat 926, 2002. To protect infants who are born alive. Available at www.gpo.gov/fdsys/pkg/PLAW-107publ207/pdf/PLAW-107publ207.pdf. Accessed March 26, 2012.
18. Meadow W, Reimschisel T, Lantos J. Birth weight-specific mortality for extremely low birth weight infants vanishes by four days of life: Epidemiology and ethics in the neonatal intensive care unit. Pediatrics 1996; 97:636–43.
19. Uhlmann RF, Pearlman RA. Perceived quality of life and preferences for life-sustaining treatment in older adults. Arch Intern Med 1991; 151:495–97.
20. President's Commission for the Study of Ethical Problems in Medicine and Biomedical and Behavioral Research. Deciding to forego life-sustaining treatment: A report on the ethical, medical, and legal issues in treatment decisions. Washington, DC: US Government Printing Office, 1983:218–9.

21. Provoost V, Cools F, Mortimer F, et al. Medical end-of-life decisions in neonates and infants in Flanders. Lancet 2005; 365:1315–20.
22. Truog RD. Tackling medical futility in Texas. N Engl J Med 2007; 357:1–3.
23. Perinatal care at the threshold of viability. Committee on Fetus and Newborn, American Academy of Pediatrics. Pediatrics 2002; 110:1024–7.
24. Pignotti MS, Donzelli G. Perinatal care at the threshold of viability: An international comparison of practical guidelines for the treatment of extremely preterm births. Pediatrics 2008; 121(1):e193–8.
25. Eichenwald EC, Stark AR. Management and outcomes of very low birth weight. N Engl J Med 2008; 358:1700–11.
26. Moster D, Lie RT, Markestad T. Long-term medical and social consequences of preterm birth. N Engl J Med 2008; 359:262–73.

18 ADVANCE DIRECTIVES

Jerome E. Kurent, MD, MPH, FAAN

LEARNING OBJECTIVES

Upon completion of this chapter, participants will be able to:

1. Compare the advantages and disadvantages of various advance directives.
2. Specify the circumstances under which advance directives become active.
3. Describe the advantages and disadvantages of appointing a surrogate decision maker with durable power of attorney for healthcare decisions.
4. Define decision-making capacity.

LEARNING RESOURCES

Key chapters in Bernat's third edition — 4, 8

Key relevant AAN documents available at www.aan.com/view/PECN

A   I   M

CLINICAL VIGNETTE

Mr. Moore, a 53-year-old man diagnosed with amyotrophic lateral sclerosis (ALS) 3 years ago, is now experiencing progressively worsening dyspnea. He has strongly indicated that he does not wish to be intubated or to be provided mechanical ventilation when he is no longer able to breathe on his own. He had intact decision-making capacity and made these decisions several months ago because he considered intubation and mechanical ventilation to be life-extending medical interventions. He maintained that an acceptable quality of life was far more important to him than extension of a burdensome life that was no longer fulfilling.

Concerned that his wife may insist that he be provided mechanical ventilation against his wishes when he is no longer able to communicate, Mr. Moore has asked how he can ensure that his wishes be honored. He wants to meet with his neurologist and his wife together to discuss the value of an advance directive (AD) in ensuring that his preferences and avoidances for medical care be honored.

QUESTIONS FOR GROUP DISCUSSION

ASSESSMENT

1. Have you ever had a patient who requested guidance regarding ADs? Did you feel prepared to advise her or to direct her to appropriate resources?
2. Have you ever encountered a circumstance in which a patient's surrogate wished to make a decision that seemed at odds with the patient's AD?
3. How rigidly should ADs be written and interpreted?

MORAL DIAGNOSIS

4. Should the neurologist document his discussion with Mr. Moore and his wife about the patient's wishes? Would such documentation have ethical or legal importance if it were the only expression of the patient's wishes (e.g., if the patient lost decision-making capacity before he could complete a written AD, or if he simply preferred not to complete such a document)?
5. Under what circumstances would an AD for healthcare decisions become "active"? If Mr. Moore had impending respiratory failure but could still communicate, to whom should his physicians talk regarding possible intubation and ventilation—him or his wife?
6. Can a patient instruct his physician to initiate treatments that are prohibited in the patient's own written and signed AD? For example, what if Mr. Moore changed his mind at the last minute and now wanted to be intubated and instructed his doctors to do so?
7. What does US federal law require hospitals to do in regard to living wills or ADs?
8. What sources of guidance regarding ADs (e.g., from hospitals or professional medical associations such as the AAN) are available for patients, healthy individuals, and surrogates?

GOAL SETTING, DECISION MAKING, AND IMPLEMENTATION

9. If an AD seems ambiguous or if the patient's clinical circumstances are not identical to the description in the patient's document, how much latitude do the surrogate decision maker and the healthcare team (HCT) have in interpreting the AD and making decisions? For example, how can the HCT best address the concerns of a nurse who thinks that the decision is contrary to the patient's wishes?
10. If Mr. Moore had an AD that stated that he did not want intubation or ventilation, what preparations would need to be made for him to have a percutaneous endoscopic gastrostomy that would require conscious sedation?
11. If Mrs. Moore suggests that she might not comply with her husband's AD, what advice could you give the patient regarding the designation of a surrogate decision maker in conjunction with the durable power of attorney for healthcare decisions?

COMMENTARY ON DISCUSSION QUESTIONS

ASSESSMENT

1. **Have you ever had a patient who requested guidance regarding ADs? Did you feel prepared to advise her or to direct her to appropriate resources?**

As noted by Bernat, ADs are of two principal types: (a) written instructional statements of a patient's wishes for treatment in different anticipated clinical situations and (b) written documents designating surrogate decision makers whose authority is activated when a patient is no longer able to make decisions.[1] The appointment of a surrogate decision maker is often accompanied by a written directive. The legally authorized surrogate with a durable power of attorney (DPOA) for healthcare decisions, depending on the state, is known variously as healthcare agent, healthcare proxy, or healthcare surrogate. "Durable" refers to the fact that such an appointment is not nullified by a patient's subsequent loss of decision-making capacity. Because the living will is more restrictive, as it is limited to patients who are terminally ill or, in many states, in a persistent vegetative state, the DPOA is considered by many to be preferable to the living will document. Many experts feel that having both documents may be redundant. When the documents conflict with each other, the living will would supersede the DPOA.

Bernat, 90, Ch. 4

Advance care planning should address the patient's understanding of the diagnosis, benefits, and burdens of potential treatments, treatment preferences and avoidances, and the likelihood of desired outcomes.[2] These issues should be addressed based upon personal values and goals of the patient. ADs are greatly underutilized as tools to help improve quality of end-of-life care.[3–5] Serious concern has also been expressed regarding their limitations and frequent inability to effect desired outcomes.[6,7] As noted by Bernat, The President's Council on Bioethics forcefully concluded that "Advance instruction directives (or living wills), though valuable to some degree and in some circumstances, are a limited and flawed instrument for addressing most of the decisions caregivers must make for those entrusted to their care."[8] The Council urged surrogate appointments as the best advance-directive mechanism,[9] particularly because surrogate appointment documents also provide the opportunity for patients to indicate specific written instructions.[10] In view of the recognized limitations of written ADs, the vital importance of effective physician–patient communication as a means to enhance advance care planning has been emphasized.[11,12]

Bernat, 92, Ch. 4

Bernat, 92–4, Ch. 4

All 50 states and the District of Columbia have statutory provisions for healthcare agents' appointments, ADs, or both. Surveys have indicated that most patients would welcome a discussion regarding ADs;

however, they expect that their physicians will initiate the discussion. Unfortunately, most practicing physicians do not take the time to have these discussions. As a result, it is estimated that only approximately 15% of the American public has completed written ADs. The obligation to obtain an AD is often relegated to a chaplain, social worker, or nurse. Many healthy individuals and patients with active disease mistakenly think that an attorney is required to complete an AD. Although an adequately informed attorney could certainly assist with completion of an AD, no law requires that a lawyer be involved. All physicians entrusted with the care of patients should be capable of having an informed discussion with their patients concerning ADs.

2. **Have you ever encountered a circumstance in which a patient's surrogate wished to make a decision that seemed at odds with the patient's AD?**

Fortunately, in most instances, a patient's designated surrogate decision maker will honor the patient's wishes as expressed in the AD and as agreed to by the surrogate. It should be clearly understood by the surrogate that she would act on behalf of the patient in respecting the specific preferences and avoidances for care when the patient loses decision-making capacity, either temporarily or permanently. If the potential surrogate expresses reservations or simply indicates an unwillingness to act according to the patient's wishes, the patient should choose a different surrogate who would reliably make medical decisions in a manner consistent with the patient's wishes. It may be helpful to designate a backup surrogate decision maker in the event that the primary surrogate cannot be located or contacted during an urgent situation. Although unlikely, the possibility does exist that the original surrogate would no longer be willing to proceed with the decision-making process. However, it is not recommended to designate two surrogate decision makers of equal authority, as this could potentially give rise to a conflicted decision-making process.

3. **How rigidly should ADs be written and interpreted?**

The AD is most useful when it conveys specific directions to the physician in the event that a patient loses decision-making capacity. It is advisable that the AD be as specific as possible, with little reliance on general directions. For example, the more general request that "no heroic measures" be provided could mean different things to different people, as the definition of "heroic" could be subject to a wide range of interpretation. Alternatively, specific requests such as "no mechanical ventilation" should be provided or that "a feeding tube placement not be permitted" are much more helpful to both the surrogate decision maker and the healthcare professionals. It is critical that the patient's designated surrogate decision maker be thoroughly familiar with the contents of the AD document, so as not to be surprised by a patient's request. Ideally, the patient should discuss specific elements of the AD with family members privately and then in collaboration with the physician prior to any potential crisis to avoid conflicts during a time of lost decision-making capacity. However, the literature does contain evidence of reluctance by surrogate decision makers to fully implement patients' wishes, especially regarding withdrawal of life-prolonging interventions.[13] Healthcare agents may occasionally be justified in overruling a patient's previously written AD.[14]

Bernat, 91–2, Ch. 4

Bernat, 176–7, Ch. 8

To optimize clinical decision making so that it respects avoidances and preferences of the patient, it will be important to establish goals of care.[15,16] Ideally, these should be defined by the patient in collaboration with the physician and in the context of specific factors related to the patient's illness. The diagnosis and prognosis, with and without implementation of various available interventions, should be discussed with the patient and, ideally, with family surrogate decision makers. For example, in the setting of an apparent life-limiting illness with an uncertain prognosis, the patient may choose a time-limited trial of aggressive potentially life-saving interventions. If the interventions fail, life-prolonging therapy may be discontinued. Palliative care or hospice may then be provided as the sole means of medical care. It is important to realize that palliative care and hospice do not mean *giving up*, but rather, the provision of aggressive pain and symptom management for the patient when cure is no longer possible.[17]

MORAL DIAGNOSIS

4. **Should the neurologist document his discussion with Mr. Moore and his wife about the patient's wishes? Would such documentation have ethical or legal importance if it were the only expression of the patient's wishes (e.g., if the patient lost decision-making capacity before he could complete a written AD, or if he simply preferred not to complete such a document)?**

In the absence of a completed AD, a well-documented written summary of the discussion concerning the patient's expressed avoidances and preferences for care would be very important. In fact, in the absence of a written directive, it could represent the *only* evidence of the patient's wishes when critical life-and-death clinical decision making is necessary and family members and the surrogate have conflicting opinions of what the patient would have wanted. The AAN Practice Parameter for care of the patient with ALS provides evidence-based management options to help facilitate decision making for the patient with ALS.[18]

Ideally, the written summary of the discussion would be signed by a second witness such as a nurse or social worker. It is not rare for an older patient with advanced systemic illness to indicate that "my family will know what to do" in the event of an acute, catastrophic health crisis. In fact, the opposite is usually true. For example, many loving and caring adult children may have differing opinions regarding what their mother would have wanted or what they individually think about how her best interests would be served. The potential for uncertainty, disagreement, and chaotic decision making by surrogate decision makers can be avoided by patients having forthright discussions with family members regarding key issues of healthcare and their preferences should they lose decision-making capacity. Inherent in this conversation is a statement of the patient's values (*values statement*). Ideally, the discussion should be followed by completion of an AD.

5. **Under what circumstances would an AD for healthcare decisions become "active"? If Mr. Moore had impending respiratory failure but could still communicate, to whom should his physicians talk regarding possible intubation and ventilation—him or his wife?**

The patient's wishes must be respected while he retains decision-making capacity and is able to communicate. From an ethical perspective, the patient's wishes cannot be overturned by a spouse, other family member, or even by a physician whose own values may be in conflict with the patient's wishes. If the attending physician, on the basis of conscientious objection, were unable to honor the patient's wishes of avoiding use of mechanical ventilation, the physician is obligated to transfer care of the patient to another physician who is willing to follow the patient's wishes. Also, the surrogate's role does not become active in decision making until the patient is no longer able to make decisions on his own behalf. Most importantly, the surrogate's role must be consistent with the patient's wishes as expressed in the AD. In Mr. Moore's case, because his wishes are so explicit, under no circumstance should he be intubated, whether under the direction of a spouse or physician. Doing so would be considered a violation of both ethical and legal principles of patient autonomy.

6. **Can a patient instruct his physician to initiate treatments that are prohibited in the patient's own written and signed AD? For example, what if Mr. Moore changed his mind at the last minute and now wanted to be intubated and instructed his doctors to do so?**

A patient may change his desires for medical care at any time. His more recent verbal directive would supersede the previously written AD and would essentially negate the written document. Under ordinary circumstances in a non-crisis situation, the written AD should also be modified to reflect the patient's revised updated request. Although it is relatively unusual for a patient to make a sudden significant change in his goals of care, if he were to do so, his wishes should be respected.

7. **What does US federal law require hospitals to do in regard to living wills or ADs?**

The Patient Self-Determination Act was passed in 1990 to encourage more hospitalized patients to complete ADs.[19,20] It requires all US

Bernat,
94–5,
Ch. 4
hospitals, skilled nursing facilities, home health agencies, and hospices that receive Medicare or Medicaid federal funding to establish a mechanism that offers patients an opportunity to discuss and complete ADs.[21]

8. **What sources of guidance regarding ADs (e.g., from hospitals or professional medical associations such as the AAN) are available for patients, healthy individuals, and surrogates?**

Most states make available standard versions of ADs, and state medical associations and professional organizations can provide practical advice regarding their completion. Although several types of ADs with varying options are available, completing more than one may give rise to conflict during a time of critical decision making. If an individual had completed two different documents, the living will would supersede the DPOA. Whereas the living will represents the individual's wishes and directives, the DPOA is implemented by the surrogate decision maker—a third party—and, therefore, is considered one step removed from the actual patient's wishes. Although the living will was historically the first AD to become available, the more recently developed DPOA is considered the preferable document by many. The living will is more restrictive because it is limited to patients who are either terminally ill or, in many states, in a persistent vegetative state. The DPOA applies to any medical condition, temporary or permanent, in which decision-making capacity has been lost. It is therefore not limited to terminal illness or persistent vegetative state.

GOAL SETTING, DECISION MAKING, AND IMPLEMENTATION

9. **If an AD seems ambiguous or if the patient's clinical circumstances are not identical to the description in the patient's document, how much latitude do the surrogate decision maker and the HCT have in interpreting the AD and making decisions? For example, how can the HCT best address the concerns of a nurse who thinks that the decision is contrary to the patient's wishes?**

If a member of the HCT feels that the patient's wishes are not being implemented and the issue cannot be resolved within the team structure, the hospital ethics committee can be an invaluable resource. On request, a member of the ethics committee can review the medical facts and medical record, and discuss the case at hand with members of the HCT. The ethics committee consultant can then provide a nonbinding opinion and important guidance in arriving at an equitable decision in support of the patient's *best interests*. Periodic
Bernat,
91–2,
Ch. 4
updates of written instructional directives can help to keep an AD contemporaneously accurate.[15]

10. **If Mr. Moore had an AD that stated that he did not want intubation or ventilation, what preparations would need to be made for him to have a percutaneous endoscopic gastrostomy that would require conscious sedation?**

It is common practice in many hospitals to temporarily suspend a patient's *do not intubate* request if the patient requires a procedure that might place him at risk for acute respiratory or cardiac complications related to that procedure. For example, placement of a percutaneous endoscopic gastrostomy tube in a severely weakened ALS patient could potentially require intubation. As part of the informed-consent process, the patient should be made aware of the risk that his respiratory drive is so weak that it is possible that he may need to be intubated during the procedure, which is an outcome he wishes to avoid. The patient should be given the choice of either letting the *do not intubate* status remain in place during the procedure or permitting the physicians to intubate him if he has respiratory arrest.

11. **If Mrs. Moore suggests that she might not comply with her husband's AD, what advice could you give the patient regarding the designation of a surrogate decision maker in conjunction with the durable power of attorney for healthcare decisions?**

It is understandable that family members may wish to base decisions on their own wishes; however, it is vitally important that the surrogate decision maker designated by the patient be willing and able to express the patient's wishes as indicated in the AD or even as expressed by the patient. It would be counterproductive and completely at odds with the spirit and intent of the DPOA and surrogate decision-making process to choose a person who could not honor the wishes of the patient for whom she were a surrogate. Although it might be unusual *not* to choose a spouse as surrogate decision maker, it may be a necessary course of action. It would also be highly advisable for Mrs. Moore to be provided opportunities to discuss her concerns regarding her unwillingness to participate as her husband's surrogate decision maker. If she still has unresolved conflicts over the decision to withhold life support for her husband, it would be advisable to identify a different surrogate decision maker to ensure that the patient's wishes would be implemented.

The DPOA can be a very useful instrument in helping to support the wishes of a patient who is in a nontraditional relationship that does not involve a married partner. An unmarried patient in a heterosexual relationship or a patient in a homosexual relationship may find some added assurance that his or her preferences can be respected by completing a DPOA and naming the partner as the proxy decision maker. Completion of this AD should also involve a discussion between the patient and proxy regarding the specifics of the document.

KEY POINTS

- The case of a patient with end-stage ALS illustrates the vital importance of establishing *goals of care*. They should be developed with the critical input of the patient and, ideally, with the support of the patient's family caregivers and affirmation of the patient's attending physician.
- Conflicts may sometimes arise between the patient and family members or between the patient and the HCT, and they must be resolved by respecting the patient's autonomy and right to determine the nature of terminal care.
- Goals of care may be implemented by means of an AD, which can indicate the patient's avoidances and preferences regarding care during loss of decision-making capacity.
- The DPOA for healthcare decisions is often considered the preferred AD and can be completed by patients with intact decision-making capacity.
- The Ethics Committee can assist in resolving conflicts in medical decision-making.

KEY WORDS

Advance directive—a written document that commonly refers to a living will and a durable power of attorney for healthcare.

Benefit–burden considerations—weighing the relative benefits of a potential therapeutic intervention versus the possible undesirable side effects. Ideally, the benefits would outweigh the burdens of a particular intervention.

Decision-making capacity—the capacity of individuals to make decisions on their own behalf, while taking into consideration the potential benefits and burdens of the decision.

Durable power of attorney (DPOA) for healthcare decisions—the legal authority granted in writing by the patient to a specifically named surrogate decision maker to make medical decisions for the patient

Goals of care—three potential goals of care include *cure, stabilization*, and *comfort only*. Benefits and burdens of each option should be considered, with decisions made primarily on the basis of patient preferences.

Quality of life at the end of life—the well-being of a dying person that is achieved through adequate pain and symptom management, avoiding inappropriate prolongation of dying, providing a sense of control, and strengthening relationships with family and loved ones.

Surrogate decision maker—person authorized to make decisions for a patient who lacks decision-making capacity; the authority may be based on an AD or a statutory hierarchy.

REFERENCES

1. Bernat, 90, Ch. 4.
2. Fried TR, Bradley EH, Towle VR, et al. Understanding the treatment preferences of seriously ill patients. N Engl J Med 2002; 346:1061–6.

3. Emanuel LL, Barry MJ, Stoeckle JD, et al. Advance directives for medical care—a case for greater use. N Engl J Med 1991; 324:889–95.
4. Gillick MR. Advance care planning. N Engl J Med 2004; 350:7–8.
5. Teno JM, Gruneir A, Schwartz Z, et al. Association between advance directives and quality of end-of-life care: A national study. J Am Geriatr Soc 2007; 55:189–94.
6. Fagerlin A, Schneider CE. Enough: The failure of the living will. Hastings Cent Rep 2004; 34(2):30–42.
7. Perkins HS. Controlling death: The false promise of advance directives. Ann Int Med 2007; 147:51–7.
8. Bernat, 92, Ch. 4.
9. President's Council on Bioethics. Taking care: Ethical caregiving in our aging society. September 2005. Available at http://bioethics.georgetown.edu/pcbe/reports/taking_care/chapter5.html. Accessed March 20, 2012.
10. Bernat, 92–4, Ch. 4.
11. Messinger-Rappaport BJ, Baum EE, Smith ML. Advance care planning: Beyond the living will. Cleve Clin J Med 2009; 76:277–85.
12. Tulsky J. Beyond advance directives: Importance of communication skills at the end of life. JAMA 2005; 294:359–65.
13. Emmanuel LL. Advance directives: Do they work? J Am Coll Cardiol 1995; 25:35–8.
14. Bernat JL, Peterson LM. Patient-centered informed consent in surgical practice. Arch Surg 2006; 141:86–92.
15. Bernat, 91–2, Ch. 4.
16. Bernat, 176–7, Ch. 8.
17. Singer PA, Martin DK, Kelner M. Quality end-of-life care. Patients' perspectives. JAMA 1999; 28:163–8
18. Miller, RG, Jackson, CJ, Kasarskis, EJ, et al. Practice parameter update: The care of the patient with amyotrophic lateral sclerosis: Drug, nutritional and respiratory therapies (an evidence-based review). Neurology 2009; 73:1218–26.
19. LaPuma J, Orentlicher D, Moss RJ. Advance directives on admission: Clinical implications and analysis of the Patient Self-Determination Act of 1990. JAMA 1991; 266:402–5.
20. Greco PJ, Schulman KA, Lavizzo-Mourey R, et al. The Patient Self-Determination Act and the future of advance directives. Ann Int Med 1991; 115:639–43.
21. Bernat, 94–5, Ch. 4.

SUGGESTIONS FOR FURTHER READING

Bernat JL. How neurologists can enhance patient-centered medicine. Neurology 2001; 56:144–5.
Bernat JL. The living will: Does an advance refusal of treatment made with capacity always survive any supervening incapacity? Med Law Int 1999; 4:1–21.
Clements JM. Patient perceptions on the use of advance directives and life prolonging technology. Am J Hosp Palliat Care 2009; 26:270–6.
Dexter PR, Wolinsky FD, Gramelspacher RP, et al. Opportunities for advance directives to influence medical care. J Clin Ethics 2003; 14:173–88.
Johnson KS, Kuchibhatla M, Tulsky JA. What explains racial differences in the use of advance directives and attitudes toward hospice care? J Am Geriatr Soc 2008; 56:1953–8.
McLean SAM. Are advance directives legally binding or simply the starting point for discussion on patients' best interests? Ethical view. BMJ 2009; 339:b4695.
Spellecy R. Reviving Ulysses contracts. Kennedy Inst Ethics J 2003; 13:373–92.
Torke AM, Moloney R, Siegler M, et al. Physicians' views on the importance of patient preferences in surrogate decision-making. J Am Geriatr Soc 2010; 58:533–8.

19

WITHHOLDING AND WITHDRAWING LIFE-SUSTAINING TREATMENT IN PATIENTS WITH DECISION-MAKING CAPACITY

Eran Klein, MD, PhD

LEARNING OBJECTIVES

Upon completion of this chapter, participants will be able to:

1. Discuss the key ethical concepts and issues involved in decisions to forgo life-sustaining treatment.
2. Identify the most salient descriptive and normative aspects of refusal of life-sustaining treatment in adults with decision-making capacity.
3. Develop strategies for assessing refusal of life-sustaining treatment in adults with decision-making capacity.

LEARNING RESOURCES

Key chapters in Bernat's third edition—1, 2, 7, 8

Key relevant AAN documents available at www.aan.com/view/PECN

A   H   O

CLINICAL VIGNETTES

CASE 1

A 71-year-old morbidly obese woman with a history of diabetes, osteomyelitis, and breast cancer is admitted to the neurology service for leg weakness. Seven years ago, Claire was treated for breast cancer with surgery, chemotherapy, and radiation. She now has a 3-day history of leg weakness (worse on the right), pain in her left leg and right arm, and vertigo with tinnitus. An MRI of the brain shows leptomeningeal enhancement of the spinal cord and brainstem, and CSF cytology shows cells consistent with her previous breast cancer. She has also developed subtle left facial droop and dysarthria. After the neurologist discusses the diagnosis and prognosis of leptomeningeal carcinomatosis with her, she is undecided about which treatment, if any, to pursue. She discusses the issue with her primary care physician and opts for limited radiation treatment to her spine for alleviation of radicular pain but refuses intrathecal or systemic chemotherapy, despite the previous favorable chemotherapeutic response of her breast cancer. She fears the side effects of chemotherapy—headache, nausea, and vomiting from chemical meningitis, and possible sepsis from osteomyelitis and myelosuppression. She now requires large doses of opiate analgesics for pain relief and dozes off during conversations. When stimulated, she says that she understands that she is forgoing treatment that might extend her life and that she will most likely die within the next 1 to 2 months.

CASE 2

Carlos, a 49-year-old physician, is admitted with self-diagnosed Guillain–Barré syndrome (GBS). Symptoms began with numbness in his toes and progressed to ascending upper- and lower-extremity weakness over several days. The CSF analysis is consistent with GBS, and EMG and NCS results show evidence of the more severe axonal variant of the disease. By the third day of his illness, he develops left facial paresis and left hypoglossal nerve paresis with intermittent dysarthria and dysphagia. He begins to have difficulty breathing, and a chest x-ray shows an elevated left hemidiaphragm. His physician begins treating him with IV immunoglobulins. He also discusses the possible need for intubation and a feeding tube. Carlos clearly states that he is amenable to intubation. However, he also states that he wishes to be extubated and allowed to die if his symptoms progress after a full course of immunoglobulins.

Carlos relates that he is married without children and that he became estranged from his parents and siblings when he immigrated to this country 25 years ago. Through tears, he adds that his wife is in the terminal stages of lung cancer. The future that he envisions—and one that he most wishes to avoid—involves a long and complicated recovery, a high likelihood of permanent disability, and probable loss of his life partner during his prolonged recovery. The neurologist advises him that this is just one possible future and that his disease might take a more benign course, but Carlos is unmoved. He would rather avoid the worst than hold out for other possibilities and asks the neurologist to promise to support him in this decision because he knows that some of those on his care team will be uncomfortable with it.

CASE 3

LuAnn is a 63-year-old woman who developed a headache and vertigo one day after chiropractic manipulation and was subsequently found on the floor at home by her caregiver, her granddaughter. She appears awake but cannot move her limbs, tongue, or lower face. She is intubated and on a ventilator. An MRI/MRA of the brain reveals a vertebral dissection with bilateral pontine infarcts and partial sparing of the ventral pons. When sedation is reduced, the neurologist explains that although the risk of mortality in locked-in syndrome is much less than previously thought, her chance of severe disability remains high. Though communication with her is difficult, by means of her preserved blink and vertical eye movements, she indicates her desire for aggressive treatment. Several days later, she develops a ventilator-associated pneumonia, and it is treated successfully with antibiotics.

As LuAnn is being discharged to a rehabilitation facility, the neurologist tries to discern the level of treatment that she wants going forward and is surprised that she wishes *not* to be treated with antibiotics if pneumonia redevelops. She explains that her granddaughter, who has been at her bedside every day, has just been accepted to study violin at a prestigious music school, which had been their mutual dream, especially since her granddaughter moved in with her. LuAnn now realizes that if she requires repeated admissions to the hospital for complications from her neurologic disability, her granddaughter will likely forfeit this opportunity and choose to take care of her instead. The money that they saved for tuition will have to be used instead to pay for LuAnn's long-term healthcare. She says that she has thought long and hard about this difficult decision and has opted to forgo future treatment and put her life in "God's capable hands."

QUESTIONS FOR GROUP DISCUSSION

GETTING STARTED
1. How does the decision to forgo life-sustaining treatment (LST) fit within the overall context of medical care?

ASSESSMENT
2. What is the concept of autonomy, and how should respect for autonomy guide a physician's response to refusals of LST?
3. What are the essential components of informed decision making?
4. Do the decisions made in the cases meet the criteria of informed refusal? If not, why not? What additional information would you want?
5. Can a person rationally decide to forgo LST? Can one be depressed and still rationally refuse LST?
6. Does a right to refuse LST extend to those with nonterminal illnesses?
7. What are the potential sources of undue influence on patients' end-of-life decisions?

MORAL DIAGNOSIS
8. Is there an ethical difference between *withholding* care and *withdrawing* care?
9. Is the distinction between "ordinary" and "extraordinary" relevant to the decision-making process for end-of-life care?

GOAL SETTING, DECISION MAKING, AND IMPLEMENTATION
10. Describe an ideal process for determining a patient's preferences for LST.

COMMENTARY ON DISCUSSION QUESTIONS

GETTING STARTED

1. How does the decision to forgo LST fit within the overall context of medical care?

Bernat, 171, Ch. 8

The freedom of adults with decision-making capacity to refuse medical treatment, including LST, has become part of the fabric of modern medical practice. This option is now assumed by many to be a legal, if not a fundamental, human right. By historical standards, this acknowledgment is a relatively recent phenomenon.[1] In bioethics, the freedom to refuse LST represents a fundamental shift away from paternalism toward patient autonomy. Although the refusal of LST is now a largely resolved issue among bioethicists, it frequently presents challenging and unsettling ethical dilemmas for clinicians involved in the care of seriously ill or dying patients. The goals of this chapter are to explore some of the more challenging problems presented by refusal of LST and to provide guidance to neurologists who encounter similar situations in clinical practice.[2]

Bernat, 188–9, Ch. 8

Decisions regarding LST involve a range of actions, from implicit to explicit, and all of these decisions require weighing interventions, their potential benefits, and the intensity of medical treatment against the possible harms that could be incurred. Most often, these decisions involve various forms of implicit consent or refusal for procedures or treatments considered to be minor, such as agreeing to regular blood draws. Sometimes they are formalized into written consent or refusal (an explicit action), such as Claire's consent for radiation therapy or Carlos's refusal of prolonged intubation. Refusal of LST falls on the explicit and more consequential end of this spectrum. These decisions stand out because LST often involves substantial burdens, and refusals of LST typically have irreversible consequences, such as respiratory failure and likely death from refusing intubation, or sepsis and likely death from refusing antibiotic treatment.

ASSESSMENT

2. What is the concept of autonomy, and how should respect for autonomy guide a physician's response to refusals of LST?

Bernat, 9–11, Ch. 1

All 3 cases involve various forms of treatment refusal. Claire refuses chemotherapy, Carlos refuses prolonged intubation, and LuAnn refuses antibiotics. From an ethical perspective, these decisions are primarily about patient autonomy. Modern medical practice in the United States recognizes that patients have a right to self-determination, or autonomy, and this right has deep roots in Western philosophy[3–5] and the law.[6] Indeed, a commitment to protecting patients from unwanted treatment has been codified in the law.[7,8]

Respect for patient autonomy, particularly at the end of life, requires more than just satisfying patient requests. Is allowing a delirious person to refuse a blood transfusion respecting autonomy? Is a patient's self-determination fostered by complying with a refusal of surgery if it is based on an inadequate understanding of the risks and benefits? The assumption that merely doing what a patient wants is sufficient to maintain patient autonomy fails to recognize the complexities of illness, modern medicine, and the rich concept of autonomy itself.

3. What are the essential components of informed decision making?

Bernat, 24–7, Ch. 2

An appropriate process of informed consent and refusal is necessary to respect patient autonomy.[9] The essential components of informed decision making include (a) provision of adequate medical information in terms that the patient can understand; (b) patient understanding of the rationale, risks, benefits, and potential outcomes of the proposed intervention and its alternatives; (c) patient decision-making capacity; and (d) voluntariness of choice.[10] Complex and rapidly changing medical conditions can make full disclosure of medical information difficult, as patients' reasoning and communication abilities can be compromised by acute illness. In addition, patients may change their minds. To the extent possible, physicians should aim for full disclosure and seek ways to enhance the other components of informed decision making.

The first criterion for an ethically acceptable informed refusal is that the patient is provided with clear medical information and that patient understanding of the interventions and their potential outcomes is verified. How much have Claire, Carlos, and LuAnn been told about their conditions, including diagnoses, prognoses, and therapies? Who has informed them and in what settings? As he is a physician, does Carlos need the same amount of information that Claire needs to make a decision? How much has Claire been told about the difference that her previous chemotherapeutic response makes to her prognosis? What has LuAnn been told about the likely complications of untreated pneumonia and the implications of this refusal on her obtaining other kinds of medical treatment? Moral and legal standards for disclosure of information vary,[10] but the goal for the physician should be to provide the patient with the kind and quantity of information that the patient can understand and act upon. Evidence that the patient understands this information would be the patient's ability to summarize the information, apply it to himself/herself, and discuss treatment options in view of this information.

The second criterion for an ethically acceptable informed refusal is that the patient possesses capacity for reasoning and communication commensurate with the decision that must be made. The capacity to reason is required to critically assess the medical information and determine preferences and desires, and the capacity to communicate is required to make the output of such reasoning known. Despite the side effects of her pain medication, are Claire's cognitive abilities preserved enough to make such an important and irreversible decision? Does she have CNS involvement from her disease that might be affecting her cognition? It is quite likely that her previous experience with breast cancer and its treatment provide her with an established framework for reasoning through the tough decisions ahead. Is Carlos' refusal an expression of clinical depression or grief, or is it a consistent expression of his deeply held convictions? How stable is LuAnn's refusal? Might her treatment preference change again tomorrow or with a modest improvement in her medical condition, such as being well enough to come off of ventilatory support, or is the decision settled in her mind such that it would endure the likely ups and downs of her current condition? At times, these important questions can be answered by simply asking patients to clarify reasons for their decisions. At other times, formal assessment of decision-making capacity conducted by psychiatrists or other trained professionals may be needed.

The final criterion is freedom from undue influence, or *voluntariness*. Patients' decisions should be their own—not the decisions of their physicians or families. Did Claire's primary care physician influence her decision about aggressiveness of care, and if so, was this appropriate persuasion based on her physician's unique knowledge of her values and preferences? Is LuAnn's decision to forgo aggressive treatment her own or that of her family? The line between permissible influence and coercion often is difficult to draw, though as will be discussed below, paradigmatic cases of persuasion, coercion, and manipulation can provide useful guidance to the clinician.[10]

4. Do the decisions made in the cases meet the criteria of informed refusal? If not, why not? What additional information would you want?

Patients should be able to give reasons for their decisions, even if these reasons are not those that other patients or the physician find convincing. Claire's case is particularly instructive. On the surface, her refusal of chemotherapy seems reasonable, but is her decision consistent with the kind of person that she is and the values that she holds? Did she express desires about end-of-life care when she was initially diagnosed with breast cancer 7 years ago that might be helpful now? What has changed in the interim, if anything, with respect to her personality, values, or interests that might be a guide? Her use of opiates for pain relief—and the temporary alterations in cognition that accompany their use—do not necessarily diminish her capacity for making this decision but do present a reason for caution. The physician should assess her decision-making capacity. Consistency of a choice is often useful in assessing the quality of decision making, as is the patient's ability to describe tradeoffs in the benefits and burdens of continuing versus limiting or withdrawing treatment.

LuAnn's case highlights the issue of stability of decisions made at the end of life because she makes a sudden change in her preferences. Many patients initially seek aggressive treatment, and their decisions to stop treatment reflect a reversal or change of heart following an internal struggle. The easiest way to determine whether the decision is fleeting or the end of a long struggle is to ask the patient. For example, if the physician's sense is that the decision is fleeting, the physician could state, "This decision seems at odds with your prior decisions. I very much wish to respect your choice, but I also want to work with you to be sure that this is the choice you're really ready to make."

5. Can a person rationally decide to forgo LST? Can one be depressed and still rationally refuse LST?

Carlos' refusal of LST raises a concern about rationality and capacity in the midst of depression. Without a longer discussion or formal psychiatric assessment, it is difficult to know whether Carlos has depression and, if so, whether it is compromising his decision-making capacity. Is his crying an appropriate expression of grief regarding his wife's terminal illness and his own new disability, or is it a sign of clinical depression? If he is exhibiting some symptoms of depression, are they severe enough to impair his judgment, given that many with depression are capable of making rational end-of-life decisions?[11] If his capacity for decision making were significantly impaired by depression, it might be reasonable not to honor his refusal temporarily while treating his depression, with the intent to reassess his wishes when he is no longer impaired.[12] One should have very compelling evidence that depression is significantly impairing a patient's judgment before overruling wishes to refuse LST.[1] Assistance from a psychiatrist and an ethics consultation service could be obtained. It is also important to recognize that after ventilatory support is started, Carlos and the medical team should have opportunities to discuss his condition and response to treatment, and to reassess whether his decision to refuse long-term ventilatory support will stand. In other words, the decision need not be rushed because his agreement to initiate ventilation affords him and the ICU team time to reconsider. In these circumstances, the ICU team should clearly identify whom Carlos wants as a surrogate decision maker.

Bernat, 182, Ch. 8
Bernat, 171, Ch. 8

Justifications for each patient's refusal of treatment could be very different. Claire may offer her desire to be pain free and die at home. Carlos may base his decision on his views of an acceptable or unacceptable quality of life. LuAnn could speak of her wish to "live on" through her granddaughter's success. What makes these refusals of treatment reasonable or unreasonable does not depend on whether they conform to reasons that most people would offer. Rather, the decision should be consistent with the patient's own value system and goals of care, and the physician can only determine if a patient's decision is consistent with a particular patient's values by getting to know that patient. It is sometimes all too easy to label as "reasonable" those decisions that are most commonly encountered in medical practice and as "unreasonable" those that are uncommonly encountered or those that differ from the personal views of the healthcare professional who is caring for the patient.

6. Does a right to refuse LST extend to those with nonterminal illnesses?

Patients do not have to have a terminal illness to refuse LST. For example, GBS is rarely fatal. It is, therefore, ethically permissible for Carlos to refuse treatment for GBS or its complications, even if it may result in his death, as long as the healthcare team has confirmed that he is making an informed decision. As case law has established, protection from unwanted treatment cannot be justifiably reserved for only patients with "terminal" illnesses.[13,14]

7. What are the potential sources of undue influence on patients' end-of-life decisions?

An individual's decision to refuse LST should be voluntary. Pressure on patients' decisions at the end of life can be substantial and come from different directions, including physicians and family members.

Physicians can exert pressure on patients in various ways.[10] Physician attempts to persuade patients are ethically permissible. *Persuasion* occurs when one person comes to believe in something through the merit of reasons advanced by another person. On the other hand, *manipulation of information* is incompatible with respect for autonomy; examples include deliberately withholding information, or presenting biased information to get a patient to agree to an intervention that a physician prefers (called framing bias). *Coercion* occurs if and only if one person (e.g., a physician) intentionally uses a credible and severe threat of harm or force to control another (e.g., a patient). For a threat to be credible, both parties must believe that the threat maker can effect the threat, or the threat maker must deceive the person into believing so. For example, a physician who informs a patient that he will keep her on the ventilator regardless of her wishes is being coercive because the physician has the power to carry out the threat.

It is important to recognize that most physicians are neither coercive nor deliberately manipulative, yet they may still influence patients more than they intend to. Some patients will follow physicians' recommendations (even if doing so differs from their own choices) because they do not want to disappoint their physicians. Thus, physicians should emphasize that patients' decisions will not adversely affect the professional physician–patient relationship. A physician may use phrases such as, "I want you to make the decision that's best for you and not necessarily because it's the decision I recommend." A physician's influence can extend from the patient's well-earned trust in the physician's judgment. For example, Claire changed her mind after discussing her diagnosis with her primary care physician. One could explore how the physician's unique knowledge of Claire led him to make his recommendation. Physicians must recognize the many ways in which they can influence patients and use that influence to help patients in making the best possible decisions.

The curative ethos that pervades medical practice can sometimes generate resistance when patients refuse LST. Clinicians are trained to cure disease and to extend the lives of their patients, and the curative ethos that arises out of this training drives much of what happens in medicine. This ethos has many positive effects, but it also sometimes leads physicians mistakenly to take death as a sign of failure. Carlos' prediction that his decision will generate discomfort on the part of some of his caregivers is evidence of this influence. The palliative care movement has been a counterweight to the curative ethos in medicine in so far as it emphasizes the important role of the clinician in providing comprehensive and compassionate care during the dying process. It seems that Claire's primary care physician has assumed this more comprehensive role. However, the reaction that Claire and LuAnn may encounter from hospital personnel to their respective decisions is indicative of the cultural ethos that still must sometimes be overcome in respecting a patient's refusal of LST.

MORAL DIAGNOSIS

8. Is there an ethical difference between *withholding care* and *withdrawing* care?

In bioethics, it is commonly accepted that no ethical distinction exists between withholding and withdrawing treatment, but this issue remains controversial for many clinicians.[15] Philosophically and legally, withholding treatment and withdrawing treatment are not considered ethically different, but many laypersons and physicians make an emotional and psychological distinction, which explains why many are more comfortable with never starting a treatment (such as ventilation) than they are with starting and then stopping it.[16] It is worth noting that in some religious traditions, particularly Orthodox Judaism, withholding treatment and withdrawing treatment are considered morally distinct. If Carlos is eventually extubated as he requests, the cause of his death would be the same (i.e., neuromuscular respiratory failure) as if he had never been intubated in the first place. The act of removing the respirator in this case (or more typically, in cases of chronically progressive conditions) may engender on the part of some practitioners feelings of responsibility for a death that would not be engendered by honoring a decision to forgo intubation in the first place. Though these feelings are common and understandable, they are not supported by a cogent ethical distinction.

9. Is the distinction between "ordinary" and "extraordinary" relevant to the decision-making process for end-of-life care?

The distinction between ordinary and extraordinary means of care, which has a rich and nuanced history in Roman Catholic casuistry,[17] is sometimes invoked in cases of refusal of LST. Casuistry (Latin, *casus* = case) is case-based reasoning used to resolve moral problems by applying theoretical rules to the case. In its most basic formulation, the distinction between ordinary and extraordinary means is used to require the provision of ordinary forms of treatment while permitting refusal or withdrawal of extraordinary treatment or interventions. Often in discussions about medical decision making, *ordinary care* is equated with "standard," "customary," or "simple" treatments, whereas *extraordinary care* is equated with "unconventional," "costly," or "technologically advanced" treatments. For example, is Claire's chemotherapy "ordinary" care because it is the most common therapy for this rare condition, even if it has limited effectiveness? Is Carlos' ventilatory support "ordinary" care because most patients with severe neuromuscular disease require intubation, or is it "extraordinary" because it requires management by specially trained health professionals? Is LuAnn's antibiotic an "ordinary" routine treatment or an "extraordinary" product of a multibillion-dollar research effort?

Appeals to the ordinary-extraordinary distinction that come out of the Roman Catholic tradition take a more nuanced approach to the terms.[18] What matters is not the sophistication of technology or the frequency of its use, but how a potential treatment fits into a particular patient's prognosis and set of values, and what future burdens and benefits it promises. Extraordinary treatments are those that involve bearing great burdens with the prospect of few benefits, while ordinary treatments do the reverse. The distinction between ordinary and extraordinary means of treatment can at times be useful, but it can also lead to confusion if not invoked with care.

GOAL SETTING, DECISION MAKING, AND IMPLEMENTATION

10. Describe an ideal process for determining a patient's preferences for LST.

Bernat, 33–4, Ch. 2

The discussion between patient and clinician regarding refusal of LST should be conducted on a model of *shared decision making*.[19] The physician brings technical expertise and firsthand experience with similar situations. The patient and family bring a unique set of values and priorities and a perspective on *this* illness at *this* time in *this* patient's life. The family should be included in the discussion as soon and as completely as the patient wishes. Involvement of family members in this process can be extremely beneficial to help them work through their own feelings, such as sorrow, fear, joy, and guilt.

TOPIC SYNOPSIS

Providing patients the opportunity to make an informed decision to start, continue, refuse, or withdraw LST is central to respecting patient autonomy. The 3 clinical cases discussed in this chapter are examples of the types of challenges that patients and clinicians face in making decisions at the end of life. Awareness of these challenges and an active commitment to promoting sound decision making are important for any practitioner who wishes to be more than just a healer of the body.

KEY POINTS

- An informed refusal of LST requires patient understanding of disclosed information and medical alternatives, decision-making capacity, and a context in which patient choice can be voluntary.
- A patient's decision to forgo LST can be a rational decision that promotes autonomy and expresses patient values.
- The distinction between withholding and withdrawing treatment, except in certain religious contexts, has limited use in decision making at the end of life.
- A model of shared decision making between clinician and patient should be the ideal that guides discussions about end-of-life treatment.

KEY WORDS

Autonomy—the freedom to make decisions in line with one's own values and self-conception.

Decision-making capacity—the capacity of individuals to make decisions on their own behalf, while taking into consideration the potential benefits and burdens of the decision.

Life-sustaining treatment—medical intervention that replaces or supports critical bodily functions.

Voluntary—arising from one's own will and unconstrained by interference.

REFERENCES

1. Bernat, 171, Ch. 8.
2. Bernat, 188–9, Ch. 8.
3. Kant I. *Foundations of the Metaphysics of Morals* (tr. Lewis White Beck). Indianapolis, IN: Bobbs-Merrill Co., Inc., 1959.
4. Mill JS. *On Liberty*. London: Penguin, 2003.
5. Bernat, 9–11, Ch. 1.
6. Schloendorff v. Society of New York Hospital, 211 N.Y. 125, 105 N.E. 92 (1914).
7. Natanson v. Kline, 186 Kansas 393, 350 P.2d 1093 (1960).
8. Cruzan v. Director, Missouri Department of Health. 497 U.S. 261, 110 S. Ct. 28441, 111L. Ed.2d. 224 (1990).
9. Bernat, 24–7, Ch. 2.
10. Beauchamp TL, Childress JF. *Principles of Biomedical Ethics, 5th ed.* New York: Oxford University Press, 2001.
11. Ganzini L, Lee MA, Heintz RT, et al. Depression, suicide, and the right to refuse life-sustaining treatment. J Clin Ethics 1993; 4:337–40.
12. Bernat, 182, Ch. 8.
13. Bouvia v. Superior Court, 179 Cal.App.3d 1127 (1986).
14. Bartling v. Superior Court, 163 Cal.App.3d 186 (1984).

15. Carver AC, Vickrey BG, Bernat J, et al. End-of-life care: A survey of U.S. neurologists' attitudes, behavior, and knowledge. Neurology 1999; 53:284–93.
16. President's Commission for the Study of Ethical Problems in Medicine and Biomedical and Behavioral Research. Deciding to forego life-sustaining treatment: Ethical, medical, and legal issues in treatment decisions. Washington, DC: US Government Printing Office, 1983.
17. Shannon TA. Nutrition and hydration: An analysis of the recent papal statement in the light of the Roman Catholic bioethical tradition. Christ Bioeth 2006; 12(1):29–41.
18. Clark P. Tube feedings and persistent vegetative state patients: Ordinary or extraordinary means? Christ Bioeth 2006; 12(1):43–64.
19. Bernat, 33–4, Ch. 2.

SUGGESTIONS FOR FURTHER READING

Brody BA. *Life and Death Decision Making*. New York: Oxford University Press, 1988.
Cassell EJ. *The Nature of Suffering and the Goals of Medicine*. New York: Oxford University Press, 1991.
Pellegrino ED. *Humanism and the Physician*. Knoxville, TN: The University of Tennessee Press, 1979.

20 WITHHOLDING AND WITHDRAWING LIFE-SUSTAINING TREATMENT IN PATIENTS WITHOUT DECISION-MAKING CAPACITY

Michael A. Williams, MD, FAAN

LEARNING OBJECTIVES

Upon completion of this chapter, participants will be able to:

1. Describe the limitations placed on surrogate decision makers who are appointed by virtue of state statute as opposed to durable power of attorney for healthcare decisions.
2. Describe a process for resolving disputes of surrogates who are at the same level of surrogate hierarchy described in state law.

LEARNING RESOURCES

Key chapters in Bernat's third edition—3, 4, 7
Key relevant AAN documents available at www.aan.com/view/PECN

A   M   O

CLINICAL VIGNETTES

CASE 1

Amy, a 22-year-old woman who has recently graduated from college and is now living with her parents, is in a motor vehicle accident and suffers a severe traumatic brain injury. Because of difficulty with intubation, mild-to-moderate hypoxic cerebral injury has also occurred. Head and spine CT shows bilateral frontal lobe contusions and traumatic subarachnoid hemorrhage and no spinal cord injury. Despite aggressive treatment, Amy has not regained consciousness after 7 days. Her eyes do not open to painful stimuli, and the best motor response is bilateral extension. Brainstem and cranial nerve reflexes are preserved, but because of aspiration pneumonitis, Amy is expected to require prolonged ventilator support. Her long-term neurologic prognosis is uncertain. The ICU team discusses tracheostomy, percutaneous endoscopic gastrostomy (PEG), and long-term care with her parents. They also inform Amy's parents that if her condition should worsen (e.g., development of a pneumonia, serious systemic infection, or cardiac arrest), the associated circulatory shock would only worsen her neurologic injuries, and they recommend that a DNR order be placed on the chart. The patient has no advance directive (AD), and her parents do not recall any conversations with her about her wishes in such a circumstance. Amy had always been active with dancing, and her career goal was to own her own dance studio. Her parents, who are her only family, disagree about the treatment. Her father believes that she could not bear to survive with severe disabilities and, as it is clear that she will not return to normal, he feels that treatment should be stopped. Her mother believes that Amy would want to persevere despite her injuries so that she could be an example and inspiration to others.

CASE 2

Marge, a 68-year-old widow who has recently retired and is living with her only daughter and son-in-law, has a subarachnoid hemorrhage from an aneurysm of the anterior communicating artery. The aneurysm is successfully treated with endovascular coiling, and hydrocephalus is treated with an intraventricular catheter. The initial prognosis is hopeful; however, vasospasm develops and is treated aggressively with the family's consent, but bilateral anterior cerebral artery territory frontal lobe infarctions and bilateral caudate head infarctions become evident on CT scans. Marge's eyes open to painful stimuli. She occasionally regards examiners but follows no commands, and the best motor response is bilateral extension. Brainstem and cranial nerve reflexes are preserved, but because of aspiration pneumonitis, Marge is expected to require ventilator support for several weeks. The ICU team discusses tracheostomy, PEG, shunt surgery, and long-term care with her family. Marge has no AD, but her daughter recalls that after her father died of a glioblastoma, her mother had told her that she would not wish to survive if she were ever in the same condition. Her family requests that all treatment, including artificial nutrition and hydration (ANH), be stopped. Several members of the ICU team question whether this request is appropriate now that Marge has shown possible signs of emerging consciousness.

QUESTIONS FOR GROUP DISCUSSION

GETTING STARTED
1. What has been your experience in helping families to make decisions for patients who lack decision-making capacity?

ASSESSMENT
2. In each case, what are the patient's condition and prognosis? Is there any uncertainty?
3. Do the patients have decision-making capacity?
4. Are the patients' preferences known? Is there any doubt or disagreement? Are the families' preferences known? Is there any doubt or disagreement?

(continued)

5. Do any issues of power or conflict in the interactions of the key actors in the cases need to be addressed?
6. In the absence of an AD, does the law limit the decisions that a family can make for a patient?

MORAL DIAGNOSIS

7. How are the moral problems in these cases being framed by the participants? Can or should this framing be reconsidered and replaced by an alternative understanding?
8. What ethical standards or guidelines exist?
9. What are the morally acceptable options for resolving the moral problems posed by the cases?

GOAL SETTING, DECISION MAKING, IMPLEMENTATION

10. How can an ethics consultation be of benefit?
11. Is judicial review needed?

EVALUATION

12. Would any changes in institutional policy or educational interventions help to prevent or resolve the moral problems posed by similar cases?

COMMENTARY ON DISCUSSION QUESTIONS

GETTING STARTED

1. What has been your experience in helping families to make decisions for patients who lack decision-making capacity?

Helping families to make decisions for patients without decision-making capacity is common in the ICU setting and in the practice of neurology. Regrettably, it is also common that such decisions are made without the assistance of a formal AD by the patient, especially among younger patients.[1] Challenges include helping families to deal with the stress and burden of surrogate decision making, negotiating conflicts within the family regarding the decision, and recognizing the limits placed by the law on such decisions. Torke et al. studied a single, large, urban, public hospital in Indiana that used an electronic medical record that captured all DNR orders and documentation of discussions, and they showed that 956 DNR orders were entered for 725 unique patients among 6,143 admissions in a 3-year period (January 1, 2004, to December 31, 2006). Of these cases, 668 had all data available for analysis; of these, the DNR order was discussed with only the surrogate in 58.2%, with only the patient in 28.6%, and with both the patient and surrogate in 13.2%.[2] The mean hospital day of DNR order was later when decisions were made by surrogates (6.6 days) than when they were made by patients (3.2 days), and it was later for shared decisions (4.4 days) than for patient decisions (3.2 days). Additionally, the adjusted hazard ratio for in-hospital death was 2.6 times higher (95% confidence interval = 1.56–4.36) for patients with surrogate decisions than for those with patient decisions. The authors' understated conclusion is, "Surrogate decision making may take longer because of the greater ethical, emotional, or communication complexity of making decisions with surrogates than with patients."[2]

ASSESSMENT

2. In each case, what are the patient's condition and prognosis? Is there any uncertainty?

In each of the cases, although the patient is still seriously ill, the immediate risk of dying seems to have passed. In fact, in both cases, the ICU teams have initiated discussions of the procedures necessary to support the patients for transfer from the ICU to a hospital ward and eventually to rehabilitation or long-term care. Thus, each patient is expected to survive in the short or intermediate term.

The prognosis for both patients is uncertain; however, differences exist. For Amy in Case 1, it would appear that the best outcome would be severe disability (i.e., awake and able to communicate in simple terms but fully dependent on assistance for all activities of daily living); however, the possibility of survival either in the vegetative or minimally conscious state is significant. As much as a year may be necessary to determine her final neurologic outcome. Amy's age and general healthy status make it more likely that she would survive long-term with these impairments as long as she receives nutrition and hydration and adequate care to prevent contractures and pressure ulcers. Given that she has no evidence of brainstem or spinal cord injury, she is unlikely to need a ventilator for a long term.

In Case 2, Marge's brain injury seems less severe, and she is already showing evidence of awareness by regarding examiners. However, with bilateral frontal lobe infarctions, if she regains consciousness, she is likely to have severe apathy or abulia, or possibly akinetic mutism, even with treatment of hydrocephalus. Thus, she is unlikely to regain independent living status. She also is unlikely to require ventilator support long-term, and as long as she receives nutrition and hydration and adequate care to prevent contractures and pressure ulcers, she can survive for many years. Although Marge is older and potentially less resilient in regard to potential complications, she is not frail and could survive rehospitalization.

3. Do the patients have decision-making capacity?

Neither patient possesses decision-making capacity at this time. Neither patient is expected to regain decision-making capacity, as Amy's diffuse cerebral injury and Marge's bilateral frontal lobe injury would impair the ability to sustain attention and to make reasoned judgments. Nonetheless, because Marge in Case 2 may be slowly regaining consciousness, the physicians should attempt periodically to assess her capacity.

4. Are the patients' preferences known? Is there any doubt or disagreement? Are the families' preferences known? Is there any doubt or disagreement?

Bernat, 88–89, Ch. 4

In Case 1, Amy's preferences are unknown. She has no AD, and to the best of her family's knowledge, she has made no statements on which to base a decision with substituted judgment.[3] Here, her parents reach

Bernat, 89–90, Ch. 4

very different conclusions regarding their daughter's best interests.[4] Her father, noting her love of dancing and other activities, believes that she would find the burdens of survival too great and the benefits too small to continue treatment. Her mother, noting that her daughter established a specific career goal at an early age, believes that she would want to persevere and be an example for others.

Conversely, in Case 2, Marge's preferences are known. Although she does not have an AD, she informed her children when her husband died of a glioblastoma that she would never wish to live in such a condition.

Bernat, 88–9, Ch. 4

Their request to stop treatment is based on the substituted-judgment standard.[3] If any doubt exists, it is only to the extent of determining whether she meant specifically that she would not want to live with a glioblastoma or, more generally, that she would not want to live with severe neurologic impairment.

5. Do any issues of power or conflict in the interactions of the key actors in the cases need to be addressed?

In Case 1, the parents disagree as to the best course of action to take for their daughter. Because they have been designated surrogate by virtue of state statute and not by durable power of attorney (DPOA) for healthcare decisions, neither of them is the sole decision maker. Most, if not all, state laws indicate a hierarchy of surrogates based on their relationship to the patient. If 2 or more surrogates at the same rank disagree and if there are no surrogates above them in the hierarchy, as in Case 1, the law usually does not give preference to one surrogate over the other.[5] Many state laws include mechanisms such as ethics consultation to resolve such disputes.

In Case 2, no issues of power or conflict are apparent.

6. In the absence of an AD, does the law limit the decisions that a family can make for the patient?

Bernat 92–4, Ch. 4

As a general rule, when patients appoint a proxy decision maker with DPOA for healthcare decisions, the proxy has the same authority that the patient had before losing decision-making capacity.[6] Therefore, the proxy with DPOA can refuse any or all treatments under any circumstance, just as the patient could.

However, because neither patient in the cases presented has an AD or a proxy with DPOA for healthcare decisions, the state statute may limit the types of decisions the family can make. In a 2006 review of statutes in the United States and the District of Columbia on withdrawal of ANH for patients in persistent vegetative state (PVS), Larriviere and Bonnie found that in more than two-thirds of the states the statute was "permissive," meaning that

> the right to withhold or withdraw ANH in PVS cases is most clearly and fully articulated—through incorporation of the clinical diagnosis of PVS, through descriptions of a state of consciousness that incorporate that clinical diagnosis, or through a definition of terminal condition that clearly encompasses PVS.[7]

On the other hand, they found 12 states with "restrictive" statutes that ban withdrawal of ANH in all cases, require a specific directive or authorization to withdraw ANH, or restrict surrogate decision making.[7]

Considering that neither patient in the cases presented is currently diagnosed with PVS and that neither is in a condition that could be described as terminal or end-stage, it is likely that a decision to withdraw ANH may *not* be allowed by state statute. Less certain is whether state statutes would restrict the families' ability to limit or withhold other life-sustaining interventions such as shunt surgery, tracheostomy, ventilation, ICU admission, or CPR. Readers are advised to become familiar with the applicable statutes where they practice medicine and to consult with legal counsel.

MORAL DIAGNOSIS

7. **How are the moral problems in these cases being framed by the participants? Can or should this framing be reconsidered and replaced by an alternative understanding?**

Case 1 is framed as a traditional benefits-versus-burdens analysis by both parents; however, they perceive the context differently in trying to ascertain their daughter's best interests. The uncertainty of her prognosis, paired with the uncertainty or disagreement about her best interests, is ethically important because in circumstances of doubt, the value of life (i.e., continuing supportive treatments) is often given preference, as it provides the opportunity to reassess the patient's condition, response to treatment, and prognosis at a future time. Thus, the decision to continue treatment can be reconsidered and reversed, whereas the decision to withdraw treatment is irreversible once the patient has died. Even though the patient's father may raise concerns about the burden of suffering by his daughter in association with her survival, she currently shows no evidence of consciousness; and although she is capable of perceiving painful stimuli and making reflex responses, she is unlikely to have conscious cognitive or affective awareness of pain and is not currently capable of suffering.[8]

To the extent that they can, surrogate decision makers must strive to set aside their own desires when attempting to describe the patient's best interests. Care must be taken in Case 1 to explore whether Amy's father is expressing *his own* desire not to see his daughter survive with severe neurologic impairment, her mother is expressing *her own* desire to see Amy survive and become an example of survival and persistence for others, or whether each is making their best attempt to ascertain Amy's best interests. Input from other members of the family or from the patient's friends could be helpful.

A first step in attempting reconciliation between Amy's parents is to explore whether they would agree to limiting future escalation of her care, such as agreeing not to initiate resuscitation for cardiac arrest or not to admit her to an ICU in case of shock, respiratory failure, metabolic abnormalities, or other life-threatening complications. The success of this approach is very context-dependent and requires skilled conversation and negotiation by an experienced attending physician.

Case 2 is, on first pass, a straightforward request by the patient's family to stop treatment because the patient's goal of care, as determined by substituted judgment, is not to survive with severe neurologic impairment. The difficulty is that Marge is no longer comatose and has begun to show definite, though intermittent, evidence of conscious awareness by regarding examiners. Research in family decisions following cardiac arrest suggests that more than two-thirds of families will decide to withdraw life-sustaining treatment (LST) if the patient's neurologic examination deteriorates or does not improve;[9] less well understood is the process by which families may decide to withdraw LST after the patient has begun to improve but is not yet transferred from the ICU.

8. What ethical standards or guidelines exist?

Guidelines for surrogate decision making in the absence of an appointed proxy with DPOA have been published by the AMA[10] and the AAN[11] and are described in most state statutes.

9. What are the morally acceptable options for resolving the moral problems posed by the cases?

In Case 1, the preferences of either parent are morally acceptable. Withdrawal of LST, including ANH is ethically permissible, and continuation of therapy with administration of ANH is also ethically permissible. Because the case must be decided based on a best-interests standard, it would be challenging to say that one choice is more preferable over the other. The dilemma in the case revolves around the appropriate surrogate more than around the choice made by the surrogate.

Although the family in Case 2 is acting on the basis of respect for patient autonomy and undisputed substituted judgment, the ethical and legal conundrum is that Marge's condition no longer matches the criteria established in most state statutes to allow a surrogate without DPOA to withdraw ANH. What other options are available to them? Although the law may prohibit them from withdrawing ANH, it does not prohibit them from limiting further escalation of Marge's care. Her current condition might best be described as the minimally conscious state, which can be a transitional state in recovery of consciousness[12]; however, her recovery of consciousness is likely to be limited, or possibly reversed if the communicating hydrocephalus is not treated with a shunt. One option for the family, therefore, is to refuse shunt surgery, tracheostomy, resuscitation, or administration of antibiotics or other therapeutic interventions but to allow provision of ANH and interventions to prevent pain and discomfort. Such an approach would be a best attempt to respect the law and honor the patient's wishes, but the continuation of ANH means that the patient could survive for days, weeks, or even a few months before succumbing to complications.

GOAL SETTING, DECISION MAKING, IMPLEMENTATION

10. How can an ethics consultation be of benefit?

In Case 1, an ethics consultation will be highly beneficial. The parents hold opposite opinions regarding their daughter's best interests. In most states, the law will not permit physicians to withdraw LST and ANH if surrogates of the same ranking in the state hierarchy disagree. Therefore, an ethics consultation is the first step in helping the parents and the ICU team to clarify and understand the patient's current condition, range of potential outcomes with and without treatment, the likelihood of the potential outcomes with and without treatment, and the patient's wishes or best interests. Until the ethics consultation process is completed, the ICU team should continue to provide full support to the patient, although invasive interventions such as PEG or tracheostomy should be delayed until the completion of the ethics consultation as long as the delay poses no serious risk of harm. Should the ethics consultation process not resolve the dispute between the parents, then they would need to go to a court of law to have a judge appoint one of them as Amy's guardian.

Marge's family in Case 2 could request an ethics consultation, posing the question whether it is ethically permissible for them to withdraw LST and ANH based on their mother's wishes even though the law may prohibit them from doing so. In many states, the statute requires the family to seek guardianship and petition a court of law to withdraw ANH and LST when the patient's condition does not match the conditions listed in the statute (terminal condition, end-stage disease, PVS). The family would present the evidence of the patient's wishes to the judge.

Additionally, in most jurisdictions, the opinion of the ethics consultation team regarding the ethical permissibility of the family's request would be given serious consideration by the judge in deciding whether to allow the family's request.

11. Is judicial review needed?

In both cases, judicial review may be needed, but for very different reasons. In Case 1, judicial review may be indicated for Amy if (a) her parents cannot resolve their opposing views of her best interests and the treatment decision they think would be best for their daughter and (b) an ethics consultation process does not help them reach consensus. In fact, it is likely that even if the ethics consultation team were to favor one parent's decision over the other, the other parent would likely object and ask for a judicial order to prevent any action from being taken until the case could be presented to the court. One of the most famous examples of a family dispute over the patient's best interests is the case of Terri Schiavo, which fortunately, is an uncommon scenario.[13–15] A judge would be asked to appoint a guardian ad litem for Amy and to interpret the law in the context of the patient's diagnosis, condition, prognosis, and uncertain wishes. A likely outcome, though by no means a guaranteed outcome, is that the judge would interpret the law and the patient's unknown wishes to conclude that the value of life prevails and that she should receive ANH and other supportive treatments.[16]

In Case 2, the purpose of judicial review would be to petition the court to allow withdrawal of ANH based on Marge's prior statements and known wishes. Here, the court's decision would likely be influenced by the evidentiary standard indicated in the state law. In some states, the standard is strict, known as "clear and convincing," which was the case in the state of Missouri at the time of the Nancy Cruzan case[17]; however, variation in the evidentiary standard still exists among state statutes for withdrawing or withholding LST.[7]

EVALUATION

12. Would any changes in institutional policy or educational interventions help to prevent or resolve the moral problems posed by similar cases?

These cases represent rare but legitimate instances when end-of-life decisions for patients without decision-making capacity *and* without ADs may need judicial intervention. In Case 1, the nature of the conflict is such that an ethics consultation is likely to be called, and barring resolution of the parents' differences after the consultation, involvement of the courts is to be expected. Hospital ethics committees and hospital legal counsel are reasonably expected to know when and how to recommend involvement of the court and the appropriate restrictions on the treating team (e.g., life-sustaining interventions should not be withdrawn until the case is resolved and permission is given). In Case 2, agreement among the family with Marge's prior verbal statements gives the appearance of substituted judgment for withdrawing life-sustaining interventions; however, the details of the state law may or may not permit such action to be taken because the patient's current condition does not meet the criteria set forth in the law for taking such action. Education among neurology, neurosurgery, and ICU healthcare professionals regarding the limits of the law is warranted, as is a review of existing hospital policy.

KEY POINTS

- Most, if not all state laws indicate a hierarchy of surrogates, based on their relationship to the patient.
- State-to-state variation in laws concerning surrogate decision making and withdrawal of life-sustaining interventions may limit the types of decisions the family or surrogate decision maker can make in the absence of an AD.
- Variation in the evidentiary standard still exists among state statutes for withdrawing or withholding LST in the absence of an AD.
- Consultation with an ethics committee can provide guidance to family and physicians alike.
- Rare but legitimate circumstances exist in which end-of-life decisions for patients without decision-making capacity and without ADs may need judicial intervention.

KEY WORDS

Decision-making capacity—the capacity of individuals to make decisions on their own behalf while taking into consideration the potential benefits and burdens of the decision.

Surrogate decision maker—person authorized to make decisions for a patient who lacks decision-making capacity; the authority may be based on an AD or a statutory hierarchy.

REFERENCES

1. Pollack KM, Morhaim D, Williams MA. The public's perspectives on advance directives: Implications for state legislative and regulatory policy. Health Policy 2010; 96:57–63.
2. Torke AM, Sachs GA, Helft PR, et al. Timing of do-not-resuscitate orders for hospitalized older adults who require a surrogate decision-maker. J Am Geriatr Soc 2011; 59:1326–31.
3. Bernat, 88–9, Ch. 4.
4. Bernat, 89–90, Ch. 4.
5. Larriviere D, Williams MA. Ethical and legal considerations in neuroscience critical care. In: Torbey MT, ed., *Neurocritical Care*. Cambridge: Cambridge University Press, 2010:308–18.
6. Bernat, 92–4, Ch. 4.
7. Larriviere D, Bonnie RJ. Terminating artificial nutrition and hydration in persistent vegetative state patients: Current and proposed state laws. Neurology 2006; 66:1624–8.

8. Williams MA, Rushton CH. Justified use of painful stimuli in the coma examination: A neurologic and ethical rationale. Neurocritical Care 2009; 10:408–13.

9. Geocadin RG, Buitrago MM, Torbey MT, et al. Neurologic prognosis and withdrawal of life support after resuscitation from cardiac arrest. Neurology 2006; 67:105–8.

10. American Medical Association. Code of Medical Ethics. Opinion 8.081, Surrogate Decision Making. Available at www.ama-assn.org/ama/pub/physician-resources/medical-ethics/code-medical-ethics/opinion8081.page. Accessed March 25, 2012.

11. Bacon D, Williams MA, Gordon J. Position statement on laws and regulations concerning life-sustaining treatment, including artificial nutrition and hydration, for patients lacking decision-making capacity. Neurology 2007; 68:1097–100. [*PECN* document M available at www.aan.com/view/PECN]

12. Giacino JT, Ashwal S, Childs N, et al. The minimally conscious state: Definition and diagnostic criteria. Neurology 2002; 58(3):349–53.

13. Peck P. Latest right-to-die case revives old debate—and important lessons for neurologists. Neurology Today 2004; 4(1):1, 24, 27.

14. Shaw G. Schiavo's legislative legacy: New look at consent, living wills, and advance directives. Neurology Today 2005; 5(6):1, 14, 21, 22.

15. Gostin LO. Ethics, the constitution, and the dying process: The case of Theresa Marie Schiavo. JAMA 2005; 293(19):2403–7.

16. Meisel A, Snyder L, Quill T, et al. Seven legal barriers to end-of-life care: Myths, realities, and grains of truth. JAMA 2000; 284(19):2495–501.

17. Orentlicher D. From the Office of the General Counsel. The right to die after Cruzan. JAMA 1990; 264(18):2444–6.

21 PERSISTENT VEGETATIVE STATE

Dan Larriviere, MD, JD, FAAN

LEARNING OBJECTIVES

Upon completion of this chapter, participants will be able to:

1. Explain the following terms and concepts: vegetative state, persistent vegetative state, minimally conscious state, advance directive, durable power of attorney for healthcare decisions, and surrogate decision maker.
2. Describe the general hierarchy of decision-making authority outlined in state laws.
3. Discuss the various standards used by surrogate decision makers to reach conclusions about patients' preferences for medical care.

LEARNING RESOURCES

Key chapters in Bernat's third edition — 2, 4, 5, 7, 8, 12

Key relevant AAN documents available at www.aan.com/view/PECN

A   M   N   O

CLINICAL VIGNETTE

A 25-year-old woman sustained severe anoxic brain injury after cardiac arrest secondary to an underlying potassium deficiency. For the first week after the event, she was in an eyes-closed, unresponsive state (i.e., coma). Thereafter, she appeared to have sleep/wake cycles but was not responsive to verbal, written, or visual stimuli. She had no advance directive (AD), and her husband was her surrogate decision maker by virtue of state statute. She had a tracheostomy and percutaneous endoscopic gastrostomy (PEG) placement for artificial nutrition and hydration (ANH). She was transferred to a nursing home one month after the cardiac arrest.

Over the next several years, her condition has not changed, despite a variety of interventions (including coma-stimulation rehabilitation, deep-brain stimulation, amphetamines, and dopamine agonists) that her husband hoped would improve her condition. Every 3 months, the same neurologist has examined her for signs of conscious awareness and found none. In addition to her husband, the patient is visited by her parents, who believe that she responds to her mother's voice by smiling and visually tracking her face. The parents have admitted that these responses are intermittent and rare, but they firmly believe that they occur and represent more than solely reflexive behavior.

Ten years after the cardiac arrest and after no further change in the patient's condition, her husband requests that the ANH be stopped so that she may be allowed to die. He believes that there is little hope that her conscious awareness will be restored, and based on 2 conversations that he had with his wife in the past, he believes that she would no longer want to live this way. The first conversation occurred when they watched a movie in which one of the characters had severe head trauma that left him in a vegetative state, to which his wife said, "I wouldn't want to go on living if I were that bad off." The second conversation occurred when a relative died after having been in a coma for a week after an anoxic injury. At that time, his wife had said, "If I'm ever at a point where I don't know what's going on around me and I won't get any better, just let me go."

Her parents are upset and plead with their son-in-law to reconsider. They believe that she has awareness. Further, they say that their daughter was a strong adherent to the Roman Catholic belief of the sanctity of life and doubt that she would ever request withholding ANH because it would be tantamount to suicide. The patient's husband disagrees, and the parents file a motion for a court injunction to prevent removal of ANH until the court can hear the case and decide whether the husband's wishes or the wishes of the parents will be honored.

QUESTIONS FOR GROUP DISCUSSION

GETTING STARTED
1. What are the patient's medical condition and prognosis?
2. What are the treatment options for the patient's condition?
3. Is the patient capable of making decisions?
4. Who is the appropriate decision maker?
5. On what basis should the surrogate make decisions on behalf of the patient?
6. What are the patient's preferences?
7. What are the preferences of the patient's family or surrogate decision makers?

MORAL DIAGNOSIS
8. Should interests other than those of the patient be considered?

GOAL SETTING, DECISION MAKING, AND IMPLEMENTATION
9. What are the ethically acceptable treatment options?

EVALUATION
10. Would the presence of consciousness alter the analysis of the treatment options or the level of evidence required to support a decision?

COMMENTARY ON DISCUSSION QUESTIONS

GETTING STARTED

1. What are the patient's medical condition and prognosis?

Bernat, 287, Ch. 12

Disorders of consciousness vary in severity.[1] Patients who have suffered severe anoxic or traumatic brain injury may progress from a state of coma—manifested by eyes-closed unresponsiveness—to the vegetative state, and then to states with varying degrees of conscious awareness. Some patients suffer injury to only the descending pontine efferent pathways, resulting in awareness and an inability to move other than by vertical eye movements, a condition known as *the locked-in* state.[2,3]

Bernat, 290, Ch. 12

Bernat, 336, Ch. 13

The patient in this case has suffered a severe anoxic injury. To the best of her neurologist's ability to determine, she is not aware of herself or her surroundings, has no meaningful responses to stimuli, and has sleep-wake cycles, consistent with the *vegetative state* (VS), and because it has persisted for more than 3 months, can be considered the *persistent vegetative state* (PVS).[4,5] Patients in VS or PVS can exhibit a variety of behaviors—vocalizations, unsustained visual pursuit, and brief movements of head or eyes toward a sound or movement—that can make it difficult to determine whether the patient has conscious awareness.[6,7]

Bernat, 289, Ch. 12

Bernat, 289, Tables 1 and 2, Ch. 12

Sometimes patients with VS evolve to the *minimally conscious state* (MCS), which is determined by the presence of awareness of self or environment; however, the MCS can be very difficult to distinguish from VS by clinical examination.[8] MCS is defined as a condition of severely altered consciousness in which minimal but definite (reproducible, if only intermittently so) behavioral evidence of awareness of self or the environment is demonstrated.[8,9] Patients in MCS may be able to follow simple commands, provide yes/no answers to questions, make intelligible verbalizations, engage in appropriate behavior (such as smiling or crying), and exhibit reproducible visual pursuit of an object.[9]

Bernat, 290–1, Ch. 12

Bernat, 290–1, Ch. 12

When examining patients to ascertain evidence for awareness of self or environment, the physician should proceed carefully and systematically. A clinical assessment scale should be used to standardize the examinations across time. These patients should be examined in a distraction-free environment, and any sedative medications should be weaned at an appropriate interval prior to the examination. Commands to follow tasks should attempt to elicit responses that lie within patients' abilities. Elevating patients to a more vertical position can improve responsiveness.[10]

Bernat, 291–3, Ch. 12

The chief critique of the current method of assessing patients for evidence of awareness is that we must rely on objective evidence to support an inference of subjective phenomena, i.e., self-awareness or environmental awareness. Critics have pointed out that awareness of self or environment may exist in a patient who does not exhibit clinical evidence for it. For example, clinical audits in one study of patients diagnosed as being in a VS found a misdiagnosis rate as high as 43%. The rate of error was attributed in part to the reliance on an intact motor ability to signal awareness of self or environment.[11]

Furthermore, even when clinical evidence to support an inference of awareness exists, careless examiners may miss it.[12] Recent research supports this argument and has deepened our understanding of the anatomic basis of consciousness. In one line of research, Laureys and colleagues demonstrated that auditory, visual, and somatosensory stimuli can activate primary sensory areas of patients in VS but do not activate the secondary cortical areas and distributed cortical networks thought to be necessary for awareness.[13] However, functional neuroimaging in MCS patients has demonstrated cortical activation with intact distributed language networks to spoken voice. Owen and colleagues demonstrated compelling evidence of conscious awareness using fMRI techniques in a 23-year-old woman who had been diagnosed as being in a VS. Six months after the study, she began showing clinical signs of awareness.[14]

Functional imaging studies are beginning to provide support for the idea that the bedside neurologic examination may, at times, be an insensitive tool to determine awareness. As the presence of awareness has implications for recovery of function, the neurologic examination may also lead to declarations of prognosis that are inaccurate. Once fMRI stimulation techniques become standardized and validated, they

Bernat, 295, Ch. 12

will likely become important ancillary tests to determine the diagnosis and prognosis of this patient population;[15] however, as of 2012, they are still considered research tools.

Prognostic factors for patients in PVS have been reported, but they are subject to some limitations. First, the data come largely from retrospective rather than prospective studies. In many of these cases, the outcomes were not clearly described. Furthermore, many patients in these studies were provided with less-than-optimal medical treatment

Bernat, 297, Ch. 12

because they were thought to have poor prognosis. This is the fallacy of the so-called self-fulfilling prophecy.[16] The Multi-Society Task Force on PVS reported that PVS carried a 70% mortality at 3 years and an 84% mortality at 5 years.[17] The chief limitation with these numbers is that they represent an experiential history rather than a natural history of

Bernat, 297, Ch. 12

PVS because life-sustaining care was withheld or withdrawn from many of these patients.[16]

Some general rules about the prognosis of patients in PVS have been formulated:

Bernat, 297, Ch. 12

1. After 1 year, recovery of awareness from traumatic PVS is rare.[16]
2. Recovery of awareness after nontraumatic (cardiopulmonary arrest, stroke) VS is rare after 3 months and *very* rare after 1 year.[16]

3. Most PVS patients recovering awareness after 6 months in traumatic PVS or after 3 months in nontraumatic PVS survive with severe disability with tetraparesis, pseudobulbar palsy, and dementia, and are incapable of independent living.[4]

The patient in the case presented has been in PVS for many years. Thus, it is extremely unlikely that she will ever regain consciousness. However, given the limitations of the bedside clinical examination to distinguish between VS and MCS, if a facility were located that was willing to conduct fMRI studies to assess for unrecognized cortical function, they might ask the attending physician to assist with a transfer of the patient. Before doing so, the attending physician should discuss the goals of care and how they relate to what the family hopes to achieve by performing the study, for even if cortical activity is found by imaging, it is highly unlikely that it has any bearing on future outcomes so long after the inciting event. In addition, even if cortical activity is found and even if one concedes the possibility that, therefore, potential for clinical improvement exists, the family would still be ethically bound by the wishes of the patient concerning additional medical treatment.

2. What are the treatment options for the patient's condition?

Patients in VS require comprehensive, holistic, and well-orchestrated medical and nursing care. Nutrition and hydration must be supplied via PEG. Most patients in VS are not ventilator dependent, and many eventually have their tracheostomy tubes removed. Some require long-term tracheostomy and are at risk for pulmonary infections. Skin breakdown is a constant risk, and frequent turning and changes of position are necessary. Passive range-of-motion exercises are necessary to prevent contractures.

Treatment with electrical or pharmacologic stimulation in an attempt to improve responsiveness may be considered for some patients. Only a few small studies have been conducted to date; therefore, these interventions should be considered investigational and not a standard of care. Studies of deep-brain stimulation of the thalamus, mesencephalic reticular formation, and the intralaminar nuclei have demonstrated variable results, making it difficult to judge efficacy of the intervention.[4] Pharmacologic interventions such as levodopa, amantadine, amphetamines, tricyclic antidepressants, bromocriptine, and anticonvulsants are unproven.[18]

Bernat, 298, Ch. 12

Although the medical care of the patient in this case is important, it is equally important to respect her prior wishes about the nature of the treatment that she would have wanted. In the United States, patients have a constitutional right to refuse medical treatment, including life-sustaining treatment (LST).[19,20]

Bernat, 301, Ch. 12

In this case, the patient had stated that she would not want medical care if she were unlikely to recover consciousness, which is extremely unlikely after 10 years. Thus, it is ethically permissible to respect her husband's instructions to withdraw ANH.

3. Is the patient capable of making decisions?

Decisional capacity refers to a patient's ability to consider relevant factors to arrive at and communicate a choice that is individually appropriate. "Capacity" is a *medical* term that refers to a clinical judgment concerning a patient's ability to make decisions, whereas "competency" is a *legal* determination by a court based on an assessment of a person's general ability to engage in transactions of daily living (e.g., forming contracts, making wills, etc.). Although capacity and competency often parallel each other, it is possible that a person with capacity for certain healthcare decisions could nonetheless be found incompetent by a court of law.

Decisional capacity is defined and assessed clinically. Patients must be able to understand information that is relevant to a decision, communicate a choice, and appreciate the nature of their situation and the consequences of their choices.[21] Special provisions should be made for patients with limited ability to communicate, e.g., eye-movement-tracking computers for patients in a locked-in state. Also, considering that level of consciousness can fluctuate (i.e., MCS), patients should be assessed at varying times of the day.

In the case presented, the patient has no clinical evidence of consciousness. By definition, she cannot possess decision-making capacity.

4. Who is the appropriate decision maker?

Almost all states allow patients to select a *proxy* to make healthcare decisions on their behalf by creating a durable power of attorney (DPOA) for healthcare decisions. Note that DPOA is not the *proxy*, but rather represents the legal authority of a proxy to make healthcare decisions for the person who wrote the DPOA. The DPOA is often a part of an AD, which is a legal document that expresses a patient's wishes to be honored should the patient become unable to express those wishes. The DPOA and the AD can each exist alone and be valid, or they can exist together. The scope of authority given to a proxy with DPOA is determined by the document. Most DPOAs give a proxy the power to make the same range of decisions that the patient could make. However, the decision-making authority of the proxy could be limited by the document; thus, the DPOA document should always be reviewed. Unless the document states otherwise, the authority of the DPOA supersedes that of all other decision makers, including spouses and blood relatives. A proxy may be verbally designated, provided that the designation is witnessed by someone other than the designee.

For patients who have not appointed a proxy with a DPOA, most state laws specify the surrogate who is to make healthcare decisions. In general, these laws designate a hierarchy based upon the surrogate's relationship to the patient. Physicians should be familiar with the laws in the states in which they practice. The usual order for selecting a surrogate is:

1. Spouse
2. Children of the patient who are above the age of majority
3. Parents of the patient
4. Adult siblings of the patient
5. Other relatives[22]

These statutes allow patients' families and the healthcare team to make decisions about medical care without going to court to obtain permission to do so.

In the absence of a DPOA, some, but not all, states recognize a same-sex domestic partner as a surrogate decision maker. Not all states recognize common-law marriage; therefore, a "common-law spouse" may not be recognized by the statute. Some states allow close friends who are not related to the patient but who may otherwise know the patient's preferences to serve as surrogate when no other persons are available or willing, provided that they sign an affidavit. In general, the law designates the person with the highest position in the hierarchy as the surrogate, provided that that person is willing to fulfill the responsibilities of that role and has decision-making capacity.

Some patients are *unbefriended*, meaning that they do not have identifiable or available family or friends to make medical decisions on their behalf. In such cases, the healthcare team must seek court appointment of a guardian *ad litem* for the patient because elective procedures such as tracheostomy or PEG do not qualify for implied consent in emergency circumstances. In some cases, because the legal process may extend beyond the time when decisions have to be made, the treating physician will assume the role of the decision maker,[23] a situation that is fraught with ethical, moral, and legal conflicts and one that is not recommended, except with the advice of hospital counsel, or ethics committee, or both. Some states, recognizing the limitations of current laws in this area, have passed legislation to assist healthcare providers in identifying alternate decision makers, such as the hospital ethics committee.[24]

In the case presented, the patient has no AD and has not assigned DPOA to anyone; therefore, the statutory hierarchy determines the appropriate decision maker. Absent a legal guardian appointed by a court, the husband is the surrogate decision maker.

5. On what basis should the surrogate make decisions on behalf of the patient?

The surrogate should adhere to treatment preferences outlined in an AD if one exists. Almost all states have laws concerning the conditions in which an AD applies and the treatment decisions allowed.[24] Most states limit the application of ADs to patients in VS, "irreversible condition," and "terminal condition," although the terminology in the statutes varies. In almost all states, patients may either refuse or request CPR and ventilation via their AD. Patients may request ANH. Most states allow patients to refuse ANH via an AD when their condition is "irreversible," "terminal," or "PVS." A few states restrict the withdrawal of ANH if the patient made no such request in an AD, and some states prohibit the withdrawal of ANH in all cases.[24]

For patients who lack ADs, surrogates should seek to make decisions that are consistent with the patient's previously stated wishes, if known. If such wishes are unknown, then the *substituted-judgment standard* should be used, in which the decision maker attempts to integrate the patient's known personal values, moral and religious preferences, and prior conversations to determine what the patient would have wanted.

If this information is unknown, the surrogate should use the *best-interest standard*, taking into account factors such as diagnosis, prognosis, risks, and benefits of the proposed treatment or intervention, and the degree of discomfort experienced by the patient. The best-interest standard can be difficult to apply because some would justify withdrawal of LST if the patient's survival would be associated with pain or other burdens, whereas others may argue that it is always in a patient's best interests to remain alive.

6. What are the patient's preferences?

The patient did not have an AD; however, her husband says that she made 2 prior statements that support his decision. In both, she indicated that she would not want to live if she were unable to interact with her environment and if she were unlikely to get any better. After 10 years, there is little reason to believe that her condition will ever improve. Her husband feels that his decision is consistent with her previously expressed wish and with her prognosis. Her parents contend that, as a Catholic, the patient would value life, regardless of how limited it might be, and as such, she would want her treatment to continue. However, the parents are unable to produce any evidence that the patient had ever voiced support of this idea. On balance, then, the weight of the evidence concerning the patient's stated preferences appears to support refusal of further care.

7. What are the preferences of the patient's family or surrogate decision makers?

The patient's parents oppose the husband's decision—in part because they believe that their daughter's religious faith tradition would prohibit withdrawal of LST. Thus, family members are in disagreement, which is not a rare occurrence. Although the healthcare team should strive for consensus within the family, not all disputes can be resolved. When one and only one surrogate of the highest rank is involved (according to state statute), the surrogate's decisions are controlling. However, when substantial disagreement exists within the family, the healthcare team should be cautious about implementing irreversible decisions, such as withdrawal of LST, before attempting to arrive at a consensus. Ethics consultations are usually sought at this point.

If consensus cannot be reached, ultimately, the decision of the highest-ranking surrogate should be honored. Family members who disagree must usually seek an injunction from a court to postpone implementation of decisions that have irreversible consequences, pending resolution of the dispute. When it becomes clear that litigation is forthcoming, the physician should seek assistance of hospital counsel and consider an ethics consult, if available. An ethics consult has several advantages under these circumstances. First, bringing in a neutral third party to hear both sides of the situation may help the parties view the facts from a different point of view and potentially be more willing to concede when it appears that they should do so. Second, if, as is likely in the present case, the ethics consultant agrees with the position of the healthcare team, another basis of support for their actions will be in the medical record. Finally, when conflicts exist among decision makers, some states (e.g., Maryland) protect physicians from claims that involve lack of informed consent or authorization if the physician acts in accordance with the decision of the ethics committee consultation.[25,26]

MORAL DIAGNOSIS

8. Should interests other than those of the patient be considered?

Although courts have uniformly upheld a patient's right to refuse LST, they have also allowed states to have requirements for the burden of proof necessary before a court will allow LST to be withdrawn. The US Supreme Court in the 1990 Cruzan decision found that the state of Missouri's requirement of "clear and convincing evidence" that the patient would want ANH withheld was constitutional because it did not violate the due process clause of the US Constitution.[27]

Thus, although the US Supreme Court recognized the right of individuals to forgo LST, it also recognized the right of states to restrict the exercise of that right. Physicians who care for patients in VS or MCS should be familiar with the laws of the state in which they practice. In cases in which a surrogate seeks to withdraw LST for a patient whose condition is not terminal, it is prudent to consult the hospital ethics committee.[28]

Bernat, 302–3, Ch. 12

Although the level of evidence to support a decision must always be critically evaluated, it is especially important to do so when family members are in dispute with each other or with the treating physician. In most cases in which the surrogate decision maker and the treating physician agree that withdrawing or withholding of LST is what the patient would have wanted, the level of evidence is rarely questioned.

However, this is not to imply, that mere agreement between the physician and surrogate allows them to make decisions that are contrary to the patient's wishes or are otherwise ethically impermissible or illegal.

GOAL SETTING, DECISION MAKING, AND IMPLEMENTATION

9. What are the ethically acceptable treatment options?

In the present case, the only ethically acceptable treatment option is to withdraw LST at the request of the patient's surrogate decision maker. Although doing so will result in the patient's death, it is consistent with prior statements made to her husband that she would not want such treatment, even if not having the therapy meant that she would die.

The practice of withdrawal of LST is considered ethically permissible within the medical profession. Professional societies such as the AAN[29] and the Society of Critical Care Medicine and American College of Chest Physicians[30] have recognized the right of patients in specific situations to forgo treatment, even if refusal may lead to death.

Continuing treatment in this case, as the patient's parents wish, would probably not result in additional suffering for the patient herself, as she is in a VS and unable to experience suffering or anguish. However, continued treatment would violate her right to refuse treatment.

EVALUATION

10. Would the presence of consciousness alter the analysis of the treatment options or the level of evidence required to support a decision?

The State of California addressed this question in the case of Conservatorship of Wendland.[31] Robert Wendland had a traumatic brain injury that left him in an MCS. His wife petitioned to have his feeding tube removed to comply with his prior statements that he would not want to live "like a vegetable." His mother opposed the action and filed the lawsuit. The California Supreme Court ruled against the wife, citing the requirement that "clear and convincing" evidence be presented about a conscious patient's wishes before LST can be withheld. The court justified its approach using 2 lines of reasoning:

a. When the consequences of an erroneous determination are particularly serious (as in the case of withdrawal of LST), it is appropriate to set the standard of proof fairly high to adjust the risk of error to favor the less perilous result. The court went on to declare that the risk of an erroneous decision to continue treatment, while potentially harmful to the patient (in terms of violating his right to refuse treatment, prolonging suffering, etc.), was at least reversible if new or better evidence came to light. The decision to withhold treatment, resulting in the death of the patient, is irreversible.[32]

b. Because the decision to withhold LST would result in the death of the patient, the patient's constitutional right to privacy was implicated. As such, if the court did not place a sufficiently rigorous evidentiary burden on the limitation of that right, the statute might be found to be unconstitutional.[33]

Although one could understand the court's reasons for invoking a rigorous burden of proof before LST could be withdrawn, it is not clear why the presence or absence of consciousness had any bearing on the level of proof required, unless there was also evidence that the presence of consciousness implied a different prognosis (which was not the case). Further, although other states have required that "clear and convincing evidence" be presented of a patient's wishes to withdraw LST, they have deemed less compelling evidence to be sufficient than was presented in the Wendland case. Clearly, one of the (erroneous) concerns expressed by the justices was the potential suffering of the conscious patient if food and hydration were withheld. More compelling, however, is the degree of ongoing suffering that the conscious patient could experience by being kept alive against his wishes.[34]

Bernat, 304–5, Ch. 12

KEY POINTS

- A few states restrict the withdrawal of ANH if the patient made no such request in an AD, and some states prohibit the withdrawal of ANH in all cases.
- The usual order for selecting a surrogate is (1) spouse, (2) children of the patient who are above the age of majority, (3) parents of the patient, (4) adult siblings of the patient, (5) other relatives.
- Because of considerable variability in the law from state to state, physicians should be familiar with the laws in the state in which they practice when helping families decide whether to withdraw ANH for patients in PVS or MCS.

KEY WORDS

Minimally conscious state—determined by the presence of awareness of self or environment; however, the MCS can be very difficult to distinguish from VS by clinical examination. MCS is defined as a condition of severely altered consciousness in which minimal but definite (reproducible, if only intermittently so) behavioral evidence of awareness of self or the environment is demonstrated.

Persistent vegetative state—state reached when the vegetative state becomes a chronic stable disorder, generally defined as after 3 months.

Surrogate decision maker—person authorized to make decisions for a patient who lacks decision-making capacity; the authority may be based on an AD or a statutory hierarchy

Vegetative state—a disorder of consciousness that is reached after one suffers a pathologic process that produces widespread dysfunction of cerebral cortical neurons, thalamic neurons, or the white matter connections between the cortex and thalamus, but that largely spares brainstem and hypothalamic neurons.

REFERENCES

1. Bernat, 287, Ch. 12.
2. Bernat, 290, Ch. 12.
3. Bernat, 336, Ch. 13.
4. Multi-Society Task Force on PVS. Medical aspects of the persistent vegetative state. Parts I and II. N Engl J Med 1994; 330(21–22):1499–579.
5. Bernat, 289, Ch. 12.
6. Bernat JL. Chronic disorders of consciousness. Lancet 2006; 367:1181–92.
7. Bernat, 289, Tables 1 and 2, Ch. 12.
8. Giacino JT, Ashwal S, Childs N, et al. The minimally conscious state: Definition and diagnostic criteria. The Aspen Neurobehavioral Conference Consensus Statement. Neurology 2002; 58:349–53.
9. Bernat, 290–1, Ch. 12.
10. Bernat, 291–3, Ch. 12.
11. Andrews K, Murphy L, Munday R, et al. Misdiagnosis of the vegetative state: Retrospective study in a rehabilitation unit. Br Med J 1996; 313:13–6.
12. Childs NL, Mercer WN, Childs HW. Accuracy of diagnosis of persistent vegetative state. Neurology 1993; 43:1465–7.
13. Laureys S, Owen AM, Schiff ND. Brain function in coma, vegetative state, and related disorders. Lancet Neurology 2004; 3:537–46.
14. Owen AM, Coleman MR, Boly M, et al. Detecting awareness in the vegetative state. Science 2006; 313:1402.
15. Bernat, 295, Ch. 12.
16. Bernat, 297, Ch. 12.
17. Ashwal S, Cranford R. Medical aspects of the persistent vegetative state—a correction. N Engl J Med 1995; 333(2):130.
18. Bernat, 298, Ch. 12.
19. Bernat, 301, Ch. 12.
20. Matter of Quinlan, 70 NJ 10, 355 A.2d 647 NJ (1976).
21. Applebaum PS, Grisso T. Assessing the patient's capacities to consent to treatment. N Engl J Med 1988; 319:1635–8.
22. See, for example, Virginia Healthcare Decisions Act, Ch 29., Sec 54.1-2982 et seq.
23. Kushel MB, Miaskowski C. End-of-life care for homeless patients: "She says she is there to help me in any situation." JAMA 2006; 296:2959–66.
24. Larriviere D, Bonnie RJ. Terminating artificial nutrition and hydration in persistent vegetative state patients: Current and proposed state laws. Neurology 2006; 66:1624–8.
25. Maryland Health Care Decisions Act. Part I. Advance Directives. § 5-609. Immunity from liability; burden of proof; presumption. Available at www.oag.state.md.us/Healthpol/HCDA.pdf. Accessed March 25, 2012.
26. 2010 Maryland Code. Health–General. Title 19, Health Care Facilities. Subtitle 3—Hospitals and Related Institutions. Part IX. Patient Care Advisory Committees. Available at http://law.justia.com/codes/maryland/2010/health-general/title-19/subtitle-3/. Accessed March 26, 2012.
27. Cruzan v. Director, Missouri Dept of Health, 497 US 261 (1990).
28. Bernat, 302–3, Ch. 12.

29. Position of the American Academy of Neurology on certain aspects of the care and management of the persistent vegetative state patient. Neurology 1989; 39(1):125–6. [*PECN* document N available at www.aan.com/view/PECN]
30. Ethical and moral guidelines for the initiation, continuation and withdrawal of intensive care. American College of Chest Physicians/Society of Critical Care Consensus Panel. Chest 1990; 97(4):949–58.
31. 28 P3d 151 (Cal. 2001).
32. 28 P3d 169 (Cal. 2001).
33. 28 P3d 169–170 (Cal. 2001).
34. Bernat, 304–5, Ch. 12.

22

END-OF-LIFE CARE FOR THE NEUROLOGICALLY IMPAIRED CHILD

Patricia Evans, MD, FAAN, FAAP

LEARNING OBJECTIVES

Upon completion of this chapter, the participants will be able to:

1. Describe the ethical issues unique to children and end-of-life decision making.
2. Discuss the differences between palliative care and end-of-life discussions.
3. Explain and incorporate into practice the early involvement of palliative care teams for children with chronic, progressive diseases.

LEARNING RESOURCES

Key chapters in Bernat's third edition—7, 8
Key relevant AAN documents available at www.aan.com/view/PECN

O

CLINICAL VIGNETTES

CASE 1

Cassie, a 2-year-old girl with severe cerebral palsy, has developed increasingly hard to control seizures in the past year. She has never been able to speak or walk, and the family has been exceptionally involved in her care and compliant with her care plan, which includes 4 antiepileptic medications and a vagal nerve stimulator. She has a percutaneous gastrostomy for her medications, fluids, and nutrition. She has been hospitalized several times with status epilepticus, each time incurring additional cerebral injury that both worsens the epilepsy and causes worsening neurologic functioning. During her last hospitalization, she received a tracheostomy, which she still has for pulmonary toilet, but she no longer requires ventilatory support. At today's visit, she does not appear to interact with examiners, as she has before. The clinic nurse asks the neurologist whether it is time to begin discussing resuscitation status and palliative care with her parents.

CASE 2

Joshua is a 15-year-old adolescent man with type 2 spinal muscular atrophy (SMA). He long ago lost the ability to sit independently and, for the last 5 years, has been on daytime and nighttime noninvasive continuous ventilation. However, in the last 6 months, his capacity to swallow, cough, and clear secretions has deteriorated. He has had pneumonia several times in the last few months. He and his family would like to review their options, including the use of a tracheotomy or to continue noninvasive ventilation as a palliative care measure.

QUESTIONS FOR GROUP DISCUSSION

GETTING STARTED
1. Have you been in the position of talking to the parents of a child with progressive neurologic illness about planning for the possibility of their child's death?

ASSESSMENT
2. Compare and contrast the cases. What are the key contextual differences?
3. How do discussions about palliative care, dying, or death in *children* with progressive illness differ from discussions about the same issues in *adults* with progressive illness?
4. Should the neurologist respond to the request of the teenager with SMA to discuss treatment options, including palliative care?

MORAL DIAGNOSIS
5. What guidelines exist for incorporating palliative care into the treatment plan for children with chronic neurologic disorders?

GOAL SETTING, DECISION MAKING, AND IMPLEMENTATION
6. What are the advantages of involving a palliative care team in the care of each of these children?
7. If the parents of the child with SMA ask the neurologist to attend the child's funeral, how could the neurologist respond? How could the response influence the parents' bereavement?

COMMENTARY ON DISCUSSION QUESTIONS

GETTING STARTED

1. Have you been in the position of talking to the parents of a child with progressive neurologic illness about planning for the possibility of their child's death?

Of the nearly 900,000 deaths that occurred during infancy, childhood, or adolescence in the United States between 1989 and 2003, 22% were attributed primarily to an underlying complex chronic condition. Well over half of these children were younger than 1 year of age. Further, more than 80% died in a hospital setting rather than at home. It follows, then, that although the individual conditions may be rare, death in children with progressive illness is not rare.[1]

It is intellectually and emotionally challenging for physicians to help parents anticipate their child's death. Physicians report various reactions to the death of a child, including self-doubt, shock, and bereavement, which may be particularly difficult for doctors who are also parents of young children.[2] One cross-sectional study using both quantitative and qualitative data found that those physicians who spend a longer time caring for their patients benefit from knowing their patients better but then have the subsequent risk of being more vulnerable to emotional distress at the time of the patient's death.[3] Particularly stressful in junior faculty and housestaff, grieving at the loss of a patient requires sensitivity on the part of the entire medical team.[4]

Although the number of formal palliative care training programs has increased over the last decade, the number of pediatric palliative care programs remains small. Well over half of American-trained and a quarter of Canadian-trained pediatric residents and fellows participate in formal palliative care training.[1,5,6] Such training has been repeatedly shown to markedly improve the quality of life and care that children receive in the final stages of illness prior to death.[1,5–10] Nevertheless, many children who would benefit from palliative care do not have access to it.

Bernat,
399–400,
Ch. 16

Bernat,
394–6,
Ch. 16

ASSESSMENT

2. **Compare and contrast the cases. What are the key contextual differences?**

In Case 1, Cassie's progressive seizures and severe neurologic impairment have progressed to the point that her death can be anticipated. Although her death is not imminent, it can be anticipated because of the progressive worsening of her health status with each hospitalization. Because of her age and cognitive impairment, her parents must make decisions for her. Although the topic can be difficult to broach, it is better to begin discussion of palliative care when her health status is stable, as opposed to waiting until she is ill and hospitalized again. By contrast, in Case 2, an intellectually normal teenager with progressive muscular dystrophy and multiple experiences with hospitalization is now beginning to contemplate whether he should live with a ventilator. The increasing difficulty that he is experiencing in secretion clearing and swallowing, as well as his inability to sit, may play a part in his and his family's decision making.

End-of-life decisions in children may provoke strong emotions and can be complicated by disagreements between family members, the medical team, hospital administrators, and legal representatives. The guiding principle is to advocate always on behalf of the child. For the young child whose wishes cannot be known, the best-interests standard applies,[11–14] as it refers to decision making when it is not

Bernat,
89–90,
Ch. 4

Bernat,
181–97,
Ch. 8

possible to know what a patient's wishes would be. Parents have a critically important role in decision making, which must be respected. However, because the doctor's first responsibility is to the patient, she is not obligated to provide needless treatment or to withhold beneficial treatment at the request of the parents.[4] The wishes of an older child or adolescent, when known, should be respected, with sensitivity given to each child's level of understanding, maturity, and insight.[15]

3. **How do discussions about palliative care, dying, or death in *children* with progressive illness differ from discussions about the same issues in *adults* with progressive illness?**

Bernat, 394–6, Ch. 16

Bernat, 159–60, Ch. 7

A longstanding sentiment is that parents should not outlive their children. As a result, the tendency in Western medicine is to be more aggressive in the care of children with a progressive illness and less aggressive in the care of adults, particularly more senior adults.[7,11,12,16–18]

Bernat, 1–23, Ch. 1

Key ethical concerns include the importance of recognizing parents as the legal decision makers on behalf of children under the age of 18 years.[7,19] Without evidence to the contrary, the presumption is that parents act in the best interests of their children.[1,20] Engaging the child herself in discussions of her illness and in those areas in which she can participate is very important. Although a young child may not have the capacity, e.g., to participate in discussions of medications, she may have a preference for which hand is used for an IV. Adjusting the level of discussion to the developmental age of the patient is an important part of ongoing care and communication for the child and the medical team.[7,16,21,22]

Bernat, 159–60, Ch. 7

4. **Should the neurologist respond to the request of the teenager with SMA to discuss treatment options, including palliative care?**

Pediatric patients have keen insight and understanding about their chronic conditions and may know more about the rigors and details of the therapies and treatment far better than the adults in their lives may know.[23] Pediatric patients have important input to add to treatment decisions, even if they do not fully understand the rationale for the medical treatment in question. Therefore, practicing tolerance for the inclusion of a child's or teen's thoughts and understanding of the process is important.[12,23–26]

Bernat, 394–6, Ch. 16

Bernat, 159–60, Ch. 7

Bernat, 1–23, Ch. 1

When considering the use of palliative care, it is important to avoid assumptions about the respective illness or its outcome prior to moving forward.[7,16,19,21,27] First, some parents and physicians may believe that life can be prolonged indefinitely in children with neuromuscular disease who are treated with technologic therapies such as noninvasive ventilation, making palliative care unnecessary.[28] However, ventilation does not extend life indefinitely for patients with neuromuscular diseases; to the contrary, noninvasive ventilation is not curative, as patients are also vulnerable to causes of death untreatable by assisted ventilation, such as progressive cardiomyopathy or catastrophic mucus plugging of the airway.[28] The Consensus Statement for Standard of Care in Spinal Muscular Atrophy recommends that clinicians and families be mindful of the potential conflict in treatment goals (palliative vs. curative) and indicates that clinicians have "a deep responsibility to present care options in an open, fair, and balanced manner."[29]

MORAL DIAGNOSIS

5. **What guidelines exist for incorporating palliative care into the treatment plan for children with chronic neurologic disorders?**

The World Health Organization provides a widely accepted definition of palliative care, attributes of which are shown in Box 22-1.[30] Palliative care is an approach that improves the quality of life of patients and their families who are facing the problems associated with life-threatening illness. It accomplishes this through the prevention and relief of suffering by means of early identification and impeccable assessment and treatment of pain and other problems—physical, psychosocial, and spiritual.[30]

BOX 22-1

World Health Organization Attributes of Palliative Care

- Provides relief from pain and other distressing symptoms.
- Affirms life and regards dying as a normal process.
- Intends to neither hasten nor postpone death.
- Integrates the psychological and spiritual aspects of patient care.
- Offers a support system to help patients live as actively as possible until death.
- Offers a support system to help a family cope during the patient's illness and in their own bereavement.
- Uses a team approach to address the needs of patients and their families, including bereavement counseling, if indicated.
- Enhances quality of life and may positively influence the course of illness.
- Is applicable early in the course of illness, in conjunction with other therapies that are intended to prolong life, such as chemotherapy or radiation therapy, and includes those investigations needed to better understand and manage distressing clinical complications.

WHO Definition of Palliative Care. Available at www.who.int/cancer/palliative/definition/en/. Accessed March 14, 2012.[30]

The American Academy of Pediatrics (AAP) endorses incorporation of palliative care for children who are dying or are at risk of dying.[11] Recognizing that palliative care for children and adults differs in some respects, the World Health Organization has a separate definition of palliative care for children:

- Palliative care for children is the active total care of the child's body and mind and involves giving support to the family.
- It begins when illness is diagnosed and continues, regardless of whether a child receives treatment directed at the disease.
- Health providers must evaluate and alleviate a child's physical, psychological, and social distress.
- Effective palliative care requires a broad multidisciplinary approach that includes the family and makes use of available community resources.
- Palliative care can be provided in tertiary care facilities, in community health centers, and even in children's homes.[30]

Specific to children with SMA, the 2007 Consensus Statement for Standard of Care in Spinal Muscular Atrophy recognizes that each case must be considered individually, that the goals of care may be difficult to clarify because the goals of quality of life and duration of life may be in conflict, and that some interventions that prolong life may also prolong suffering without reducing the burden of the disease.[29]

The discussion of palliative care with the parents of the child in Case 1 will have to broach the topic of either continuing or stopping artificial nutrition and hydration via the feeding tube. The AAP finds that "the provision of medically provided fluids and nutrition is morally optional if it does not provide a net benefit to the child."[31] At the same time, the symbolic importance of feeding and the values possessed by individual families mean that some families may wish to continue artificial nutrition and hydration, while others may not. The AAP finds that parents should be allowed discretion to make this decision and recommends that the wishes of parents to continue artificial nutrition and hydration for ethical, religious, cultural, or medical reasons should be honored.

GOAL SETTING, DECISION MAKING, AND IMPLEMENTATION

6. **What are the advantages of involving a palliative care team in the care of each of these children?**

Palliative care teams counsel, provide disease-specific information, and arrange hospice care, respite care, and other support. Parents of a terminally ill child face many emotional, physical, financial, and spiritual challenges and fatigue.[12] When palliative care teams are present, families typically report that every aspect of care appears improved, including better communication among family and medical team members, better understanding about respite care, and better understanding about the specific illness or trauma in question. All respondents mentioned that the presence of a palliative care team was important for family members as they grieved the loss of their child.[12] The AAP provides guidelines on developing palliative care teams, with the stated goal that the team is available to add quality of life to each child's remaining quantity of life, however long or short the time may be.[11]

Sadly, the ability to obtain either healthcare or palliative care when needed is often linked to economic status and race.[32] Children from poor families are at higher risk for having severe chronic conditions, being uninsured, and lacking a usual source of care.[33–38] This inaccessibility extends to palliative and end-of-life care, with the end result being that patients from families with economic hardship are less likely to die at home with less access to palliative care, either in the hospital or at home.[32] Minority patients in particular have limited access to pain management, a critical component of palliative care.[32]

Although the level of pain among seriously ill inpatients does not vary according to race, minority patients with cancer pain are less likely to receive adequate pain management in nursing-home and outpatient settings. Research has shown that although pain from terminal cancer is experienced similarly regardless of race or socioeconomic class, minority patients not infrequently are treated less aggressively for their pain needs in institutional settings than are non-minority patients.[32,39,40] These trends are also well documented outside the United States. Of 24 European countries, pediatric palliative care may be described as being well developed only in the United Kingdom.[41] According to a 2007 study, only 12% of terminally ill children in Canada receive support from palliative care programs.[6]

7. If the parents of the child with SMA ask the neurologist to attend the child's funeral, how could the neurologist respond? How could the response influence the parents' bereavement?

Efforts to support families after a child's death can vary, but typically most efforts are appreciated by families. Studies have shown that families place great importance on the presence of physicians and staff at memorial services for recently deceased children for whom the teams have cared. Additionally, parents typically express appreciation for cards, phone calls, and attendance at a funeral service.[42–45] Such studies also underscore how the involvement of the team at the time of a child's death can provide important elements of comfort and closure to a grieving family. Indeed, the team's participation in memorial services, sending cards, and making calls can be important both for the child's family and for the team members as they work through feelings of loss that they may have.[32]

TOPICAL SYNOPSIS

End-of-life decision making in children requires different considerations than it does in adults. Decisions for children, who are considered never-competent (that is, not ever comprehending or articulating their thoughts and wishes regarding end-of-life issues), should be made with the best-interest standard. Older children who can make their wishes known and may be considered mature minors can be involved in their own decisions. Children with terminal illness and their families benefit greatly when a well-trained multidisciplinary palliative care team is involved. In all cases, the medical team is the most effective when it is prepared to spend sufficient time simply listening to a families' needs and wishes, and being empathetic to the wide range of issues that living with a terminally ill child can present.

KEY POINTS

- When possible, children or adolescents should be encouraged to provide their preferences to treatment options.
- *Palliative care* and *end-of-life discussions* are separate concepts. Palliative care refers to implementation of comfort rather than curative measures, regardless of how long an individual may have prior to death. By contrast, end-of-life discussions are usually centered on where and how an individual wishes to die.
- Families appreciate the involvement of staff members in memorials for their children and typically express sadness if medical team members are not present at memorial services or other forms of remembrances.

KEY WORDS

Best-interests standard—a standard for surrogate decision making that asks how a reasonable person would balance the anticipated burdens borne as a result of a proposed course of treatment against the benefits that accrue from it. As infants and young children fall into the category of "never-competent," in the sense that they are not able to make their wishes known, parents and/or surrogate decision makers must act on behalf of the child's best interest.

Cerebral palsy—a group of disorders that are characterized by being nonprogressive, noncontagious motor conditions that cause physical disability. Severity may range from being very mild to being severe enough to be an indirect cause of death because of involvement of the pulmonary and other affected systems.

End-of-life care—may refer in the most narrow sense to care delivered to patients in the last hours or days of life, or may refer more broadly to care rendered to patients whose terminal illness has become advanced.

Palliative care—an approach that improves the quality of life for patients facing life-threatening illness (as well as their families) through the prevention and relief of suffering by addressing pain and other symptoms, whether physical, psychosocial, or spiritual.

Spinal muscle atrophy—a group of inherited diseases that cause muscles to lose function. The progressive muscle deterioration causes weakness and, in more severe forms, is ultimately fatal.

REFERENCES

1. Feudtner C, Feinstein JA, Satchell M. Shifting place of death among children with complex chronic conditions in the United States, 1989–2003. JAMA 2007; 297 (24):2725–32.
2. Meier D, Back A, Morrison R. The inner life of physicians and care of the seriously ill. JAMA 2001; 286(23):3007–14.
3. Redinbaugh E, Sullivan A, Arnold R, et al. Doctors' emotional reactions to recent death of a patient: Cross-sectional study of hospital doctors. BMJ (Clinical Research Ed) 2003; 327(7408):185.
4. Committee on Fetus and Newborn, American Academy of Pediatrics. Noninitiation or withdrawal of intensive care for high-risk newborns. Pediatrics 2007; 119(2):401–3.
5. Michelson KN, Ryan AN, Jovanovic B, et al. Pediatric residents' and fellows' perspectives on palliative care education. J Palliat Med 2009; 12(5):451–7.
6. Widger K, Daview D, Drouin DJ, et al. Pediatric patients receiving palliative care in Canada. Arch Pediatr Adolesc Med 2007; 161:597–602.
7. Bernat, 394–6, Ch. 16.
8. Bernat, 399–400, Ch. 16.
9. Junger S, Pestinger M, Elsner F, et al. Criteria for successful multiprofessional cooperation in palliative care teams. Palliat Med 2007; 21:347–54.
10. Thompson LA, Knapp C, Madden V, et al. Pediatricians' perceptions of and preferred timing for pediatric palliative care. Pediatrics 2009; 123:e777–82.
11. Committee on Bioethics and Committee on Hospital Care, American Academy of Pediatrics. Palliative care for children. Pediatrics 2000; 106(2 pt 1):351–7.
12. Steele R, Davies B. Impact on parents when a child has a progressive, life-threatening illness. Int J Palliat Nurs 2006; 12:576–85.
13. Bernat, 89–90, Ch. 4.
14. Bernat, 181–97, Ch. 8.
15. Freye DR. Care of the dying adolescent: Special considerations. Pediatrics 2004; 113:381–8.
16. Bernat, 159–60, Ch. 7.
17. Meisel A. Seven legal barriers to end-of-life care: Myths, realities, and grains of truth. JAMA 2000; 284:2495–501.
18. Weir RF, Peter C. Affirming the decisions adolescents make about life and death. Hastings Cent Rep 1997; 27:29–41.
19. Bernat, 1–23, Ch. 1.
20. Feudtner C. Collaborative communication in pediatric palliative care: A foundation for problem-solving and decision-making. Pediatr Clin North Am 2007; 54(4):583–607.
21. Godkin MD, Faith K, Upshur RE, et al. Project examining effectiveness in clinical ethics (PEECE): Phase 1—descriptive analysis of nine clinical ethics services. J Med Ethics 2005; 31:505–12.
22. Scheirton LS. Determinants of hospital ethics committee success. HEC Forum1992; 4:342–59.
23. Levetown M and Committee on Bioethics. Communicating with children and families: From everyday interactions to skill in conveying distressing information. Pediatrics 2008; 121:e1441–60.
24. Dubler NN, Leibman CB. *Bioethics Mediation: A Guide to Shaping Shared Solutions*. A United Hospital Fund book. Nashville, TN: Vanderbilt University Press, 2011.
25. Schlam L, Wood JP. Informed consent to the medical treatment of minors: Law and practice. Health Matrix: J Law Med 2000; 10:141–74.
26. Kuther TL. Medical decision making and minors: Issues of consent and assent. Adolescence 2003; 38:343–58.

27. Fletcher JC, Spencer EM, Lombardo PA. *Fletchers' Introduction to Clinical Ethics, 3rd ed.* Hagerstown, MD: University Publishing Group, 2005.
28. Birnkrant DJ, Noritz GH. Is there a role for palliative care in progressive pediatric neuromuscular diseases? The answer is "yes"! J Palliat Care 2008; 24(4):265–87.
29. Wang CH, Finkel RS, Bertini ES, et al. Consensus statement for standard of care in spinal muscular atrophy. J Child Neurol 2007; 22(8):1027–49.
30. WHO Definition of Palliative Care. Available at www.who.int/cancer/palliative/definition/en/. Accessed March 14, 2012.
31. Diekema DS, Botkin JR. Committee on Bioethics. American Academy of Pediatrics. Forgoing medically provided nutrition and hydration in children. Pediatrics 2009; 124:813–22.
32. Linton JM, Feudtner C. What accounts for differences of disparities in pediatric palliative and end-of-life care? A systematic review focusing on possible multilevel mechanisms. Pediatrics 2008; 122:574–82.
33. Montgomery L, Keily J, Pappas G. The effects of poverty, race, and family structure on US children's health: Data from the NHIS, 1978 through 1980 and 1989 through 1991. Am J Public Health 1996; 86(10):1401–5.
34. Newacheck P. Poverty and childhood chronic illness. Arch Pediatr Adolesc Med 1994; 148(11):1143–9.
35. Newacheck P, Stein R, Bauman L, et al., Research Consortium on Children with Chronic Conditions. Disparities in the prevalence of disability between black and white children. Arch Pediatr Adolesc Med 2003; 157(3):244–8.
36. Singh G, Yu S. US childhood mortality, 1950 through 1993: Trends and socioeconomic differentials. Am J Public Health 1996; 86(4):505–12.
37. Stevens G, Seid M, Mistry R, et al. Disparities in primary care for vulnerable children: The influence of multiple risk factors. Health Serv Res 2006; 41(2):507–31.
38. Ward E, Jemal A, Cokkinides V, et al. Cancer disparities by race/ethnicity and socioeconomic status. CA Cancer J Clin 2004; 54(2):78–93.
39. Cleeland C, Gonin R, Baez L, et al. Pain and treatment of pain in minority patients with cancer: The Eastern Cooperative Oncology Group Minority Outpatient Pain Study. Ann Intern Med 1997; 127(9):813–6.
40. Cleeland C, Gonin R, Hatfield A, et al. Pain and its treatment in outpatients with metastatic cancer. N Engl J Med 1994; 330(9):592–6.
41. Dangel T. The status of pediatric palliative care in Europe. J Pain Symptom Manage 2002; 24(2):160–5.
42. Macdonald ME, Liben S, Carenvale FA, et al. Parental perspectives on hospital staff members' acts of kindness and commemoration after a child's death. Pediatrics 2005; 116:884–90.
43. deCinque N, Monterosso L, Dadd G, et al. Bereavement support for families following the death of a child from cancer: Practice characteristics of Australian and New Zealand paediatric oncology units. J Paediatr Child Health 2004; 40:131–5.
44. Holland J. Management of grief and loss: Medicine's obligation and challenge. J Am Med Women's Assoc 2002; 57:95–6.
45. Macnab A, Northway T, Ryall K, et al. Death and bereavement in a paediatric intensive care unit: Parental perception of staff support. Paediatr Child Health 2003; 8:357–62.

23 PALLIATIVE CARE

Robert M. Taylor, MD, FAAN

CLINICAL VIGNETTES

CASE 1

Mr. Thomas is a 62-year-old man who is in the ED with a 6 cm right thalamic hemorrhage with left-to-right shift and intraventricular extension. His past medical history includes previous myocardial infarction, congestive heart failure, and emphysema. The neurology resident initially recommends aggressive treatment with intubation, hyperventilation, management of intracranial pressure, and surgical evacuation. However, the neurosurgery resident believes that the prognosis is poor and recommends comfort care because "there's nothing that we can do for the patient," and even an intraventricular catheter for the hemorrhage would only be "delaying the inevitable." The neurology attending and resident meet with the patient's wife, son, and daughter, who express concern that Mr. Thomas was already frail and might suffer with aggressive treatment. They believe that he would not want to live severely debilitated. Mr. Thomas has no written advance directive (AD).

CASE 2

Mrs. Evans is a 75-year-old woman with inoperable colon carcinoma who, 3 days after exploratory surgery and a diverting colostomy for a nearly obstructive colon mass, woke up from sleep with right hemiparesis and aphasia. Although she was not a candidate for thrombolytic therapy, she was transferred to the neurology service. She is widowed and has one daughter who has durable power of attorney for healthcare decisions. Following surgery but before the stroke, the patient and her oncologists agreed on DNR code status. Her stroke symptoms have partially resolved, and she has partial expressive aphasia and moderate right hemiparesis. She comprehends speech and can communicate with occasional paraphasias, but she has significant dysphagia. She cannot maintain adequate oral intake of fluids or nutrition, and a percutaneous endoscopic gastrostomy (PEG) tube is being considered. Before the stroke, her survival from her cancer was estimated at 6 months.

CASE 3

Mr. Harris is a 69-year-old man with advanced Parkinson disease who was admitted to the hospital for aspiration pneumonia and decreased mental status. He had been living at home with his wife and had been ambulating with a walker. His clinical status has deteriorated recently, and he has had mild dysphagia. He was treated with intravenous fluids and antibiotics, and a nasogastric tube was inserted for medications, nutrition, and hydration. After 10 days, Mr. Harris remains encephalopathic, severely dysphagic, and moderately dyspneic, although the chest X-ray is clear. He is confused and mildly delirious. The medicine service and the patient's wife want to know his neurologic prognosis. Mrs. Harris advises that he has no AD and never wanted to discuss his treatment preferences, but she feels that, in his current condition, he would not want resuscitation or mechanical ventilation, nor would he want a PEG for tube feedings.

QUESTIONS FOR GROUP DISCUSSION

GETTING STARTED
1. Have you ever been consulted for prognostication in cases like those presented? How comfortable are you in this role?

ASSESSMENT
2. How certain is each patient's prognosis? What are the treatment options for each patient?
3. Who is the appropriate surrogate decision maker?
4. On what criteria should the surrogates base their decisions?
5. What information do decision makers need to ensure that their decisions are informed?
6. What policies exist at your institution? What guidelines are available from professional organizations?

(continued)

MORAL DIAGNOSIS

7. How would you rank the ethical problems in each case?
8. How do the ethical principles of respect for patient autonomy, nonmaleficence, beneficence, and justice apply to each of these cases?
9. Should neurologists make specific recommendations? Explain your reasoning. How should recommendations be made?

GOAL SETTING, DECISION MAKING, AND IMPLEMENTATION

10. What are the ethically permissible options? Are any options ethically preferred or ethically impermissible? If so, explain.
11. Are there barriers to resolution of these cases? How does the culture at your institution influence the process of resolving cases like those presented?

COMMENTARY ON DISCUSSION QUESTIONS

GETTING STARTED

1. Have you ever been consulted for prognostication in cases like those presented? How comfortable are you in this role?

Bernat, 37–8, Ch. 2

Neurologists are often asked to provide prognostic information for patients and families.[1] Circumstances often make it difficult to provide an accurate prognosis, even though this is often what families want. This conundrum places a great deal of responsibility on neurologists, and for many, it is an unwelcome and uncomfortable responsibility. A 1998 survey of internists who were experienced in end-of-life care found that approximately 60% felt poorly prepared for prognostication and found it stressful and difficult. In addition, 80% believed patients and families expected too much certainty, and half believed that they would be "judged adversely" for errors.[2] It is probable that neurologists share these concerns.

The cases presented provide a range of diagnoses and prognoses and give some idea of the spectrum of palliative care. Palliative care is defined by the World Health Organization as

> an approach that improves the quality of life of patients and their families facing the problems associated with life-threatening illness, through the prevention and relief of suffering by means of early identification and impeccable assessment and treatment of pain and other problems, physical, psychosocial, and spiritual.[3]

The American Association of Hospice and Palliative Medicine defines palliative care even more broadly, stating:

> The goal of palliative care is to prevent and relieve suffering and to support the best possible quality of life for patients and their families, regardless of the stage of the disease or the

need for other therapies. Palliative care is both a philosophy of care and an organized, highly structured system for delivering care. Palliative care expands traditional disease-model medical treatments to include the goals of enhancing quality of life for patient and family, optimizing function, helping with decision making and providing opportunities for personal growth. As such, it can be delivered concurrently with life-prolonging care or as the main focus of care.[4]

Bernat, 155, Ch. 7 Palliative care would be appropriate for the patients in all 3 cases presented.[5] It is ideally provided by an interdisciplinary team, typically including a nurse or nurse practitioner, a social worker, a chaplain, a pharmacist, and representatives from other disciplines. Such a team can best provide comprehensive support for patients and families who are struggling with complex and emotionally wrenching decisions. Whenever possible, such a team should be included in caring for patients who are critically ill or are at risk of dying.

ASSESSMENT

2. How certain is each patient's prognosis? What are the treatment options for each patient?

In Case 1, the neurosurgery resident is probably correct that the team has no medical options to offer Mr. Thomas because the hematoma is large, intraventricular hemorrhage is present, and the patient is comatose, all of which are poor prognostic signs. Further, Mr. Thomas has significant cardiac disease, ischemic cardiomyopathy, history of congestive heart failure, and emphysema. Even if he were to survive, he would have aphasia and right hemiparesis and would probably require 24-hour care.

In Case 2, Mrs. Evans' prognosis is primarily related to the inoperable colon cancer. If she did not have the cancer, the prognosis from the stroke would be favorable. However, because of dysphagia, she requires a PEG tube to achieve adequate nutrition and hydration. If she chooses not to have a PEG, and if the dysphagia does not resolve, she would be forgoing artificial nutrition and hydration, as it would be unsafe for her to try to take oral sustenance because of the risk of aspiration pneumonitis.

The prognosis of Mr. Harris in Case 3 is perhaps the most uncertain. On one hand, with continued aggressive supportive treatment, he might recover from pneumonia to his previous functional status. He could also worsen, despite continued aggressive treatment. The presence of delirium is an unfavorable prognostic factor. Thus, a middle path of not escalating therapy but continuing supportive treatments may permit Mr. Harris to stabilize or recover. This approach requires frequent re-evaluation of the patient's progress in relation to the burdens of continuing treatments, as well as discussions with the patient's wife to decide whether to continue or stop treatment and to help her with the emotional burden of the process.

3. Who is the appropriate surrogate decision maker?

In Case 2, the first step is to determine whether, despite her partial aphasia, Mrs. Evans has decision-making capacity. If she does, she is entitled to make her own decisions. She should be asked whether she wants her daughter to help her. Families can help patients to understand the implications of their decisions and can provide emotional support.

In Cases 1 and 3, Mr. Thomas and Mr. Harris have overt impairment of cognition (coma and delirium), and neither has an AD. Many states have laws that indicate who should be the proxy decision maker for a patient who has not designated one in an AD. Most of the laws describe a hierarchy, and the person with the highest ranking is designated the proxy. Problems arise when the proxy is not the person whom the patient would have chosen—for example, the life partner of a gay man or a lesbian. If a conflict arises between the patient's life partner and the proxy decision maker designated by law, an ethics consultation can help to identify the morally preferable decision maker. However, such problems can often be prevented by encouraging patients with "nontraditional" relationships to assign a durable power of attorney for healthcare decisions. In Cases 1 and 3, the surrogates would be the patients' wives.

4. On what criteria should the surrogates base their decisions?

Bernat, 87, Ch. 4

It is important to help surrogates to understand that their role is to help to make decisions based on their understanding of the patient's preferences, as opposed to their own preferences.[6] An AD, if it exists, provides a framework for understanding the patient's preferences or goals of care, especially if the patient has discussed these preferences previously with the surrogate. In the absence of an AD or other enduring documentation (e.g., audio or video recording), the patient's preferences should be surmised by the proxy based on the patient's values, moral and religious outlook, prior conversations, etc. to determine what the patient would have wanted in this circumstance—a process known as *substituted judgment*.[7] When the healthcare team explores patient preferences and goals of care with families, it is helpful to ask a question, such as, "If he were able to talk to us, what do you think would be his biggest concern, or what would be most important to him?"

Bernat, 88–90, Ch. 4

Using the *best-interests standard*, the proxy, unable to determine what the patient would want, bases the decision on what seems best from a medical point of view.[7] This standard is also sometimes called the *reasonable-person standard* because it is based on what a "reasonable" person would probably want done in such circumstances.

In Case 1, it is clear that, based on his prior statements and the dire clinical situation and poor prognosis, Mr. Thomas would not want aggressive intervention, and he should be provided comfort measures and palliative care. Mr. Harris' preferences in Case 3 are uncertain. Further discussion with his wife is needed.

Asking the patient and family their understanding of the situation can help the physician to identify any misunderstandings and to build on the family's current knowledge of the circumstances. Research suggests that permitting the family to talk more is correlated with improved satisfaction.[8] The family's concerns and emotions should also be considered and addressed.

Patients, families, and healthcare teams often become entangled in discussions of treatments (e.g., intubation, CPR, antibiotics) before they have established the goals of care, which can be conceptualized as the range of acceptable or unacceptable medical conditions or outcomes of care from the patient's perspective. Once the goals of care are understood, the physicians can then explain whether the goals can be reached and the treatments that will be necessary to reach them.[9]

The physician's role is to help the patient or proxy to understand which goals are achievable and the burdens that might be associated with striving for the goals.[10] For example, if Mrs. Evans in Case 2 were to say that the most important thing for her was to have additional time with her daughter, as long she did not suffer, then the PEG tube would make sense for her. If instead, her biggest concern was to avoid prolonging the dying process and maintaining her comfort, then declining the PEG tube and a referral to hospice would make more sense. In Case 1, if the family said that the goal was for Mr. Thomas to have his prior level of function and independence, the neurologist should explain that, based on the outcomes research of similar patients, this is not achievable because of the severity of the hemorrhage. Patients often also have the goal of not suffering or not surviving in a coma or vegetative state (as is often indicated in ADs). With such patients, orienting the care plan toward palliation would help to meet their goals of care.

Bernat,
33,
Ch. 2

5. What information do decision makers need to ensure that their decisions are informed?

The physician should explain the patient's condition, response to treatment, treatment options, and the range of outcomes. The degree of certainty or uncertainty of the prognosis should also be shared.

In Case 1, Mr. Thomas' family should be advised of the probability of a poor outcome, even with aggressive treatment. As it is likely that he will die, physicians should say so gently and in plain language, as euphemisms or avoidance of the so-called "D-words" (die, death, dying) can be confusing. For example, the physician could say, "The brain hemorrhage is so severe that even with our very best treatment, it is likely that he will die." It is also important to be mindful of how the option of palliative care is presented. It is incorrect and inappropriate to say, "there's nothing we can do," as providing for both the patient's comfort and the family's comfort is an active intervention. Further, families often perceive "there's nothing we can do" as an indication of abandonment or of devaluing the patient and family.

For Mrs. Evans in Case 2, the likely outcomes and the risks of inserting or not inserting the PEG tube should be explained. Asking her and her daughter to restate their understanding in their own words (i.e., the teach-back method) can help to ensure that their decision is informed.

Mrs. Harris, in Case 3, should be told the complexity and uncertainty of her husband's prognosis. Clarifying her husband's values and goals is essential. If he wanted measures to maintain his ability to interact with family and friends, even if he were in a nursing home, then it would be appropriate to continue nasogastric tube feedings and increase his medications for Parkinson disease. Depending on his response, he might advance to taking oral nutrition and medications; if not, then comfort care can be provided.

6. **What policies exist at your institution? What guidelines are available from professional organizations?**

Most institutions have policies for end-of-life decisions, identifying surrogate decision makers, ethics consultation, palliative care, and more. These policies are usually found in policy manuals or on the hospital's website.[11] The AAN and the AMA have published guidance.[12,13]

Bernat, 124, Ch. 5

MORAL DIAGNOSIS

7. **How would you rank the ethical problems in each case?**

In Case 1, the ethical problems might be ranked as (a) identifying the surrogate, (b) establishing the basis for knowing Mr. Thomas' preferences and goals of care, and (c) determining whether aggressive intervention or palliative care is most consistent with his goals.

In Case 2, the ethical problems might be (a) establishing whether Mrs. Evans has decision-making capacity in light of her partial aphasia, (b) determining her daughter's proper role in the process based on the patient's capacity or preferences, (c) establishing the goals of care and treatment options.

In Case 3, the ethical problems include (a) identifying the surrogate, (b) establishing the basis for knowing Mr. Harris' preferences and goals of care, (c) reviewing the uncertainty of his prognosis at this early stage, (d) determining whether continued aggressive intervention or palliative care is most consistent with his goals, and (e) determining how long to provide interventions before concluding that they are ineffective if he does not respond.

8. **How do the ethical principles of respect for patient autonomy, nonmaleficence, beneficence, and justice apply to each of these cases?**

Respect for patient autonomy means that, within broad limits, competent patients have the right to accept or refuse medical treatment.[14] In neurology, patients often lack decision-making capacity and are incapable of being autonomous because they are unconscious,

Bernat, 9, Ch. 1

unable to express their wishes (e.g., aphasia), or unable to understand their circumstances or to reason (e.g., dementia or delirium). In this circumstance, their autonomy is protected by having a surrogate decision maker. Further, their prior autonomy and wishes are protected and respected by means of ADs and the surrogate decision-making process.

Bernat, 11–12, Ch. 1

Nonmaleficence and beneficence are complementary principles.[15] Contrary to popular belief, nonmaleficence does not mean to "do *no* harm," as nearly all interventions in healthcare entail some degree of risk or harm. Therefore, nonmaleficence means to avoid or to minimize harm or burdens to the extent possible while providing beneficial interventions (i.e., beneficence).

Bernat, 13, Ch. 1

Justice has two components.[16] The first is *equity* or *fairness*, which means to treat all persons with medically similar cases similarly. For example, persons with similar medical conditions should not be treated differently because of differences in race or socioeconomic background. Conversely, the only justifiable reason to treat patients differently is on the basis of their individual medical circumstances. The second component of justice is *distributive justice*, which means to provide a fair distribution of resources among all patients. Appeals to distributive justice are sometimes made in the ICU for patients with prolonged or expensive hospitalization, with the rationale that the resources they are utilizing could better be used for others. However, physicians are obligated to advocate for the best interests of their own patients and not for the best interests of "other" patients, and ad hoc decisions to limit or withdraw treatment on the basis of distributive justice are inappropriate. The application of the principle of distributive justice should be based on institutional policies for allocation of scarce resources, as might be indicated in times of disaster or mass casualties. Distributive justice is also a legitimate consideration in distributing truly limited resources, such as allocating organs for transplantation.

9. Should neurologists make specific recommendations? Explain your reasoning. How should recommendations be made?

Bernat, 31, Ch. 2

Physicians sometimes fear that making recommendations is tantamount to paternalism, i.e., the practice of making decisions for the patient without considering the patient's wishes,[17] which violates the principle of autonomy. However, not making recommendations may compromise respect for autonomy because the decisions of the patient or proxy would be uninformed or less informed. It is reasonable, ethical, and perhaps obligatory for physicians to make recommendations based on their understanding of the medical circumstances and the patient's preferences and goals of care. Autonomy is respected by allowing the patient or proxy to decide whether to accept or reject the physician's recommendation.

GOAL SETTING, DECISION MAKING, AND IMPLEMENTATION

10. What are the ethically permissible options? Are any options ethically preferred or ethically impermissible? If so, explain.

In Case 1, Mr. Thomas' medical condition and goals of care lead away from aggressive intervention. For some families, it is discomforting not to try to intervene. A short trial of aggressive treatment would be reasonable and ethically permissible to determine whether Mr. Thomas is capable of responding to interventions, but they should be undertaken with the understanding that the physician would meet with the family within a short time to review the patient's response and decide whether to continue or to reorient the care plan toward palliative care. However, given the family's belief that Mr. Thomas would not want to live with a severe disability, the ethically preferable option is to provide comfort measures only. Many would argue that it would be ethically impermissible, based on the patient's stated goals, to undertake prolonged aggressive treatment that might lead to survival in a vegetative state or condition of severe disability.

In Case 2, it is ethically permissible to insert or not insert the PEG tube as long as Mrs. Evans' decision is informed and uncoerced and she has decision-making capacity. Neither option is more ethically preferable than the other, and neither is ethically impermissible.

In Case 3, depending on Mr. Harris' goals of care, several options would be ethically permissible, ranging from aggressive treatment to palliative care. Because his wishes are not well clarified, more of the burden of decision making falls to his wife. Ambivalence and uncertainty are natural in such circumstances, and the team should support the wife through the decision-making process. When ambivalence and uncertainty exist, it can be helpful to undertake a trial of treatment and to let the patient's clinical response guide subsequent decisions to continue or limit treatment. The presence or absence of clinical improvement during the trial period may help families and physicians to reach a common understanding of the patient's prognosis.

11. Are there barriers to resolution of the case? How does the culture at your institution influence the process of resolving cases like those presented?

In each of these cases, an ethically satisfactory solution was reached through discussion and negotiation with the patient or family. Unfortunately, this is not always the case, and there are many potential barriers to resolution.[18] The explanation of diagnosis, prognosis, and treatment options may be inadequate, which can cause confusion for the family. The patient or proxy may have unrealistic expectations. The patient or proxy may not trust the physicians, for any number of reasons, including poor communication, prior experiences, or cultural or religious factors. The physician may have excessively rigid ideas about ethically acceptable options and be unwilling to negotiate with the patient or proxy.

Bernat, 160, Ch. 7

Many institutions now have palliative care services and units, which may make it easier to transition patients from aggressive therapies to a more palliative approach. Conversely, the lack of a palliative care service may make such a transition more difficult. Biases inherent to the culture of some hospitals, departments, or divisions may influence decisions.

KEY POINTS

- Striving to understand the patient's goals of care, based on discussion with the patient or family, is a necessary step in determining which course of treatment is most appropriate for a patient with serious illness.
- If a patient lacks decision-making capacity, it is essential to determine the proper surrogate decision maker and to help him or her to understand the basis on which to make treatment decisions.
- For seriously ill patients, it is important to optimize patient comfort and provide emotional support for the family, regardless of other treatment decisions.

KEY WORDS

Goals of care—the range of acceptable or unacceptable medical conditions or outcomes of care from the patient's perspective.

Nonmaleficence—the avoidance or minimalization of harm or burdens to the extent possible while providing beneficial interventions (i.e., beneficence).

Palliative care—an approach that improves the quality of life for patients facing life-threatening illness (as well as their families) through the prevention and relief of suffering by addressing pain and other symptoms, whether physical, psychosocial, or spiritual.

Surrogate decision maker (or proxy)—person authorized to make decisions for a patient who lacks decision-making capacity; the authority may be based on an AD or a statutory hierarchy.

REFERENCES

1. Bernat, 37–8, Ch. 2.
2. Christakis NA, Iwasyna TJ. Attitude and self-reported practice regarding prognostication in a national sample of internists. Arch Int Med 1998; 158:2389–95.
3. WHO Definition of Palliative Care. Available at www.who.int/cancer/palliative/definition/en/. Accessed March 25, 2012.
4. American Academy of Hospice and Palliative Medicine. Statement on clinical practice guidelines for quality palliative care. Available at www.aahpm.org/Practice/default/quality.html. Accessed March 25, 2012.
5. Bernat, 155, Ch. 7.
6. Bernat, 87, Ch. 4.
7. Bernat, 88–90, Ch. 4.
8. McDonagh JR, Elliott TB, Engelberg RA, et al. Family satisfaction with family conferences about end-of-life care in the intensive care unit: Increased proportion of family speech is associated with increased satisfaction. Crit Care Med 2004; 32:1484–8.

9. Larriviere D, Williams MA. Ethical and legal considerations in neuroscience critical care. In: Torbey MT, ed., *Neurocritical Care*. Cambridge, UK: Cambridge University Press, 2010:308–18.
10. Bernat, 33, Ch. 2.
11. Bernat, 124, Ch 5.
12. American Academy of Neurology. AAN Position Statements. Available at www.aan.com/view/PECN. Accessed March 25, 2012. [*PECN* documents H, M, O]
13. American Medical Association. Code of Medical Ethics. Available at www.ama-assn.org/ama/pub/physician-resources/medical-ethics/code-medical-ethics.page?. Accessed March 25, 2012.
14. Bernat, 9, Ch. 1.
15. Bernat, 11–2, Ch. 1.
16. Bernat, 13, Ch. 1.
17. Bernat, 31, Ch. 2.
18. Bernat, 160, Ch. 7.

24 PHYSICIAN-ASSISTED SUICIDE

Michael P. McQuillen, MD, MA, FAAN

LEARNING OBJECTIVES

Upon completion of this chapter, participants will be able to:

1. Describe the differences between withholding or withdrawing life-sustaining treatment, sedation for the imminently dying, and physician-assisted suicide.
2. Discuss the *moral* differences between withholding or withdrawing life-sustaining treatment, palliative care (including palliative sedation), physician-assisted suicide, and euthanasia.
2. Describe the principles of palliative care and how they apply to the care of patients at the end of life.

LEARNING RESOURCES

Key chapters in Bernat's third edition—3, 4, 7, 8, 9

Key relevant AAN documents available at www.aan.com/view/PECN

A   H   M   O   P

CLINICAL VIGNETTES

CASE 1

Mrs. Wood, a 48-year-old woman, had an episode of left-body heminumbness 10 years ago and an episode of blurred, double vision 5 years ago, each lasting a month or so. Three years ago, a slowly progressive quadriparesis developed, eventually complicated by shortness of breath. She carries the diagnosis of myelopathy caused by multiple sclerosis (MS); however, because she recently moved to a new community from out of state, her new neurologist has not yet received her prior records and scans.

Mrs. Wood is brought to the hospital in a semiconscious state, with very shallow breathing. Her arterial pO_2 is 40 and pCO_2 is 70. She is intubated, placed on a ventilator, and regains consciousness as her blood gases normalize, at which point she asks, "What are all that equipment and this machine for?" When the neurologist explains the purpose of the ventilator, she then asks, "Will I need it for the rest of my life?" When told—truthfully—that given her clinical course to this point, that might be possible, she says, "Then stop it. I don't want it!" When told that she might die if ventilation is withdrawn, she responds, "That's alright. I don't want to live the rest of my life like this."

CASE 2

Mr. Burr is a 32-year-old man who, for the past 7 years, has carried a diagnosis of amyotrophic lateral sclerosis (ALS), confirmed clinically by EMG, bloodwork, and muscle biopsy, and he returns to clinic for a regular checkup. Since his last visit 3 months ago, his speech has become less clear; he now requires assistance in all aspects of daily living (washing, dressing, toileting, feeding); it has become more difficult for him to swallow; and he is sleeping poorly, getting short of breath when supine, and unable to get into a comfortable, pain-free position. With some difficulty, he says that this is no life for him, despite the aid and assistance that the social worker and his family have provided; he can even hear his wife crying herself to sleep in the next room most nights. As the neurologist completes the exam, Mr. Burr says "Doc, I want this all to end. Will you help me?" When asked to elaborate, he says that he wants a prescription for enough sedation that he will go to sleep and never awaken to the "horror" of his existence again.

QUESTIONS FOR GROUP DISCUSSION

ASSESSMENT

1. What is each patient asking the physician to do? Are there medically important differences in their clinical circumstances? Is there an ethically important difference between the requests?
2. Do any of the diagnoses impair the decision-making capacity of the patient? Does certainty of diagnosis make any difference?
3. Does the presence of depression automatically mean that a patient's request to limit or withdraw life-sustaining treatment (LST) should not be honored because of impaired decisional capacity?
4. Would it matter if the patients in the cases presented had previously told others that they would want all LST measures?

MORAL DIAGNOSIS

5. Assuming that the patients in these cases are both at or near the end of their lives, how can a physician assist them to die?
6. What are the moral differences between withholding treatment, withdrawing treatment, palliative care (including palliative sedation), physician-assisted suicide (PAS), and euthanasia?

GOAL, DECISION MAKING, AND IMPLEMENTATION

7. What ethical principles should guide decision making in settings such as these? If these principles are in conflict, how do you rank the importance of the competing principles?
8. What help is available for challenging cases such as these?

COMMENTARY ON DISCUSSION QUESTIONS

ASSESSMENT

1. **What is each patient asking the physician to do? Are there medically important differences in their clinical circumstances? Is there an ethically important difference between the requests?**

   Mrs. Wood in Case 1 was placed on a ventilator in the midst of a medical emergency (respiratory failure), an action that is ethically justifiable on the basis of implied consent for emergency treatment. In the absence of an advance directive and when the delay necessitated by the process of learning of the patient's wishes from others would harm the patient or result in the patient's death, it is justifiable to initiate emergency treatment. The continuation of ventilator support, with all that it entails (tracheostomy, etc.), involves a series of elective procedures, each of which requires consent, which the patient can now give or withhold because she has recovered consciousness and, presumably, is competent to do so. When offered a tracheostomy and continued ventilator support, she refuses the one and asks the physician to withdraw the other.

   Mr. Burr in Case 2 is not only refusing to go on ventilator support, but is also asking the physician to prescribe a medication that would sedate him to the point at which he would *never* awaken—which raises the question of whether he is requesting PAS or palliative sedation.

   Medically, Mrs. Wood is *presumed* to have MS for which treatment options are available.[1] Conversely, there is no known effective treatment—certainly no known cure—to offer a patient with a *confirmed* diagnosis of ALS, such as Mr. Burr.[2]

   Mrs. Wood is asking that a burdensome treatment be removed, as she does not want to spend the rest of her life on a ventilator. In Cruzan v. Director, Missouri Department of Health, the US Supreme Court found that a competent person has a liberty interest under the Due Process Clause in refusing unwanted medical treatment.[3] Although Mrs. Wood *may* die without ventilator support, it is not *certain* that she will die without it. The action of removing the ventilator *causes* her burden to be removed; her death, *if* it happens, is an unintended effect of the action.[4] On the other hand, the nature of the request of Mr. Burr is ambiguous and unresolved. In the context of dyspnea and somatic pain, his request for "enough sedation that he will go to sleep and never awaken to the 'horror' of his existence again" could be interpreted as *palliative sedation*, which Bernat describes as the "purposeful sedation of the suffering, dying patient to unconsciousness or near-unconsciousness by administering barbiturates or benzodiazepines when doing so becomes the only means of achieving comfort care."[5] Alternatively, if Mr. Burr seeks a prescription with the intent of ending his life, as opposed to relieving his suffering, then the request is either for (a) *physician-assisted suicide*, or assisted

Bernat, 161, Ch. 7

killing, which Bernat defines as an act in which "at the request of a competent patient, a physician provides the necessary medical means for the patient to commit suicide, and the patient subsequently follows the physician's instructions to employ these medical means to take her own life,"[6] or, if the physician must administer the drugs because the patient's ALS prevents him from doing so himself, for (b) *voluntary active euthanasia*, which is an act that "a physician performs at the request of a competent dying patient, most commonly a lethal injection, to directly kill the patient."[6]

Bernat, 200, Ch. 9

2. Do any of the diagnoses impair the decision-making capacity of the patient? Does certainty of diagnosis make any difference?

The accuracy of the medical diagnoses in both cases is an essential component of addressing the ethical issues in each of them. Case 1 involves a relatively young person with a diagnosis that was made elsewhere, for which there currently are no records. Even if it is MS, new treatment options are frequently emerging.[1] Thus, the first question to ask is whether the diagnosis is, indeed, MS. Could the earlier episodes of heminumbness and diplopia have been due to another disease or condition? Could a treatable lesion at the cervicomedullary junction be causing her progressive myelopathy? MRI of the brain and spinal cord is warranted.

For the sake of discussion, presume that the studies confirm the diagnosis of MS. The patient presumably has the capacity to make medical decisions for herself. However, because MS can cause cognitive impairment, her decision-making capacity is a matter that should be explored and validated.[7] In addition, MS is often associated with depression,[8] the presence of which may impair decision-making capacity. Assuming that Mrs. Wood has the capacity to make medical decisions for herself and is not seriously depressed, then she is asking for withdrawal of a treatment (mechanical ventilation), the medical benefit of which has been demonstrated, even though it is probable that she will die without it. Is it reasonable to explore the issue of *why* she would make that choice? In short, is she asking for something (withdrawal of her ventilator) *in order that* she die or that she be relieved of unwanted burdens?

As for Case 2, in that ALS may be associated with frontotemporal dementia,[9] one could ask whether Mr. Burr's decision-making capacity is impaired. Therefore, like Case 1, the question is whether comorbid depression is impairing Mr. Burr's decisional capacity.

3. Does the presence of depression automatically mean that a patient's request to limit or withdraw LST should not be honored because of impaired decisional capacity?

With regard to Case 1, although Mrs. Wood's desires are explicit and unambiguous, the suddenness and discomfort of being on a ventilator may give her a sense of pessimism. However, her view may be justified, considering that she may not come off of the ventilator for months, if ever. At the very least, she needs emotional support. Often, it is ethically permissible to defer acting on a patient's request to withdraw LST until the influence of depression on the request can be thoroughly evaluated. Psychiatric colleagues may be helpful in identifying whether depression is impairing decision-making capacity and, if so, how to best treat it. If depression is not impairing capacity, or if depression is treated and capacity restored, the request can then be considered informed and autonomous and, as such, ought to be respected.

With regard to Case 2, emotional distress—including depression—is common in ALS. Pseudobulbar affect may confuse the issue and make testing for depression more challenging. Moreover, the clinical benefits of treating depression and pseudobulbar affect are not well studied in ALS—making the certainty upon which a choice can be affirmed as informed and autonomous all the more difficult.[10]

4. Would it matter if the patients in the cases presented had previously told others that they would want all LST measures?

Although it is generally preferable for the past and current wishes of a patient to be consistent, patients are nonetheless entitled to change their minds, and they often do so based on their own experience with their illness and the benefits or burdens of its treatment. Some patients switch from not wanting LST to wanting it, whereas others switch from wanting such therapies to forgoing them. Regardless of the direction of the switch, if a patient has decision-making capacity and the decision is informed, then it is ethically permissible even to withdraw ventilatory support. The important issue is not necessarily whether a patient has a change of heart, but whether the patient's decision is stable. Affirming a decision as stable is difficult when the patient is ambivalent. It is difficult to give an exact amount of time that must pass or number of encounters that must occur before a decision can be affirmed as stable. However, it must be recognized that the longer the delay and the larger the number of unwanted burdens or discomforts the patient may be experiencing, the harder it may be to recognize and affirm the presence of a stable decision. The healthcare team must exercise both judgment and timeliness in determining when a decision is stable.

MORAL DIAGNOSIS

5. Assuming that the patients in these cases are at or near the end of their lives, how can a physician assist them to die?

The terms "assisted dying" and "assisted death" were originally euphemisms for PAS and, regrettably, can be mistaken to mean palliative care. As such, Bernat recommends that these terms be abandoned.[11] In ethical analysis of actions that could be considered—PAS, palliative care, or end-of-life care—precision with terminology is essential. If the

Bernat, 201, Ch. 9

wrong action or wrong intent is the premise for analysis, then the ethical reasoning can be faulty. The principal ethical issue is when—under what circumstances—it is ethically permissible or ethically impermissible to take a particular action.

The terms ethically permissible or impermissible can be applied to the *action* taken, the *consequences* of the action, or the *intent* of the person taking the action. It is generally accepted that it is wrong for one human being to intentionally take another human being's life, with the possible exception of justifiable self-defense, where the intention is to protect oneself from an attacker. In like manner, it is generally accepted that it is right for one human being to respect and care for and about other human beings.

6. **What are the moral differences between withholding treatment, withdrawing treatment, palliative care (including palliative sedation), PAS, and euthanasia?**

With regard to *withholding* and *withdrawing* unwanted treatment based on the instructions of an adult with decisional capacity, the consequence of *both* actions can be the same (the death of the patient), and it is widely accepted that no significant ethical or moral difference exists between the two. The major difference is medical—if treatment is withheld, it will never be known whether it might have worked.[12] However, psychologically, it is often harder to *withdraw* than to *withhold* a treatment.

When a patient's disease cannot be cured, physicians may only be able to provide symptomatic treatment—this is the essence of *palliative care*.[13] Neurologists and other physicians who treat patients with chronic disease have the opportunity to *care* for their patients, even when they cannot *cure* them—as once put, "There are times in life when one can do nothing except stand there—but for God's sake, *do* stand there!"[14] It is worth stating, however, that just as caring for patients and being with them as they are dying are key practices of virtuous physicians, palliative care is a recognized subspecialty, the practice of which entails planning and palliative interventions in addition to empathy and counseling. Palliative sedation, or sedation for the imminently dying, is ethically justifiable because appropriately administered doses of sedatives do not shorten life.[15] As well, a 1996 AAN position statement on palliative care states (in a reference to alert patients with progressive and incurable neuromuscular diseases suffering with anxiety and dyspnea) that

> to relieve these symptoms, it is appropriate to sedate such patients, even to the point of unconsciousness, if necessary and requested. Because the goal of such treatment is to relieve suffering, it is entirely justified and appropriate, even if it unintentionally hastens the patient's death.[16]

Palliative care should not be delayed or deferred until a patient's death is imminent, as the aim of palliative care is to relieve symptoms. Palliative care measures can and should be implemented alongside curative treatments, and palliative care issues can and should be discussed with the patient.

The experience in Oregon is that more than 50% of patients with ALS say that they would consider requesting PAS,[17] and a disproportionately high percentage (8%) of those dying as a result of PAS have had ALS.[18] Though physicians have been forbidden to kill for centuries, some would now argue, on the basis of compassion and respect for the patient's autonomy, that this is what a caring physician *should* do,[19,20] whereas others continue to emphasize that *doctors must not kill*.[21] In 1998, the AAN adopted a policy "vigorously opposing physician-assisted suicide, euthanasia, and any other actions by neurologists that are directly intended to cause the death of patients," and further stated that "even if such actions by physicians should become legally acceptable, the Academy emphasizes that this will not make them morally or ethically acceptable *ipso facto*."[22]

GOAL SETTING, DECISION MAKING, AND IMPLEMENTATION

7. **What ethical principles should guide decision making in settings such as these? If these principles are in conflict, how do you rank the importance of the competing principles?**

Bernat, 9–14, Ch. 1

Bernat, 203–4, Ch. 9

The most widely accepted ethical principles that are used to guide decision making in situations such as those described in the cases presented are autonomy, beneficence, nonmaleficence, and justice. Although in many clinical situations, *autonomy* predominates the other principles, ethical analysis should consider all of the principles.[23,24] Important applications of these principles include the *benefits–burden* analysis; the concept of *intentionality;* and its corollary, the *principle of the double effect*.[4]

If patient autonomy is the primary factor influencing end-of-life care in Cases 1 and 2, one should determine each patient's decision-making capacity, whether their illness or other factors (e.g., depression) compromise that capacity, whether they understand the likely consequences of their decision, and finally, what the wishes of each patient are.

Bernat, 52, Ch. 3

Physicians also possess ethical values and principles, including autonomy. With rare exceptions, physicians are not obliged to participate in actions that violate their own principles; however, in doing so, physicians remain obligated to show respect for patients and not to abandon them. Thus, if a patient requests PAS or euthanasia and the physician finds these actions morally objectionable, the physician may respectfully refuse the patient's request (conscientious objection or refusal).[25] In most situations, the physician should offer to continue treating the patient or providing palliative care until the patient establishes a relationship with another physician (nonabandonment).

8. **What help is available for challenging cases such as these?**

In these types of situations, physicians can often seek assistance from a hospital ethics committee.[26] The members of such a multidisciplinary committee are sensitive to the impact of such decisions on all parties concerned and involved in the care of the patient, including the patient and her physician; the patient's family and friends; nursing staff; other physicians, residents, and students; and ancillary staff. In collaboration with the hospital's risk management office, an ethics committee can also help to ensure that any legal constraints are honored. Finally, the committee can serve to mediate any open or hidden conflicts that may come to light during the care of the patient.

Social and spiritual care services, as well as hospice and bereavement care specialists, can provide invaluable assistance in situations such as these. Finally, guidelines and standards of care that can be helpful in providing quality end-of-life care to patients such as those described in this chapter have been developed and promulgated by several organizations, including the AAN,[27] the ALS Association,[28] and the National Multiple Sclerosis Society.[29]

KEY POINTS

- PAS occurs when, at the request of a competent patient, a physician provides the necessary medical means for the patient to commit suicide, and the patient follows the physician's instructions and employs these medical means to take her own life.
- The AAN opposes PAS, euthanasia, and any other actions by neurologists that are directly intended to cause the death of patients.
- Palliative sedation—the purposeful sedation of a suffering, dying patient to unconsciousness or near-unconsciousness when doing so is the only means of relieving the patient's suffering—is considered ethically permissible when properly administered.

KEY WORDS

Double effect—the results of an action with 2 expected results—one intended, the other merely permitted—with neither dependent upon the other.

Palliative care—an approach that improves the quality of life for patients facing life-threatening illness (as well as their families) through the prevention and relief of suffering by addressing pain and other symptoms, whether physical, psychosocial, or spiritual.

Physician-assisted suicide—an action taken by a physician whose direct and only purpose is to end the life of a patient.

REFERENCES

1. Goodin DS, Frohman EM, Garmany, Jr. GP, et al. Disease-modifying therapies in multiple sclerosis: Subcommittee of the American Academy of Neurology and the MS Council for Clinical Practice Guidelines. Neurology 2002; 58:169–78.
2. Miller RG, Jackson CE, Kasarskis EJ, et al. Practice parameter update: The care of the patient with amyotrophic lateral sclerosis: Drug, nutritional, and respiratory therapies (an evidence-based review). Neurology 2009; 73:1218–26.
3. Cruzan v. Director, Missouri Dept of Health, 497 US 261 (1990).
4. Sulmasy DP. Commentary: Double effect—intention is the solution, not the problem. J Law Med Ethics 2000; 28:26–9.
5. Bernat, 161, Ch. 7.
6. Bernat, 200, Ch. 9.
7. DeSouza EA, Albert RH, Kalman B. Cognitive impairments in multiple sclerosis: A review. Am J Alzheimers Dis Other Demen 2002; 17:23–9.
8. Patten SB, Newman S, Becker M, et al. Disease management for depression in an MS clinic. Int J Psychiatry Med 2007; 37:459–73.
9. Phukan J, Pender NP, Hardiman O. Cognitive impairment in amyotrophic lateral sclerosis. Lancet Neurol 2007; 6:994–1003.
10. Krause JS, Saunders LL, Newman S. Posttraumatic stress disorder and spinal cord injury. Arch Phys Med Rehabil 2010; 91:1182–7.
11. Bernat, 201, Ch. 9.
12. Beauchamp TL, Childress JE. *Principles of Biomedical Ethics, 5th ed*. New York: Oxford University Press, 2001:454.
13. Voltz R, Bernat JL, Domenico G, et al., eds. *Palliative Care in Neurology*. New York: Oxford University Press, 2004:476.
14. Daley JM, SJ, *personal communication*.
15. Russell JA, Williams MA, Drogan O. Sedation for the immanently dying: Survey results from the AAN Ethics Section. Neurology 2010; 74:1303–9.
16. The American Academy of Neurology Ethics and Humanities Subcommittee. Palliative care in neurology. Neurology 1996; 46:870–2.
17. Ganzini L, Johnston WS, McFarland BH, et al. Attitudes of patients with amyotrophic lateral sclerosis and their care givers toward assisted suicide. N Engl J Med 1998; 339:967–73.
18. Hedberg K, Hopkins D, Kohn M. Five years of legal physician-assisted suicide in Oregon. New Engl J Med 2003; 348:961–4.
19. Quill TE. Death and dignity: A case of individualized decision making. N Engl J Med 1991; 324:961–4.
20. Goldblatt D. The gift. When a patient chooses to die. Perspect Biol Med 2006; 49:537–41.
21. Pellegrino ED. Compassion needs reason too. JAMA 1993; 270:874–5.
22. The Ethics and Humanities Subcommittee of the American Academy of Neurology. Assisted suicide, euthanasia, and the neurologist. Neurology 1998; 50:596–8.
23. Bernat, 9–14, Ch. 1
24. Bernat, 203–4, Ch. 9.
25. Bernat, 52, Ch. 3.
26. Lo B. *Resolving Ethical Dilemmas. A Guide for Clinicians, 3rd ed*. Philadelphia: Lippincott Williams & Wilkins, 2005:307.
27. Carver AC, Vickrey BG, Bernat JL, et al. End-of-life care: A survey of US neurologists' attitudes, behavior, and knowledge. Neurology 1999; 53:284–93.
28. The ALS Association's Patient Bill of Rights for People Living With ALS, and other resources. Available at www.alsa.org. Accessed March 22, 2012.
29. Brandis M, Reitman NC. Talking about palliative care, hospice, and dying. Washington, DC: National Multiple Sclerosis Society, 2009. This resource and others are available at www.nationalmssociety.org. Accessed March 22, 2012.

SUGGESTIONS FOR FURTHER READING

Foley K, Hendin H, eds. *The Case Against Assisted Suicide. For the Right to End-of-Life Care*. Baltimore: The Johns Hopkins University Press, 2002:371.

Poser CM, Paty DW, Scheinberg L, et al., eds. *The Diagnosis of Multiple Sclerosis*. New York: Thieme-Stratton Inc., 1984:253.

In re Quinlan, 70 NJ 10, 355 A2d 647, *cert denied sub nom. Garger v New Jersey*, 429 US 922, 1976.

In 1997, the Robert Wood Johnson Foundation embarked upon a national program entitled "Promoting Excellence in End-of-Life Care." One of its first efforts, a consensus document, entitled "Completing the Continuum of ALS Care," was developed in association with the ALS Association and published in 2004. Further information available at www.alsa.org.

25 BRAIN DEATH

Jennifer Berkeley, MD, PhD

LEARNING OBJECTIVES

Upon completion of this chapter, participants will be able to:

1. Identify aspects of brain-death testing that engender medical and moral ambiguities.
2. Describe the ethical and medical rationale for performing brain-death examinations in a timely manner.

LEARNING RESOURCES

Key chapters in Bernat's third edition—10, 11

Key relevant AAN documents available at www.aan.com/view/PECN

A

Q

CLINICAL VIGNETTE

CASE 1

A 54-year-old woman is admitted to the ICU with an aneurysmal subarachnoid hemorrhage. She is awake and alert and, when asked about advance directives, states in the presence of her husband that she wants everything done to save her life. A cerebral angiogram identifies a complex left middle cerebral artery bifurcation aneurysm that cannot be treated with endovascular coiling. She undergoes surgical clipping of the aneurysm. After extubation, she is alert and oriented in the ICU. On postop day 5, she exhibits new word-finding difficulty and a right-side drift. The TCD study is consistent with vasospasm. She is treated with triple-H therapy, including vasopressors, to raise the mean arterial pressure. Her exam improves, with fluent language and symmetric strength.

Then, suddenly, the patient has a severe headache and becomes unconscious. CT scan shows new subarachnoid blood and cerebral edema. Cerebral angiogram shows severe vasospasm that is not amenable to endovascular intervention. Despite maximum medical treatment, her neurologic examination worsens, with progressive loss of cranial nerve reflexes. At 3 a.m., her pupils are fixed and dilated, and no brainstem reflexes are present. Mannitol and hyperventilation are ineffective. The patient's husband is notified. He understands that her death is imminent but cannot bring himself to withdraw ICU support and decides to wait for the declaration of brain death.

At 6 a.m., the first brain-death exam reveals no evidence of neurologic function. At 10 a.m., unbeknownst to the ICU team, the routine daily TCD is performed. At noon, the second brain-death exam, including an apnea test, confirms brain death. The ICU attending informs the patient's husband. However, before the ICU team can introduce the transplant coordinator, the ICU attending receives the TCD results, which show high velocities in a pattern consistent with anterograde flow. The ICU attending concludes that because of evidence of cerebral circulation, the diagnosis of brain death must be withdrawn and the patient should be re-examined in 6 hours. The ICU residents, nursing staff, and transplant coordinator strongly disagree; they urge the ICU attending to withhold this information from the patient's husband and to proceed with plans to discuss organ donation with him.

CASE 2

A 29-year-old man is admitted to the ICU on a Friday night following a severe traumatic brain injury that he suffered while bicycling without a helmet. CT scan shows severe contusions and diffuse cerebral edema. Neurosurgical interventions other than placement of an intracranial pressure monitor are not indicated, and despite maximal medical therapy, his intracranial pressure rises to 90 mmHg. By 10 a.m. on Saturday, his pupils are fixed and dilated, and no brainstem reflexes are present.

The patient's wife, who has been at the hospital, is notified. She understands that his death is imminent and would like his suffering to end, but because he had previously made her promise "never to pull the plug on me," she decides to wait for the declaration of brain death. She asks about organ donation, as she knows her husband had wanted to donate one of his kidneys to a coworker. The transplant coordinator speaks to her about options for transplanting all of his organs, and she agrees to do this.

The ICU attending performs the first brain-death exam at 1 p.m., which reveals no evidence of neurologic function. Hospital policy requires that 2 brain-death exams be performed at least 6 hours apart and that at least one of the exams be performed by a neurology or neurosurgery attending. The neurologist is called at 2 p.m. and is asked to perform the second exam at 7 p.m., but the neurologist replies that it is not urgent, as the patient cannot be harmed by the delay, and refuses to come in to examine the patient until the next day. The transplant coordinator and the patient's wife separately complain to the ICU attending about the delay, but the ICU attending cannot persuade the neurologist to come in. The neurologist arrives the next day at noon, performs the second exam, and pronounces death at 12:45 p.m. Because the patient became hemodynamically unstable during the wait, the transplant coordinator informs his wife that many of the organs may not be suitable for transplantation.

QUESTIONS FOR GROUP DISCUSSION

GETTING STARTED

1. Have you experienced brain-death testing that does not go smoothly? Were the unusual circumstances caused by medical, family, or institutional barriers?

ASSESSMENT

2. In each case, what are the patient's medical condition and prognosis?
3. Is there uncertainty regarding the diagnosis?
4. Do any institutional factors contribute to the moral problems in Case 2?
5. In the setting of brain death, should interests other than those of the patient and family be considered?

MORAL DIAGNOSIS

6. How are the moral problems in these cases framed by the participants?
7. In Case 1, is it ethically or legally permissible to ignore the TCD results or withhold them from the patient's husband?
8. Are there laws, institutional policies, or consensus guidelines that help to clarify the diagnosis of brain death or the process of declaring brain death?
9. What are the professional obligations of neurologists regarding the diagnosis of brain death?
10. What are the morally acceptable options for resolving the moral problems posed by each case?

GOAL SETTING, DECISION MAKING, AND IMPLEMENTATION

11. Would an ethics consult have been helpful in providing clarity and guidance on the moral issues presented in Case 1?

EVALUATION

12. How did the care received by the patient in each case match standards of good practice? What might have been done to improve the care of the patient?
13. Might changes to institutional policy help to prevent or resolve the moral problems posed by similar cases?

COMMENTARY ON DISCUSSION QUESTIONS

GETTING STARTED

1. Have you experienced brain-death testing that does not go smoothly? Were the unusual circumstances caused by medical, family, or institutional barriers?

Although the clinical criteria for the declaration of brain death appear straightforward, unusual situations often occur in the performance of brain-death testing in real life. For instance, patient-specific issues such as laboratory abnormalities may interfere with testing. In 2010, the AAN released guidelines for determining brain death that stipulate that "there should be no severe electrolyte, acid-base, or endocrine disturbance (defined by severe acidosis or laboratory values markedly deviated from the norm)," but precise cutoffs for abnormal laboratory values were not specified.[1] In a critically ill patient, it is often not possible to correct every laboratory abnormality. Thus, the question becomes, which abnormal lab values should be corrected before brain-death testing is performed? Reasonable and well-meaning physicians may answer that question quite differently. The laboratory abnormalities that are most important to correct (such as hyponatremia and hyper/hypocalcemia) are those that may negatively affect the neurologic exam and lead to the false declaration of brain death. Laboratory abnormalities not known to cause a loss of neurologic function, such as hypernatremia, are not as important to correct.

Another example of vague guidance is the AAN's recommendation that brain-death testing may proceed once "a certain period of time has passed since the onset of the brain insult to exclude the possibility of recovery (in practice, usually several hours)." Often, the physician is under an unacknowledged pressure to complete brain-death testing as soon as possible. Doing so permits closure for the family and medical staff, a discussion with the family by the local organ procurement organization about organ donation,[2] and freeing an ICU bed in often overcrowded hospitals. Thus, physicians may feel pressured to perform brain-death testing sooner than they may feel is appropriate, or when laboratory values are significantly abnormal. By recognizing this outside pressure, a physician may feel more comfortable taking a step back and asking herself whether she is rushing to perform the brain-death testing to satisfy such demands or because it is medically appropriate. A physician should feel comfortable in refusing to perform the testing until the patient's medical condition is appropriate.

Brain-death testing may also be complicated by family issues and requests. In Case 2, the family was eager for the brain-death testing to be completed. However, a more common scenario is that families ask for brain-death testing to be delayed. The reasons to request a delay vary, but often the reason is so that other members of the family may come to see the patient before death is declared.[3] Given the emotional circumstances of brain death, most hospitals should be as accommodating as possible and tolerate some delay. However, families who are interested in organ donation should also be informed that delays may diminish the likelihood of successful transplantation. Some families are unable to comprehend the concept of brain death or to cope with the associated loss and may request that the process of brain-death declaration be delayed indefinitely. Except for circumstances in which religious belief precludes the declaration of brain death, indefinite

Bernat,
272,
Ch. 11
delays are not possible.[4] Families should be provided with appropriate emotional support to cope with their loss, but brain-death testing should proceed.[5]

ASSESSMENT

2. In each case, what are the patient's medical condition and prognosis?

Bernat,
257,
Ch. 11
In both cases, the patients' medical conditions are clear. Neither patient's examination shows evidence of any neurologic function, and because of the catastrophic nature of the injuries and the absence of confounding factors, no anticipated neurologic recovery is anticipated. Both patients meet the clinical criteria for brain death, yet neither is declared initially because of technicalities in the process of determining brain death. Brain death is defined as "the irreversible cessation of all brain function, including the brainstem."[6,7] To declare brain death, an examiner must (a) know the cause of the brain injury and that the injury is catastrophic and irreversible, and then (b) perform a detailed neurologic exam assessing a patient's responsiveness to external stimuli. When an examiner is unable to perform the entire neurologic exam, ancillary tests may be used to assess brain activity (EEG) or cerebral blood flow (TCD, nuclear medicine flow study), which are used as surrogate markers of brain activity.

3. Is there uncertainty regarding the diagnosis?

Bernat,
261–2,
Ch. 11
In Case 1, the results of the clinical brain-death exam conflict with the TCD results. When a complete clinical brain-death exam can be done, ancillary studies are unnecessary and usually are not ordered.[8] Yet, in the unusual circumstance in Case 1, the TCD study that was unintentionally ordered and completed shows results that are disparate with the clinical exam. Thus, the physician is left with uncertainty as to whether the clinical exam (consistent with brain death) or the TCD study (showing cerebral blood flow) more accurately reflects the patient's condition. Evidence of cerebral blood flow is inconsistent with the diagnosis of brain death.

In Case 2, there is no uncertainty regarding the diagnosis; the only issue is the delay in making the diagnosis.

4. Do any institutional factors contribute to the moral problems in Case 2?

Staffing patterns in the hospital certainly contributed to the delay in declaration of brain death in Case 2. The hospital policy stated that 2 exams must be completed at least 6 hours apart and that one must be performed by a neurologist or neurosurgeon; however, a neurologist was not available in the hospital at the 6-hour mark when the second exam was to be completed. In this case, the treating team might have anticipated that the neurologist would not be available late in the afternoon on a weekend and considered having the neurologist perform the first exam and the intensivist perform the second later in the day. However, many hospitals do not have 24/7 neurology or intensivist coverage. Neither the AAN guidelines nor most state laws specify that brain-death exams must be completed by a physician of a certain specialty, only that the physician be competent to perform the exam. Thus, hospitals with limited coverage by specialists may consider broadening their brain-death policies so that physicians who are capable of performing brain-death testing are available at all times.

5. **In the setting of brain death, should interests other than those of the patient and family be considered?**

A patient who is near brain death (whether or not testing has begun) has such a devastating injury that neurologic recovery is deemed impossible. In such cases, several parties—among them, the patient, the family, the surrogate decision maker, the healthcare team, the hospital, and society (possible donor recipients, other critical patients who require ICU beds)—may have interests that require exploration.

A declaration of brain death enables a patient to become an organ donor. A single brain-dead donor can directly save up to 7 lives via organ donation and help many more recipients through tissue donation.[9] A timely declaration of brain death ensures the greatest likelihood of successful organ transplantation. Nonetheless, organ donation is often a time-consuming process that may require a patient to remain in the ICU for as long as 24 to 48 hours while testing and matching occur. Maintaining a patient in this critical condition utilizes significant resources and keeps an ICU bed occupied. A conflict may arise if another critically ill patient were to require an ICU bed at a time when the only bed that could become available is the one occupied by the brain-dead patient.[10] This conflict may be more acute in a situation in which the patient is near brain death but the family has not yet decided on organ donation or has declined it. In neither case would it be permissible to accelerate the declaration of brain death in order to save another patient. The ICU team's obligation is to the patient already in the ICU bed, and the team cannot change the standard for declaring brain death simply to accommodate another patient.

Bernat, 13, Ch. 1

In Case 1, the TCD data cannot be ignored so that the declaration of brain death can be made, either for the purpose of pursuing organ donation or for opening an ICU bed for another patient. For a patient who is not a potential organ donor, it might be acceptable to offer the family the opportunity to withdraw life-sustaining interventions rather than wait for a declaration of brain death, but this must not be done in a manner that rushes the family or that causes them to learn that the ICU team thinks that another patient needs the ICU bed more than they do. In Case 2, the prolonged delay in making the declaration of brain death may have delayed the organ-donation process. Yet, the delay was clearly against the family's wishes. Further, if the patient were ultimately deemed unsuitable for donation because of the delay, then the delay would have caused an ICU bed to remain unavailable to other critically ill patients for longer than necessary. Thus, the neurologist's assertion that no harm would result from delaying the second brain-death examination to a convenient time is a false one.[4]

Bernat, 272, Ch. 11

MORAL DIAGNOSIS

6. How are the moral problems in these cases framed by the participants?

Case 1 involves two conflicts. One is the medical/scientific conflict between the results of the clinical exam, which are consistent with brain death, and the results of the TCD study, which are not. In this case, the attending has not succumbed to the pressure to declare brain death when she does not feel that the evidence supports the diagnosis. Given that brain death is a clinical diagnosis based on the evaluation and judgment of the attending physician, the attending may delay the declaration until he feels the diagnosis is correct.

The second conflict is the one within the care team as to whether to inform the patient's husband of the conflicting test results. The residents, nursing staff, and transplant coordinator all argue in favor of withholding the TCD results so that brain death can be declared in a timely manner. A timely declaration of brain death enables closure for the family, allows the transplant coordinator the opportunity to discuss organ donation with the patient's husband, and if organ donation is refused, opens an ICU bed for another critically ill patient. The attending physician, on the other hand, feels bound by the knowledge that the patient's TCD results do not confirm brain death. Thus, she cannot declare dead a patient whom she does not feel meets the criteria for brain death.

In Case 2, the neurologist who refused to come in to perform the exam is framing the case only in terms of the patient whom he believes cannot be harmed by the delay. However, the physician, healthcare team, and the patient's spouse are concerned about the patient's autonomy as well as the potential benefit to others by virtue of timely brain-death determination and subsequent organ donation.

7. In Case 1, is it ethically or legally permissible to ignore the TCD results or withhold them from the patient's husband?

Given that the TCD results conflict with the results of the brain-death test, they cannot be ignored. The argument that the test was supposed to be canceled and not performed does not nullify the results once they are known. The attending physician responsible for the declaration of brain death must be confident that all data point to the same conclusion, and in this case, they do not. The patient's husband had already been told the results of the clinical brain-death exam, and he must also be informed of the TCD results. It should be made clear that this does not change the prognosis and that the patient will most likely be declared brain dead later in the day.

8. **Are there laws, institutional policies, or consensus guidelines that help to clarify the diagnosis of brain death or the process of declaring brain death?**

The Uniform Determination of Death Act (UDDA), approved in 1981 by the National Conference of Commissioners on Uniform State Laws, states:

> An individual who has sustained either (1) irreversible cessation of circulatory and respiratory functions, or (2) irreversible cessation of all functions of the entire brain, including the brain stem, is dead. A determination of death must be made in accordance with accepted medical standards.[6]

This act has been enacted in 36 states, the District of Columbia, and the US Virgin Islands. Information about specific state laws governing the determination of death is available from braindeath.org.[11] Many state laws are no more explicit than the UDDA, allowing individual institutions latitude to derive their own policies.

Many institutions have used guidelines released by the AAN as a basis for their brain-death policies. The first such guidelines were published in 1995 and recommended that 2 brain-death exams be performed, separated by a period of time (usually 6 hours).[12] In 2010, The AAN released revised guidelines that suggest that a single brain-death examination is adequate in most situations.[1] Many institutions have not updated their policies to reflect these newest AAN guidelines. Even though healthcare institutions use published guidelines as a basis for their policies, relatively little standardization exists among them; therefore, the procedure for declaring brain death may differ among hospitals. A survey of *US News and World Report* top-ranked institutions for neurology/neurosurgery reveals wide variability in institutional policies and adherence to AAN guidelines.[13]

Furthermore, even in institutions where detailed brain-death policies exist, adherence to the policy is variable. One study exploring the completeness of brain-death documentation showed that a mean of only 11 of 15 elements of the brain-death examination were documented in the medical record. Use of a computerized template/checklist increased documentation compliance to a mean of 14.9 of 15 elements.[14] To improve compliance, the latest AAN guidelines recommend the use of a template/checklist for the documentation of brain-death testing.[1]

9. **What are the professional obligations of neurologists regarding the diagnosis of brain death?**

Neurologists and neurosurgeons are considered to have expertise in the diagnosis of brain death, as learning to do so is a required component of residency training.[15] Some state laws and some institutional policies require neurologist or neurosurgeon involvement in brain-death determination.[13] However, this expertise is by no means limited to neurologists. Many state laws and the AAN guidelines state that any physician may declare brain death so long as that physician is familiar with brain-death criteria and is competent to perform the exam.[1] Thus, hospitals that require a neurologist/neurosurgeon for the declaration of brain death should explicitly define for specialists who are on call the expectations of an acceptable delay for brain-death testing.

10. What are the morally acceptable options for resolving the moral problems posed by each case?

In Case 1, the patient's husband should be told of the conflicting TCD test results and how these results confound the declaration of brain death. The team may want to ignore or conceal the TCD results to spare the husband any further difficult decisions; however, this rationale does not overcome the requirement for honesty and the consideration of all known data to make the determination of death. The attending physician must have an honest discussion with the patient's husband to explain the dilemma and discuss options for proceeding as expeditiously as possible.

The reason that the patient in Case 1 was undergoing brain-death testing was that the husband had been unwilling to withdraw LST until declaration of brain death. This option should be offered again. However, the husband should also understand that withdrawal of life support may limit the patient's ability to become an organ donor. In this case, as often occurs, the topic of organ donation had not yet been broached with the patient's husband, as the team and transplant coordinator were awaiting the declaration of brain death. When a family may be weighing the options of withdrawing life support versus waiting for a patient to be declared brain dead, a discussion of organ donation is warranted. In ordinary circumstances, a discussion of organ donation is "decoupled" from the discussion of brain death. This decoupling, along with the presence of a trained representative from an organ procurement organization, has been shown to increase consent for donation.[16] Recent studies have shown that while the discussions of brain death and organ donation should not be simultaneous, the patient's physician may be involved in the discussion regarding donation.[10,17] In fact, families have often developed a relationship with the physician and may be more receptive to the prospect of donating organs when coming from a trusted source.

Bernat, 13, Ch. 1

In this case, if the husband were to opt to continue with brain-death testing, other options may expedite the process. The attending physician may decide to consult a colleague as to the best way to resolve the discrepancy between the clinical exam and the TCD results; options may include repeating the TCD, performing a secondary ancillary test that also evaluates cerebral blood flow (a conventional angiogram or a nuclear medicine flow study), or waiting a defined period of time and repeating the clinical exam and apnea test. Ultimately, the physician who is making the declaration of brain death should feel confident that it is the correct diagnosis.

In Case 2, the determination of brain death was delayed because of the unavailability of the neurologist. Many hospitals do not have 24/7 neurology/neurosurgery coverage; thus, this situation is not unusual.

In fact, a study of brain-death examinations shows that the average interval between the 2 brain-death exams is 19.9 hours in small hospitals (<750 beds).[18] Furthermore, the same study showed that in all hospitals (including large teaching hospitals), brain-death examination is performed 26% less frequently on weekends than on weekdays and that the interval between brain-death examinations is 12% longer on weekends than on weekdays.[18]

In Case 2, a follow-up call to the neurologist is warranted to explain that the patient is a possible organ donor and that waiting until the next day may preclude successful organ donation. His comment that the patient will not be harmed by the delay is not true, as the patient's wish to donate his kidney may be affected. However, this patient had a neurosurgeon involved in his care. A call could have been made to the neurosurgeon, who is also eligible by hospital policy to perform brain-death testing. In hospitals where a neurologist or neurosurgeon is on call, expectations for prompt declaration of brain death should be clarified. Hospital policies should make contingencies for lack of neurology/ neurosurgery coverage, perhaps by credentialing other physicians to perform brain-death testing.

GOAL SETTING, DECISION MAKING, AND IMPLEMENTATION

11. Would an ethics consult have been helpful in providing clarity and guidance on the moral issues presented in Case 1?

An ethics consult may be quite helpful in a scenario such as that in Case 1. Although the attending physician is ultimately responsible for making the declaration of brain death, she should not dismiss the concerns of the residents, nurses, and transplant coordinator. An ethics consultation will allow everyone's concerns to be voiced and may help the team to arrive at a mutually satisfactory solution. In addition, in Case 1, the consult would have been helpful in framing why it is not permissible to withhold information about the TCD from the patient's family. This case is ultimately about honesty and professionalism on the part of the healthcare team.

EVALUATION

12. How did the care received by the patient in each case match standards of good practice? What might have been done to improve the care of the patient?

In Case 1, the patient was treated according to the standards of care. The only aspect of care that could be changed for future patients is that once a decline in exam is noted and brain death seems imminent, the routine TCD studies should be canceled. If this study had not been performed in Case 1, the confounding test result would have never been an issue. This conflict between the clinical and TCD study might cause some to question the reliability of the clinical brain-death exam. However, in the 2010 updated AAN guidelines, a review of the literature revealed no reports of patients who met the clinical criteria for brain death recovering their neurologic function.[1] Thus, there are no recommendations that flow studies be obtained on all patients who meet clinical criteria for brain death. The disparity seen in this case may call into question the reliability of TCDs as a confirmatory test for brain death. Reliable TCDs require technical expertise, are not widely available, and are therefore not considered by the AAN to be a preferred ancillary test for the determination of brain death.[1]

No specific guidelines exist regarding an acceptable *maximal* interval between brain-death exams. In Case 2, the interval between the exams was 23 hours. A survey of 88 hospitals in New York state showed a mean interval of 19.2 hours, a median of 18.5 hours, and a range of 3 to 50 hours. Only 10 of the 88 hospitals had a mean interval of less than 10 hours. On weekends, the mean interval increased to 21.9 hours.[18] Thus, the delay in this case was not significantly outside of the standard of care; however, the delay that occurred was avoidable.

It is also unknown whether the delay in the declaration of brain death prevented successful organ donation. Discrepancies are found in the literature as to whether a prolonged interval from brain death to organ donation affects donation rates. A 2011 study showed that a prolonged interval between exams decreased organ donation rates. However, most of the organs lost to donation were attributed to family refusal to consent to donation, as opposed to poor organ viability.[18] (In Case 2, consent was not an issue, as the patient's wife had consented to donation prior to the declaration of brain death.) The same study showed that a prolonged interval between brain-death exams is associated with a slight increase in the percentage of patients who had cardiac arrest before donation could occur: 2.9% in patients with the shortest interval between exams (<6 hours) and 3.3% in patients with a 21- to 40-hour interval between exams. The rate of failed organ recovery (12.9%) was not different between the groups, suggesting that the delay did not adversely affect organ viability.[18] A second study confirmed that a prolonged interval from brain death to organ procurement was not associated with decreased organ procurement rates or increased numbers of organs unable to be transplanted because of poor organ viability.[19] The issues of (a) decline in rate of family consent for donation with a prolonged interval and (b) lack of reported cases of recovery of neurologic function between the first and second exams partially contributed to the AAN's 2010 recommendation that only a single brain-death exam is necessary.[1]

In addition to jeopardizing successful organ donation, a delay in the declaration of brain death may be detrimental for other reasons. Families are often seeking closure to a difficult period, and the patient's wife in Case 2 clearly expressed that the delay was against her wishes. The consulting neurologist did not consider the patient's or family's wishes in his decision not to perform the brain-death exam in a timely manner.

13. **Might changes to institutional policy help to prevent or resolve the moral problems posed by similar cases?**

The 2010 AAN guidelines for the determination of brain death recommend only one brain-death exam. Many institutions have already, or are currently, revising brain-death policies to adhere to these updated guidelines. However, some states continue to require 2 brain-death exams separated by a period of time, and they have variable requirements for neurospecialist involvement. In institutions where a neurospecialist is required for brain-death determination, institutional policy should set clear expectations for the timeliness of the exam. Contingencies should also be established for those times when a specialist is unavailable. In states where a neurospecialist is not required to declare brain death, institutions without 24/7 neurology/neurosurgery coverage should consider carefully whether to create a credentialing process to allow physicians in other specialties to declare brain death. A credentialing process would help to ensure that all physicians entrusted with the high-stakes task of declaring a patient brain dead are competent to do so. The literature shows a wide variability in performance and documentation of brain-death exams and that neurologists and neurosurgeons are no better at documenting exam findings than are other specialists.[20] With only a single brain-death exam, it is especially important that the exam be performed correctly; thus, both neuro and other specialists would benefit from a formal process to ensure their knowledge of the procedure for the declaration of brain death.

KEY POINTS

- Because brain-death policies vary from state to state and hospital to hospital, providers should know their institutions' requirements for the declaration of brain death.
- The declaration of brain death may be complicated by both medical and ethical ambiguities.
- In 2010, the AAN revised their recommendations. Rather than 2 brain-death examinations, a single exam is now recommended to avoid unnecessary delays and to possibly improve consent rates for organ donation.

KEY WORDS

Brain death—irreversible cessation of all clinical brain function, including the brainstem.

Donation after cardiac death—also known as "non-heart-beating" donation, is the removal of organs from a patient following the removal of LST and determination of death by the absence of pulsatile cardiac activity for a defined period of time (usually 3–5 minutes) that is determined by local standards.

Organ procurement organizations—private nonprofit organizations that are responsible for increasing donor registration in their service areas and for coordinating the donation process in their service area hospitals.

REFERENCES

1. Wijdicks EF, Varelas PN, Gronseth GS, et al. Evidence-based guideline update: Determining brain death in adults: Report of the Quality Standards Subcommittee of the American Academy of Neurology. Neurology 2010; 74:1911–18. [*PECN* document Q available at www.aan.com/view/PECN]
2. US Department of Health and Human Services. Health Resources and Services Administration. Organ Procurement and Transplantation Network. Available at http://opotxfind.hrsa.gov/Search_OPO_OTC.aspx. Accessed March 22, 2012.
3. Williams MA. When is postponing removal of the ventilator after the diagnosis of brain death justifiable? Lahey Clin Med Ethics J 2011; 18(2):3, 8.
4. Bernat, 272, Ch. 11.
5. American Academy of Neurology. Code of Ethics. Section 3.5, The Brain-Dead Patient. [PECN appendix document A also available at www.aan.com/view/PECN]
6. Uniform Law Commission. The National Conference of Commissioners on Uniform State Laws. Determination of Death Act. Available at www.nccusl.org/Act.aspx?title=Determination-of-Death-Act. Accessed March 22, 2012.
7. Bernat, 257, Ch. 11.
8. Bernat, 261–2, Ch. 11.
9. US Department of Health and Human Services. US Government information on organ and tissue donation and transplantation. Available at www.organdonor.gov/index.html. Accessed March 22, 2012.
10. Bernat, 13, Ch. 1.
11. Determination of Death Act by state. Available at www.braindeath.org/law.htm. Accessed March 22, 2012.
12. Practice parameters for determining brain death in adults (summary statement). The Quality Standards Subcommittee of the American Academy of Neurology. Neurology 1995; 45:1012–14.
13. Greer DM, Varelas PN, Haque S, et al. Variability of brain death determination guidelines in leading US neurologic institutions. Neurology 2008; 70:284–9.
14. Stockwell JA, Pham N, Fortenberry JD. Impact of a computerized note template/checklist on documented adherence to institutional criteria for determination of neurologic death in a pediatric intensive care unit. Pediatr Crit Care Med 2011; 12:271–6.
15. ACGME Program Requirements for Graduate Medical Education in Neurology, 2010. Available at www.acgme.org/acWebsite/downloads/RRC_progReq/180_neurology_07012010.pdf. Accessed March 22, 2012.
16. von Pohle WR. Obtaining organ donation: Who should ask? Heart Lung 1996; 25:304–9.
17. Williams MA, Lipsett PA, Rushton CH, et al. The physician's role in discussing organ donation with families. Crit Care Med 2003; 31:1568–73.
18. Lustbader D, O'Hara D, Wijdicks EF, et al. Second brain death examination may negatively affect organ donation. Neurology 2011; 76:119–24.
19. Inaba K, Branco BC, Lam L, et al. Organ donation and time to procurement: Late is not too late. J Trauma 2010; 68:1362–6.
20. Mathur M, Petersen L, Stadtler M, et al. Variability in pediatric brain death determination and documentation in southern California. Pediatrics 2008; 121:988–93.

SUGGESTION FOR FURTHER READING

Wijdicks EFM. *Brain Death*. New York: Oxford University Press, 2011.

26 ORGAN DONATION

Michael A. Williams, MD, FAAN

LEARNING OBJECTIVES

Upon completion of this chapter, participants will be able to:

1. Describe the application of the "dead donor rule" for organ donation after brain death or cardiac death.
2. Describe an ethical justification for allowing a patient to occupy an ICU bed until brain death occurs, even though this may prevent other patients from receiving ICU services.
3. Discuss how to resolve a conflict between patient autonomy and healthcare professional autonomy when members of the healthcare team express conscientious objection to participating in a patient's care.

LEARNING RESOURCES

Key chapters in Bernat's third edition — 1, 3, 8, 11

Key relevant AAN documents available at www.aan.com/view/PECN

A   Q

CLINICAL VIGNETTE

A 40-year-old man is admitted to the ICU after hemorrhage from a previously unknown pontocerebellar vascular malformation. At the hospital where he is initially treated, neurosurgery on-call coverage is not available. He is intubated and medical management of intracranial pressure is initiated. The CT scan shows parenchymal hemorrhage in the pons and midbrain, intraventricular extension of blood with obstructive hydrocephalus, and crowding of the cerebellum and medulla in the foramen magnum. By the time he is transferred to a hospital with a neuro-ICU, where an intraventricular catheter (IVC) is inserted to treat the hydrocephalus, 3 hours pass.

The neurologic examination is dire. No motor, brainstem, or cranial nerve reflexes can be elicited, and he has no spontaneous respirations. No improvement is seen despite aggressive treatment for 24 hours. Follow-up CT shows severe brainstem and cerebellar edema and adequate treatment of hydrocephalus, with no evidence of cerebral hemispheric infarction or edema.

An EEG shows diffuse bilateral 1–2 cps slowing and no response to stimuli. Brainstem auditory-evoked potentials cannot be elicited, and somatosensory-evoked potentials cannot be recorded above the cervicomedullary junction, consistent with interruption of major white matter tracts.

Representatives of the organ procurement organization (OPO) have been notified of the patient's condition, consistent with hospital policy and US federal regulations, and it is known that the patient has indicated that he wishes to donate his organs.[1,2] Because EEG activity is present and the patient does not meet criteria for brain death, the ICU team and OPO representative prepare to discuss with the family the topic of organ donation after cardiac death (DCD). In fact, the patient is considered an ideal candidate for DCD because he has been in superb health and has suffered no injury to other organ systems. Further, because he has no ventilatory drive, cardiac pulsatility is likely to cease no more than 10 or 15 minutes after extubation. A rapid death in this setting limits the warm ischemic period of the organs to be transplanted, which increases the likelihood that they will function in the transplant recipients.[3]

The ICU team informs the patient's family, including his wife, his parents, and his 2 sisters, that his prognosis is grave. Although tearful, they are not surprised at this news, and even though the patient does not have an advance directive, all of them agree that he had previously made it known that he would not want to be kept alive in such a condition. They also say that the patient was a strong and vocal advocate of organ donation because his best friend in college had benefited from donation made by the family of a teenager who died of traumatic brain injury. Therefore, they ask if his organs can be donated. The ICU team and the OPO representative begin to describe the process of DCD, and when the family learns that fewer organs can be transplanted in the context of DCD than in the context of brain death, they ask that the IVC be removed so that brain death can develop, which will allow more organs to be donated. As a group, they insist that the patient's wishes would be to donate all of his organs. The OPO representative and the ICU attending physician agree with this goal.

Several members of the ICU team, including the ICU nurse manager, express concerns that permitting brain death to develop would be an unwarranted and possibly illegal manipulation of the patient's condition that would be seen as causing the patient's death; they state that they will not proceed until the hospital attorney and ethics committee can be consulted. They are also concerned that by waiting for brain death to develop, an ICU bed will be unavailable for other patients. They argue that the family should either proceed with DCD or withdraw life-sustaining interventions, consistent with the patient's wishes.

QUESTIONS FOR GROUP DISCUSSION

GETTING STARTED
1. Have you experienced families making unusual or unexpected requests in the process of organ donation? How have these been handled?

(continued)

ASSESSMENT
2. What is the patient's condition and prognosis? Is there any doubt or disagreement?
3. Does the patient have decision-making capacity?
4. Are the patient's preferences known? Is there any doubt or disagreement? In the absence of an advance directive, does the law limit the decisions that the patient's wife can make for him? Are the family's preferences known? Is there any doubt or disagreement?
5. Do any competing interests exist?
6. Do any issues of power or conflict in the interactions of the key actors in the case need to be addressed?

MORAL DIAGNOSIS
7. How are the moral problems in this case being framed by the participants? Can or should this framing be reconsidered and replaced by an alternative understanding?
8. Is there precedent in organ donation for the family's request to remove the IVC and wait for brain death? What ethical standards or guidelines exist?

GOAL SETTING, DECISION MAKING, AND IMPLEMENTATION
9. How can ethics consultation be of benefit?
10. What are the morally acceptable options for resolving the moral problems posed by this case? What are the merits of alternative options for resolving the moral problems in the case?

EVALUATION
11. What changes in institutional policy or educational interventions might help to prevent or resolve the moral problems posed by similar cases?

COMMENTARY ON DISCUSSION QUESTIONS

GETTING STARTED

1. Have you experienced families making unusual or unexpected requests in the process of organ donation? How have these been handled?

The experience of families during the ICU stay of a patient with severe brain injury, possible brain-death determination, and requests for organ donation significantly influences not only their memories of the ICU stay, but also their decision whether to proceed with organ donation.[4,5] A common scenario is that the family asks to delay withdrawal of ventilator and hemodynamic support until family members can travel to see the patient.[6] The procedures involved in organ donation requests and in supporting the patient for possible organ procurement are very detailed and protocolized; however, changes in these protocols are sometimes necessary to accommodate family requests, especially when the family has expressed interest in donating organs.

ASSESSMENT

2. **What is the patient's condition and prognosis? Is there any doubt or disagreement?**

   The clinical assessment is straightforward, and all involved parties are in agreement that the patient's prognosis is grave and that even if he were kept alive with long-term ventilation and artificial nutrition and hydration, the brainstem injury would prevent him from ever recovering consciousness.

3. **Does the patient have decision-making capacity?**

   No. He is comatose and, by definition, cannot possess decision-making capacity.

4. **Are the patient's preferences known? Is there any doubt or disagreement? In the absence of an advance directive, does the law limit the decisions that the patient's wife can make for him? Are the family's preferences known? Is there any doubt or disagreement?**

   The patient's wishes not to be kept alive under such circumstances are also not in dispute, as all members of his family indicate that he had spoken of this, albeit, mainly in the context of wishing to donate his organs should he ever be comatose and expected to die. His wife, who is his surrogate by virtue of state statute (as opposed to durable power of attorney for healthcare decisions), is making decisions that are supported by all members of the family. Thus, the patient's preferences and the family's preferences are not in conflict. Although state statutes may limit the scope of decisions that can be made by a surrogate in the absence of durable power of attorney in the context of persistent vegetative state, particularly in regard to artificial nutrition and hydration,[7] the condition of the patient in this case is best described as terminal, as his death is imminent regardless of the actions taken by the healthcare team. Thus, it is unlikely that the law would prohibit the patient's wife from deciding to have the IVC removed.

5. **Do any competing interests exist?**

   Members of the ICU team have raised concern about the scarce resource of ICU beds. They worry that other future patients may be deprived of needed ICU care, as the length of time needed for brain death to develop after removal of the IVC cannot be predicted and could take as long as a week, or possibly longer, because the patient's cardiorespiratory and renal function would have to be maintained as optimal as possible to ensure organ viability for transplantation.

6. **Do any issues of power or conflict in the interactions of the key actors in the case need to be addressed?**

   The ICU attending physician and the ICU nurse manager do not agree that the family's request to remove the IVC should be honored.

The manner in which they identify and attempt to resolve their conflict has the potential either to escalate the conflict or to keep it managed. Additionally, some members of the team have expressed objection to participating in the patient's care if the IVC is removed because of the belief that this would constitute expediting the patient's death.

MORAL DIAGNOSIS

7. How are the moral problems in this case being framed by the participants? Can or should this framing be reconsidered and replaced by an alternative understanding?

The analysis of the case depends both on moral framing and on the tension between ethical principles. The argument against honoring the family's request is framed so that the request is seen as going beyond the limits of respect for patient autonomy by asking the ICU team to deliberately remove the IVC to cause brain death to occur. How is this different, the team argues, from shooting the patient in the head to hasten brain death? Would this not be a violation of the "dead donor rule," which indicates that the patient's death should not be hastened by organ procurement? The issue of the professional autonomy of the involved healthcare professionals is also at stake, as some members of the team have indicated that they will raise conscientious objection to participating in the patient's care. They also argue on the basis of social justice and allocation of scarce resources that an ICU bed should not be used for an indeterminate and possibly prolonged period of time to wait for the patient to die, as it would prevent other patients from being admitted to the ICU. The appropriate balance is to use the ICU bed only as long as is needed to proceed with DCD.[8]

Bernat, 176–9, Ch. 8

The argument in favor of honoring the family's request is framed in terms of respecting the patient's autonomy and wishes, not only to donate organs, but also to have unwanted medical treatments (i.e., the IVC) removed. The patient's goal, they argue would be to make it possible to donate as many of his organs and as much of his tissue as possible to benefit others. This argument is based on respect for patient autonomy, social justice, and allocation of scarce resources—in this case, transplanted organs and tissues.[8–10] By allowing brain death, this patient's organs can benefit 8 other persons (2 lungs, 2 kidneys, 1 liver, 1 heart, 1 pancreas, 1 intestine),[11] whereas with DCD, only 3 or 4 persons can benefit from solid-organ donation (2 kidneys, 1 liver, possibly the pancreas). Further, the success rate of liver transplantation in DCD is significantly lower.

Bernat, 176–9, Ch. 8
Bernat, 9–11, Ch. 1
Bernat, 64–7, Ch. 3

The argument in favor of the family's request cannot ignore consideration of the potentially prolonged use of the ICU bed while waiting for brain death to occur. It is, in fact, possible that even with the removal of the IVC, the development of hemispheric cerebral edema leading to hemispheric cerebral infarction may take several days.

Further, the determination of hemispheric cerebral infarction (or death) would require ancillary methods to demonstrate either circulatory arrest (e.g., transcranial Doppler, cerebral arteriography, or radionuclide flow study) or absence of hemispheric function (e.g., EEG for electrocerebral silence). If brain death does not develop rapidly, the potential burdens of waiting include the use of the ICU bed and the prolonged stress or grief for the family and the healthcare professionals involved in the patient's care.

8. Is there precedent in organ donation for the family's request to remove the IVC and wait for brain death? What ethical standards or guidelines exist?

Conceptually, the family's request to remove the IVC and wait for brain death is not any different from the process of DCD. In DCD, even though the decision has been made to withdraw LST, the patient is supported while preparations are made to take the patient to the operating room, where the ventilator and hemodynamic support are then deliberately removed to allow the patient to die.[12,13] Only after cardiac death has occurred are the organs procured for transplantation.

The same procedural and ethical framework applies in this patient's case, except that the withdrawal of LST is staged. The withdrawal of the IVC would occur first, as it is necessary to allow brain death to occur, which is equivalent to withdrawal of the ventilator and hemodynamic support in DCD to allow cardiac death to occur. The dead-donor rule is not violated because the patient is pronounced dead by cerebral criteria, and organs are not removed until after brain death has been declared.[14] The remainder of the organ-procurement process then proceeds as it does for all patients who donate organs after brain death.

Bernat, 270-1, Ch. 11

GOAL SETTING, DECISION MAKING, AND IMPLEMENTATION

9. How can ethics consultation be of benefit?

Bernat, 119-23, Ch. 5

An ethics consultation is useful in a case like this.[15] Although it might be tempting for the attending physician to ignore the concerns raised by the nurse manager and other members of the team, to do so would be disrespectful, if not dismissive, of their concerns. The ethics consultation process would allow all members of the healthcare team, the family, and the OPO to express their views, and as a group, they may find alternative approaches or compromise that they would not have been able to achieve on their own.

10. What are the morally acceptable options for resolving the moral problems posed by the case? What are the merits of alternative options for resolving the moral problems in the case?

First, the family's request to remove the IVC to allow brain death to develop is ethically permissible, based on longstanding ethical and legal principles that allow patients to reject or have removed unwanted treatment, even if doing so leads to the patient's death.[16] No requirement exists that all life-sustaining interventions be removed simultaneously; in fact, the stepwise limitation or withdrawal of life-sustaining interventions is ubiquitous in ICU practice. Therefore, it is also permissible to delay honoring the patient's wish to have LST removed in order to achieve the patient's primary goal of donating organs to help others.

Conscientious objection is also ethically permissible. Should members of the ICU team feel strongly that they cannot participate in this patient's care, their wishes should be honored; however, out of respect for the family's feelings and in deference to the ethical permissibility of the family's decision, the family should not be made aware of the opinions of those who disagree or their reasons. Further, conscientious objection must be balanced by the principle of nonabandonment, which means that the obligation of the ICU and the ICU team to care for the patient and the patient's family must be met before any healthcare professionals can be permitted to refuse to participate in the patient's care.[17]

Bernat, 51–2, Ch. 3

Contingency plans should be made in the event that brain death does not develop as rapidly as the family hopes. The family, the ICU team, and the OPO representative should discuss in advance how long they can reasonably wait. Should brain death not develop within this time frame, or should it appear that the patient's cardiorespiratory status is becoming unstable to the extent that organ viability may be compromised, they should be prepared to proceed with DCD as a backup plan.

EVALUATION

11. What changes in institutional policy or educational interventions might help to prevent or resolve the moral problems posed by similar cases?

A case such as the one presented provides an opportunity to re-evaluate and potentially expand institutional policies regarding organ donation. Involved stakeholders would include representatives of the ICU, the ethics committee, the OPO, the transplant team (if present in the institution), and pastoral care, among others. The lessons learned from responding to the family's request, analyzing the ethical permissibility of their request, and increasing the number of persons benefited by organ donation in this scenario can lead to formal protocol modifications for determining whether, when, and how to offer families the option of waiting for brain death to occur or proceeding with DCD.

KEY POINTS

- When a patient's death is imminent (as in the case presented), state law does not prohibit removal of an IVC.
- Organ donation after brain death can benefit up to 8 recipients, whereas with DCD, only 3 or 4 recipients may benefit.
- Conscientious objection must be balanced by the principle of nonabandonment.

KEY WORDS

Brain death—irreversible cessation of all clinical brain function, including the brainstem.

Donation after cardiac death—also known as "non-heart-beating" donation, is the removal of organs from a patient following the removal of LST and determination of death by the absence of pulsatile cardiac activity for a defined period of time (usually 3–5 minutes) that is determined by local standards.

Organ procurement organizations—private nonprofit organizations that are responsible for increasing donor registration in their service areas and for coordinating the donation process in their service area hospitals.

REFERENCES

1. Title 42 CFR 482.45. Public Health. Condition of participation: Organ, tissue, and eye procurement. Available at www.ecfr.gpoaccess.gov/cgi/t/text/text-idx?c=ecfr&sid=54a69a091f844ed732026907fbdfa856&rgn=div8&view=text&node=42:5.0.1.1.1.3.4.13&idno=42. Accessed March 26, 2012.
2. US Department of Health and Human Services. Health Resources and Services Administration. Organ Procurement and Transplantation Network. Available at http://optn.transplant.hrsa.gov/. Accessed July 30, 2012.
3. Bernat JL, D'Alessandro AM, Port FK, et al. Report of a national conference on donation after cardiac death. Am J Transplant 2006; 6(2):281–91.
4. Siminoff LA, Gordon N, Hewlett J, et al. Factors influencing families' consent for donation of solid organs for transplantation. JAMA 2001; 286(1):71–7.
5. Simpkin AL, Robertson LC, Barber VS, et al. Modifiable factors influencing relatives' decision to offer organ donation: Systematic review. BMJ 2009; 339:b991.
6. Williams MA. When is postponing removal of the ventilator after the diagnosis of brain death justifiable? Lahey Clin Med Ethics J 2011; 18(2):3,8.
7. Larriviere D, Bonnie RJ. Terminating artificial nutrition and hydration in persistent vegetative state patients: Current and proposed state laws. Neurology 2006; 66(11):1624–8.
8. Bernat, 176–9, Ch. 8.
9. Bernat, 9–11, Ch. 1.
10. Bernat, 64–7, Ch. 3.
11. US Department of Health and Human Services. US Government information on organ and tissue donation and transplantation. Available at www.organdonor.gov/index.html. Accessed March 26, 2012.
12. Institute of Medicine Committee on Non-Heart-Beating Organ Transplantation II. The Scientific and Ethical Basis for Practice and Protocol, which resulted in the publication: *Non-Heart-Beating Organ Transplantation. Practice and Protocols*. Washington, DC: National Academy Press, 2000.
13. Donatelli LA, Geocadin RG, Williams MA. Ethical issues in critical care and cardiac arrest: Clinical research, brain death, and organ donation. Seminars in Neurology 2006; 26:452–60.
14. Bernat, 270–1, Ch. 11.
15. Bernat, 119–23, Ch. 5.
16. American Academy of Neurology. Code of Professional Conduct. 3.1, The Dying Patient. [*PECN* appendix document A also available at www.aan.com/view/PECN]
17. Bernat, 51–2, Ch. 3.

27 GENETIC TESTING IN HUNTINGTON DISEASE

Allison W. Willis, MD

LEARNING OBJECTIVES

Upon completion of this chapter, participants will be able to:

1. Describe the ethical issues associated with presymptomatic testing for neurologic disease.
2. Identify the social, financial, and public health factors that should be considered when contemplating presymptomatic testing for an untreatable or fatal neurodegenerative disease.
3. Discuss the ethical considerations that are involved in the distribution of scarce health resources and describe the role of the physician in such situations.
4. Incorporate into their practices a method for deciding when presymptomatic or prenatal testing for neurodegenerative disease is appropriate and establish a protocol for presymptomatic testing that approaches ethical and public health equipoise.

LEARNING RESOURCES

Key chapters in Bernat's third edition—17

Key relevant AAN documents available at www.aan.com/view/PECN

A   R   S

CLINICAL VIGNETTES

CASE 1

Donna is a 47-year-old woman self-referred because she wishes to pursue presymptomatic testing for Huntington disease (HD). "I'm tired of wondering. I want to find out and plan accordingly." When Donna was 17, her father died from colon cancer at age 50 but had been diagnosed clinically with HD at age 45. Two years ago, Donna's older sister was diagnosed with HD by a positive gene test after she had developed unexplained behavioral symptoms.

Donna states that she wants to know her genetic status so that she can make social and financial plans. She says that if she were to test positive, she would travel instead of returning to school, choose her company's early retirement option, and arrange for long-term nursing care. She has a partner, and they have begun to contemplate marriage. She feels that a negative result "would be the greatest wedding gift I could give him."

On taking Donna's history, the neurologist learns that Donna has a 2-year history of depressed mood and irritability that had been ascribed to menopause. On examination, she has tongue impersistence (inability to sustain tongue protrusion for 30 seconds, a sign of chorea) and mild generalized chorea of which she is unaware.

CASE 2

Annette is a 55-year-old divorced woman who returns to her neurologist for a follow-up visit. Five years ago, she developed cervical dystonia with head tremor, followed by progressive gait problems and dementia that was thought to be Parkinson disease with dementia or Lewy body dementia. After obtaining a history of early-onset dementia with psychosis in two maternal aunts and observing mild chorea in addition to the dystonia on examination, her neurologist recommended HD gene testing; the result was positive with 53 CAG repeats, and Annette is here to discuss the test results. She is accompanied by her 35-year-old identical twin sons, Gavin and Patrick. Gavin is a newly married, successful corporate attorney who hopes to become a partner at the law firm where he works. Patrick is married with three children and an assistant professor of history at a university.

Upon hearing the test results, Patrick states that he wants to be tested as soon as possible. Gavin is opposed to this idea, saying, "Since neither of us is symptomatic, there is no reason to ruin our lives." He knows that even if he is not tested, his twin brother Patrick's test results would reveal his own status against his wishes. He fears that this knowledge would jeopardize his chances of being offered partnership at the firm.

CASE 3

Kate is a 19-year-old newly married woman whose paternal grandfather was recently diagnosed with HD after 8 years with an illness characterized by involuntary movements and cognitive decline. She is interested in testing so that she can make informed childbearing choices. If she tests positive for HD, she plans not to become pregnant. Kate and her father were estranged for many years because of his substance abuse. However, with his recent completion of a rehabilitation program, they have begun to mend their relationship. Her father, who has no symptoms of HD, does not want to be tested and does not want to know his status. Kate's neurologic examination is normal. Thus, either she is presymptomatic or she does not have HD.

QUESTIONS FOR GROUP DISCUSSION

GETTING STARTED

1. Have you ever faced an ethical dilemma in genetics testing? How do ethical considerations in genetic testing differ from ethical considerations in other clinical situations?

ASSESSMENT

2. Is HD DNA testing appropriate in each of the cases presented? Why or why not?
3. What information about HD genetic testing is important for a neurologist to know and discuss with a candidate prior to offering the HD DNA test?
4. Identify and discuss the relevant contextual, demographic, lifestyle, and family relationship factors in Cases 2 and 3. Whose interests compete with those of the patient?
5. Discuss the ethical dilemmas present in Cases 2 and 3 and offer ethically permissible solutions.
6. In what instances would it be ethically permissible not to offer HD DNA testing?

MORAL DIAGNOSIS

7. What are the ethical guidelines for HD genetic testing in adults?

GOAL SETTING, DECISION MAKING, AND IMPLEMENTATION

8. Suppose that Patrick in Case 2 proceeds with testing. If negative, should his identical twin, who declined testing, be told? If Kate in Case 3 tests positive, should her father be told?
9. Six months after Patrick's negative test, Gavin's wife calls the neurologist's office. She is pregnant and "just needs to know if the baby will be okay." She promises never to tell Gavin and offers to supply a sworn, notarized affidavit of her intent to keep this information confidential. What should the neurologist's response be?

COMMENTARY ON DISCUSSION QUESTIONS

GETTING STARTED

1. Have you ever faced an ethical dilemma in genetics testing? How do ethical considerations in genetic testing differ from ethical considerations in other clinical situations?

The primary difference between regular clinical testing and genetic testing is that the test results sometimes provide information about other members of a person's family, e.g., parents, children, and siblings, including identical twins.[1] Thus, genetic information, if inappropriately disclosed, can result either in unwanted knowledge on the part of family members who wish not to know their status, or in a violation of patient confidentiality if the patient has requested that the information not be shared with others. This latter circumstance can result in conflicts of autonomy between family members.[2]

ASSESSMENT

2. **Is HD DNA testing appropriate in each of the cases presented? Why or why not?**

In all 3 cases, the *optimal* choice respects autonomy, protects all involved parties from harm, and minimizes economic and social burden. However, achieving all of these goals is very difficult in practice, and the ethical analysis will differ according to the context of each case. HD testing in Case 1 would generally be considered ethically acceptable and medically appropriate. Donna's intent is to use the information to make future financial and personal decisions, and there is no evidence of coercion. Further, the family history of HD is already known, and she is seeking confirmatory testing. It would be important to inform Donna of the significant exam findings that may represent early symptomatic HD, as her response and feelings about that information may affect her decision to proceed with genetic testing.

Cases 2 and 3 are both complicated by a need to consider an additional person's genetic information and privacy. As in Case 1, the patients have a reason to be tested, are not coerced, and have a right to know their genetic status. However, in each scenario, the patient's relative would also be affected by the results of the patient's genetic test, and the relative does not wish to know this information.

The physician's primary duty is to the patient—to Patrick in Case 2 when he returns for a pretest evaluation and counseling visit and to Kate in Case 3. It is not necessary to obtain legal or ethical approval from the relatives of either patient, although it would be prudent to counsel both of them regarding the nature of genetic information and its implications for their families.

3. **What information about HD genetic testing is important for a neurologist to know and discuss with a candidate prior to offering the HD DNA test?**

The neurologist should discuss with each patient the basic features of HD and HD gene testing in an easily understood manner prior to performing the test. Discussion should begin with a description of the features of HD and its clinical course. Principles such as autosomal-dominant transmission and the concept that HD is caused by triplet repeat expansion may be more easily explained using diagrams. Included in the discussion should be an explanation of penetrance (proportion of persons with an abnormal allele who express a trait associated with the allele) and anticipation (earlier age of symptomatic onset with each succeeding generation with a heritable disorder, especially with triplicate repeats as seen in HD). The patient should be made aware of the high sensitivity and specificity of the HD gene test as it relates to the test's predictive value. It is also helpful to provide material from nationally recognized resources, such as the Huntington's Disease Society of America[3] or the Huntington Study Group.[4] A genetic counselor can be an invaluable resource as a neurologist educates and prepares a patient or consults for HD genetic testing.

4. **Identify and discuss the relevant contextual, demographic, lifestyle, and family relationship factors in Cases 2 and 3. Whose interests compete with those of the patient?**

In Cases 2 and 3, familial interests compete with those of the patient. Specifically, Gavin feels that he and his brother will experience societal prejudice or discrimination if the HD genetic test is abnormal. Genetic discrimination is defined as "discrimination directed against an individual or family based solely on an apparent or perceived genetic variation from the 'normal' human genotype."[5] HD is a disease with prominent psychiatric and cognitive manifestations that are often initially obscure, but the potential exists for those who have the disease to experience significant impact on their professional performance, interpersonal relationships, and general well being.[6,7] A 2009 survey of asymptomatic persons at risk for HD in Canada found that nearly 40% had perceived discrimination, most often involving insurance coverage (29.2%), among family members (15.5%), and in social settings (12.4%).[8] Gavin may also fear his own ability to cope with a positive test result, and this sentiment should not be taken lightly, given the significant psychologic stress associated with HD presymptomatic testing, the fact that mood disorders are more prevalent in families with a history of HD, and the persistence of psychologic stress regardless of the test result.[9–11]

The fragile relationship between Kate and her father in Case 3 contributes to the ethical quandary. The neurologist should discuss with Kate how she will handle her father's insistence that he not know his genetic status.

5. **Discuss the ethical dilemmas present in Cases 2 and 3 and offer ethically permissible solutions.**

Because of their family history, each of the twins in Case 2 and Kate's father in Case 3 have a 50% chance of having an abnormal HD gene test, and in each case, a positive presymptomatic test for the patient is also a positive test for the twin or father.[12] This situation represents a significant ethical dilemma for the clinician in which the right of the patients to know their own genetic status competes with the right of their relatives not to know their HD genetic status. Physicians' primary duty is to their patients. Withholding testing because of the objection of a relative would violate the patient's autonomy. Although refusing a patient's request to be tested because of a relative's objection cannot be ethically justified, it is reasonable to take the time to discuss the implications of the testing with the patient and family before proceeding.

In Case 2, ethical guidelines are in place to protect Gavin from the social consequences he fears.[13–15] Therefore, it is ethically permissible to test the twin who desires to know his HD status.

In Case 3, testing would provide Kate information that would allow her to make informed reproductive choices, such as prenatal testing or adoption. Because she is the patient requesting the testing, her interests should prevail over her father's, and the neurologist should proceed with the testing. However, the neurologist should either refer Kate to a genetic counselor or discuss with her how to respect her father's wish not to know his status.

6. In what instances would it be ethically permissible not to offer HD DNA testing?

In general, it is not ethically permissible to perform presymptomatic or symptomatic HD DNA testing of competent patients against their wishes when the test is requested by a third party, such as a family member or an insurance company. Nor is it ethically permissible to obtain the testing without the patient's knowledge or consent, as this would constitute deception.

It is generally agreed that presymptomatic testing of a minor is ethically inappropriate because no effective treatment exists for HD and testing a minor violates the minor's right not to know.[16,17] In this situation, presymptomatic testing can be offered once the minor reaches the age of majority and has received appropriate presymptomatic genetic counseling. Although it is commonly thought that genetic testing of adolescents before the age of majority provides only harm and no benefits, qualitative analysis of interviews of 18 persons who were tested between the ages of 12 and 25 suggests that both benefits and harms are associated with positive test results, negative test results, and the process of genetic testing, even for HD.[18]

MORAL DIAGNOSIS

7. What are the ethical guidelines for HD genetic testing in adults?

Ethical guidelines for performing predictive genetic testing were first outlined by Thomas in 1982.[19] The Huntington's Disease Society of America has also published guidelines.[12] As stated by Bernat, HD genetic status assessment via DNA testing when performed within a genetic counseling program satisfies ethical standards because (a) the DNA test for HD has minimal potential to harm the patient, as a false-positive or false-negative result is virtually impossible (i.e., the positive and negative predictive values approach 1), (b) presymptomatic testing is performed only on adults with voluntary informed consent, (c) the test is not intended to be performed at the request of other persons or parties, (d) safeguards are in place to ensure patient confidentiality and privacy, and (e) testing is intended to be accompanied by a comprehensive program of pre-test and post-test counseling for patients and their families.[20]

Bernat, 413, Ch. 17

GOAL SETTING, DECISION MAKING, AND IMPLEMENTATION

8. **Suppose that Patrick in Case 2 proceeds with testing. If negative, should his identical twin, who declined testing, be told? If Kate in Case 3 tests positive, should her father be told?**

The primary moral elements in these scenarios involve the right to privacy and autonomy. Primarily because of privacy and confidentiality obligations to the patient, the physician should not disclose the test results to anyone else, including family, without the patient's consent. A secondary reason not to divulge this information is respect for the family member's right not to know the test results of the patient. Although it might be tempting to think that a "negative result" for Patrick would be good news for Gavin, a negative result does not eliminate psychological burden.[18] Bernat points out that studies reveal persistent psychological burden accompanying a negative test result, suggesting that some patients suffer "survivor guilt."[21,22] In both cases, the clinician should make it known to all parties involved that the desire to not know is reasonable and will be respected, regardless of the result of the genetic test.

Bernat, 414, Ch. 17

9. **Six months after Patrick's negative test, Gavin's wife calls the neurologist's office. She is pregnant and "just needs to know if the baby will be okay." She promises never to tell Gavin and offers to supply a sworn, notarized affidavit of her intent to keep this information confidential. What should the neurologist's response be?**

The fact that Gavin's wife has called to get the information means that Patrick has withheld the information from her, which is ethically equivalent to an instruction to the physician not to share the information. Patrick's right to privacy should be respected and maintained. Moreover, there is no legal document that Gavin's wife can provide that could ethically justify such an action. The breach of confidentiality is only sanctioned in a few medical circumstances, such as when a patient voices intent to harm another. The appropriate response would be to explain to Gavin's wife why the test results cannot be revealed. Although it might be tempting to provide her with general HD genetic risk counseling or to inform her of family planning options, the neurologist has no physician–patient relationship with her. Thus, it would be best to provide her with information and for her and her husband to schedule an appointment for genetic counseling.

KEY POINTS

- Genetic testing, particularly for adult-onset neurodegenerative disease, potentially raises social, familial, financial, and public health issues that must be recognized and ethically addressed by the treating neurologist.
- The role of the neurologist in these scenarios is to uphold the ethical principles of beneficence and autonomy and privacy of the person who chooses testing, even though doing so may cause conflict between practical desires to avoid redundant testing in affected family members and personal desires to alleviate potential suffering in those who do not know their status.
- Implementing a standard methodology for neurodegenerative genetic testing, with specific approaches for symptomatic, presymptomatic, and prenatal testing, can aid the clinician in providing morally acceptable and ethically appropriate care.

KEY WORDS

Autonomy—the ethical principle that a patient has a right to choose to accept or refuse diagnostic testing or treatment.

Genetic discrimination—discrimination directed against an individual or family based solely on an apparent or perceived genetic variation from the "normal" human genotype.

Presymptomatic genetic testing—a method for identifying persons carrying the HD gene before symptoms appear.

REFERENCES

1. Knoppers BM, Strom C, Wright CE, et al. Professional disclosure of familial genetic information. Am J Hum Genet 1998; 62:474–83.
2. Ensenauer RE, Michels VM, Reinke SS. Genetic testing: Practical, ethical, and counseling considerations. Mayo Clin Proc 2005; 80:63–73.
3. Huntington's Disease Society of America. Available at www.hdsa.org. Accessed March 11, 2012.
4. Huntington Study Group. Available at www.huntington-study-group.org/. Accessed March 11, 2012.
5. Billings PR, Kohn MA, de Cuevas M, et al. Discrimination as a consequence of genetic testing. Am J Hum Genet 1992; 50:476–82.
6. Julien, CL, Thompson JC, Wild S, et al. Psychiatric disorders in preclinical Huntington's disease. J Neurol Neurosurg Psychiatry 2007; 78:939–43.
7. Ho AK, Sahakian BJ, Brown RG, et al. NEST-HD Consortium. Profile of cognitive progression in early Huntington's disease. Neurology 2003; 61(12):1702–6.
8. Bombard Y, Veenstra G, Friedman JM, et al. Perceptions of genetic discrimination among people at risk for Huntington's disease: A cross-sectional survey. BMJ 2009; 338:b2175.
9. Bird TD. Outrageous fortune: The risk of suicide in genetic testing for Huntington disease. Am J Genet 1999; 64:1289–92.
10. Paulsen JS, Hoth KF, Nehl C, et al. Critical periods of suicide risk in Huntington's disease. Am J Psychiatry 2005; 162:725–31.

11. Wiggins S, Whyte P, Huggins M, et al. The psychological consequences of predictive testing for Huntington's disease. N Engl J Med 1992; 327:1401–5.
12. United States Huntington's Disease Genetic Testing Group. Genetic testing for Huntington's disease: Its relevance and implications. New York: Huntington's Disease Society of America, 2003. Available at www.hdsa.org/images/content/1/1/11884.pdf. Accessed March 21, 2012.
13. Rothstein MA. Genetic privacy and confidentiality: Why they are so hard to protect. J Law Med Ethics 1998; 26(3):198–204.
14. Adams J. Confidentiality and Huntington's chorea. J Med Ethics 1990; 16(4):196–9.
15. American Medical Association. Code of Medical Ethics. Opinion 2.131, Disclosure of Familial Risk in Genetic Testing. Available at www.ama-assn.org/ama/pub/physician-resources/medical-ethics/code-medical-ethics/opinion2131.page. Accessed March 21, 2012.
16. Richards FH. Maturity of judgment in decision making for predictive testing for nontreatable adult-onset neurogenetic conditions: A case against predictive testing of minors. Clin Genet 2006; 70(5):396–401.
17. Clarke A. The genetic testing of children. In: Chadwick R, Shickle D, Ten Have H, et al., eds. *The Ethics of Genetic Screening.* The Netherlands: Kluwer Academic Publishers, 1999:231–47.
18. Duncan RE, Gillam L, Savulescu J, et al. "You're one of us now": Young people describe their experiences of predictive genetic testing for Huntington disease (HD) and familial adenomatous polyposis (FAP). Am J Med Genet Part C Semin Med Genet 2008; 148C:47–55.
19. Thomas S. Ethics of a predictive test for Huntington's chorea. BMJ 1982; 284:1383–5.
20. Bernat, 413, Ch. 17.
21. Bernat, 414, Ch. 17.
22. Hakimian R. Disclosure of Huntington's disease to family members: The dilemma of known but unknowing parties. Genet Test 2000; 4:359–64.

28 OPIATE TREATMENT OF CHRONIC NONMALIGNANT PAIN

Peter Lars Jacobson, MD, FAAN

LEARNING OBJECTIVES

Upon completion of this chapter, participants will be able to:

1. Describe the ethical obligation and duty to treat patients with chronic pain.
2. Define addiction, physical dependence, pseudoaddiction, and tolerance.
3. Identify the important components of the informed consent–treatment contract.
4. Identify the barriers to treatment of patients with chronic pain.

LEARNING RESOURCES

Key chapters in Bernat's third edition—2, 3

Key relevant AAN documents available at www.aan.com/view/PECN

A

S

CLINICAL VIGNETTE

A 45-year-old man describes severe "pressure" headaches that have increased during the past year. They begin in the cervical region and, with activity, extend into the occipital and frontal regions, last for 6–12 hours, reach 9–10 on the pain scale, and have increased in frequency from 2–3 per month to 10–12 per month. The patient was involved in a motor vehicle accident 4 years ago that caused fractures of the cervical spine. Burning paresthesias of the left arm are controlled with gabapentin, and depression is being treated with psychotherapy and fluoxetine.

Recent MRI and CT of the cervical spine show healed fractures with evidence of posttraumatic arthritis, including ligamentous laxity with a 2-mm shift of the odontoid and stepoffs at C_3–C_4 and C_5–C_6 on flexion and extension. EMG shows old left C_6 radicular findings and a chronic radiculopathy of the left brachial plexus. A rheumatologist has diagnosed posttraumatic cervical spondylosis and recommended opioid treatment; although the consultation note expresses concern about opioid diversion, it provides no details. The neurologic examination shows reduced cervical spine range of motion; atrophy of the left pectoralis, deltoid, and triceps; and decreased left triceps reflex. The occipital nerves are tender to touch bilaterally, and multiple trigger points are palpable in the neck and scapular region on the left.

The patient denies any history of substance abuse or analgesic overuse and insists to the neurologist that his current pain treatment (NSAIDs and tramadol) is inadequate and that he needs something stronger. As the neurologist does not want to contend with another "drug-seeking" patient, he cites concerns about scrutiny by the US Drug Enforcement Administration (USDEA) and possible problems with the state medical board and, despite the patient's documented neurologic, neurosurgical, and orthopedic sources of pain, refuses to treat the patient.

QUESTIONS FOR GROUP DISCUSSION

GETTING STARTED

1. Have you ever treated or evaluated patients with chronic nonmalignant pain? Do you ever have negative thoughts about treating such patients, or do you feel comfortable in handling a treatment plan?

ASSESSMENT

2. Define addiction, tolerance, and physical dependence.
3. What is pseudoaddiction?
4. What is the patient's medical condition?

MORAL DIAGNOSIS

5. When is it justified to refuse to treat patients with chronic nonmalignant pain? Is the physician justified to fear scrutiny by the USDEA and possible problems with the state medical board?
6. Do physicians have an ethical obligation to believe patients' statements regarding their pain? What are the consequences of labeling patients with pseudoaddiction as "drug seekers"?

GOAL SETTING, DECISION MAKING, AND IMPLEMENTATION

7. Is this patient capable of decision making?
8. Who is the decision maker for informed consent?
9. What are the elements of valid informed consent in treating patients with pain?
10. How can opioids be incorporated in the treatment plan?
11. Would a treatment contract help the patient and the physician?

EVALUATION

12. What changes in institutional policy, feasible changes in the clinical environment, or educational interventions might help to prevent or resolve the moral problems posed by similar cases?

COMMENTARY ON DISCUSSION QUESTIONS

1. **Have you ever treated or evaluated patients with chronic nonmalignant pain? Do you ever have negative thoughts about treating such patients, or do you feel comfortable in handling a treatment plan?**

   Neurologists routinely evaluate and treat patients for chronic nonmalignant pain. Pain medicine is a certified subspecialty of neurology; however, medical students, residents, and practicing physicians have historically received minimal training in pain medicine.[1–3] Fortunately, training in pain management is now a required component for all neurology graduate medical programs.[1] For decades, patients with pain have been poorly treated.[3] In that pain level has become the "fifth" vital sign, evidence of substandard care of patients with chronic nonmalignant pain highlights a sad legacy.[1–6] The areas of pain medicine and headache medicine are subspecialities of neurology certified by the American Board of Psychiatry and Neurology and by the United Council of Neurologic Subspecialities, and neurologists should be competent in the evaluation and multidisciplinary approach to the treatment of patients with chronic pain.[3,7,8]

   Negative feelings on the part of medical professionals toward patients with chronic nonmalignant pain are not unusual. A study of the staff members in EDs in Calgary, Canada, demonstrated a hostile environment for patients with pain.[5] Approximately 4%–5% of patients were responsible for more than 30% of ED visits[5]; this subgroup had significant psychiatric and addiction issues. After the findings of the study were shared with medical staff (physicians, nurses, social workers, and pharmacists), such patients were referred to the appropriate specialists. Subsequently, the attitudes among the medical staff toward patients with pain became significantly more positive.[5]

ASSESSMENT

2. **Define addiction, drug tolerance, and physical dependence.**

   Addiction is a chronic neuropsychologic disease that has genetic, environmental, and psychosocial components.[1,6] Associated behavior can be reflected in impaired control with drug (and multiple drug) abuse, compulsive drug use, drug cravings, and continuous drug use despite physical and psychosocial harm to the patient.[1,2,6] Addiction worsens a patient's quality of life.

   Drug tolerance is the body's need to have progressively higher doses of a medication to obtain the same response,[1,2,6] and with long-term opioid therapy, it is expected. The need for an increase in the dosage of medication may result from tolerance over several months, but a clinical change in the patient's condition must be assessed by history and examination.

Physical dependence is the body's physiologic requirement of a drug to avoid a withdrawal syndrome[1,2,6] and can occur after daily use for a prolonged period. Opioid-withdrawal syndrome can produce marked autonomic effects (sweating, diarrhea, and mood shifts) and is an expected risk of long-term use of opioids.

3. What is pseudoaddiction?

Pseudoaddiction is the undertreatment of severe pain, which elicits behavior in the patient that looks like "drug-seeking." Patients with pseudoaddiction may sometimes have the autonomic symptoms of physical dependence. Appropriate dosing of medication and monitoring of the patient are successful strategies for correcting this behavior pattern.[6]

4. What is the patient's medical condition?

The patient has suffered over the past year with headaches that have increasingly intensified in pain, and he has not had an effective treatment plan. Posttraumatic cervical arthritis with ligamentous instability, brachial plexopathy, cervical radiculopathy, possible depression (pending medical records from psychiatrist), and occipital neuralgia have been documented by history, examination, EMG, and imaging. The patient denies any history of substance abuse or addiction. The most likely diagnosis is undertreated pain, and although the patient's requests for narcotics may be perceived as drug-seeking they probably represent pseudoaddiction.

MORAL DIAGNOSIS

5. When is it justified to refuse to treat patients with chronic nonmalignant pain? Is the physician justified to fear scrutiny by the USDEA and possible problems with the state medical board?

Treatment for chronic nonmalignant pain is justified if a comprehensive neurologic history and examination are performed by the neurologist and if the patient signs the informed consent–treatment contract form (detailed at Question 11 below) in the presence of a witness. Both neurologist and patient have autonomy in decision making when they both have capacity to understand the risks and benefits. If the neurologist cannot document and monitor the patient treated with opiates on a regular basis, then the physician has an ethical obligation to refer the patient to another pain specialist to avoid harm to the patient.[9] Doing so protects the patient and the neurologist.

Bernat, 52, Ch. 3

A barrier to therapy is the physician's fear of the USDEA and medical boards. Should this reason be used to refuse to treat this patient? The answer is "no."[1,3] The Federation of State Medical Boards has published a revised policy that supports medically indicated pain control with good monitoring and documentation.[6] A main concern of the USDEA is medication diversion, which can be avoided by strict compliance with the treatment plan and contract.[2,6,7]

6. **Do physicians have an ethical obligation to believe patients' statements regarding their pain? What are the consequences of labeling patients with pseudoaddiction as "drug seekers"?**

Bernat, 51–6, Ch. 3

Physicians do have an ethical obligation to believe patients' statements about their pain unless they have medical evidence to the contrary.[10] Once patients who genuinely require narcotics for pain treatment are wrongly labeled as "drug seekers," they will continue to suffer with pseudoaddiction; this act would be harmful and unethical.

GOAL SETTING, DECISION MAKING, AND IMPLEMENTATION

7. **Is this patient capable of decision making?**

The patient in this case has no evidence of communication problems or impaired thought and thus has decision-making capacity. If the neurologist has any concerns about a patient's ability to understand the risks and the benefits of the treatment plan, consultation with psychiatry would be potentially helpful to assess competence and capacity.

8. **Who is the decision maker for informed consent?**

In this case, the patient is the decision maker for informed consent.

9. **What are the elements of valid informed consent in treating patients with pain?**

The *threshold elements* of informed consent include capacity or competence, voluntariness, and vulnerable populations. The *information elements* are disclosure, health literacy, primary language of the patient, recommendation and possible alternatives, and an attempt to avoid the use of therapeutic privilege. The *consent elements* involve the patient wanting to follow the informed-consent process, and the utilization of this process provides an opportunity to establish doctor–patient rapport.

Bernat, 24–7, Ch. 2

Voluntariness in valid informed consent means no undue influence or coercion in the consent process.[11] The physician has undue influence on a physically dependent patient by the physician's potential treatment, thus another provider (e.g., a nurse) should review the consent and answer any questions. Patients need to understand that their care will not be compromised by their decision. Another physician can be contacted if necessary. Excessive manipulation through physician behavior and any threat of abandonment of the patient should be avoided.

10. **How can opioids be incorporated in the treatment plan?**

The Ethics, Law, and Humanities Committee of the AAN has described a structured approach to humane and comprehensive treatment of patients with chronic nonmalignant pain, which includes neurologic history and examination coupled with analysis of essential diagnostic tests.[8] Comprehensive evaluations, diagnoses, treatment plans, medication histories, monitoring histories, and outcomes should be documented in detail to reduce risk of side effects, medication diversion, and potential reduced quality of life for these patients.[1,3,4,8]

Based on previous attempts to control the patient's pain with gabapentin, fluoxetine, and NSAIDS, opioids would be a definite possibility in the complete treatment plan. Opioids are recommended for patients with pain levels exceeding 3 to 4[1-3]; this patient has pain levels of 9 to 10. A key factor in follow-up visits will be the patient's quality of life. If the quality of life is improving, opioids, with dosages and responses monitored closely, may be a component in the multidisciplinary treatment plan.[1,2,8]

The goal of opioid treatment is an improvement in the patient's ability to function, a reduction in headache, and a reversal of the patient's secondary suffering that includes depression, social isolation from the family and community, and fear of continued pain.[12] These benefits must be assessed with the risks of opioid therapy, which include the potential of tolerance, addiction, and direct medication side effects (e.g., nausea, constipation, analgesic hypersensitivity), as well as the patient's compliance with required follow-up visits and strict enforcement of the treatment contract (see discussion at Question 11).[7] Before opioid therapy is started, these issues should be reviewed with the patient and family. A comprehensive informed consent–treatment contract must be signed by the patient and witnessed by the physician and a staff member.[7]

11. Would a treatment contract help the patient and the physician?

For the patients' safety, every patient who is considered for opioid therapy for chronic pain should have a treatment contract with strict compliance.[7] At a minimum, the following elements should be included in a treatment contract:

1. Have a signed valid informed consent.
2. Require the use of a single pharmacy with its name, address, and telephone number.
3. Permit refills only during office hours.
4. Describe and show the patient the prescription flowchart that will remain in the patient's chart.
5. Indicate that only one physician will be prescribing opioids and any controlled substances.
6. Require that the patient maintain follow-up visits to monitor therapeutic response and possible adjustments in the treatment regimen.
7. Require periodic random drug screens.
8. Require notification to the physician's office when the patient receives a prescription for a controlled substance by another physician in an acute medical situation.
9. Require agreement by the patient for immediate referral to a drug rehabilitation program or possible dismissal from the physician's care for violations of the signed contract.
10. Give one copy of the witnessed and signed contract to the patient and place the other copy in the patient's medical record.[1,7]

EVALUATION

12. **What changes in institutional policy, feasible changes in the clinical environment, or educational interventions might help to prevent or resolve the moral problems posed by similar cases?**

    The ethics committee of a hospital can be consulted with the issues on the management of patients with pain who are being treated in various areas of the facility, including burn units, pain management clinics and consults, psychiatric units. Having served on the Ethics Committee of the University of North Carolina Hospitals, this author can attest that systematic approaches in policy can be of great service to patients, physicians, and staff. Although many situations are unique, a framework is helpful to begin the thought process. Education of physicians and staff on the proper approach can be essential to avoid miscommunication with patients and their families, which can lead to conflicts. Ethical communication is therapeutic to all parties involved.

TOPICAL SYNOPSIS

In this hypothetical case, the neurologist has a duty to treat the patient who is in pain. The treatment plan may include opiate therapy as one element of the comprehensive multidisciplinary approach to patient care. The appropriate responses include informed consent–treatment contract, monitoring plan, documentation, and consults with specialists within the multidisciplinary approach to chronic nonmalignant pain.

KEY POINTS

- The neurologist has an ethical obligation and duty to treat chronic pain that leads to suffering.
- Opioid therapy, with the appropriate monitoring and safeguards, is an option for a multidisciplinary treatment plan for chronic nonmalignant pain.
- If opioid therapy is utilized, the informed consent–treatment contract is essential for patient safety and physician monitoring and evaluation.
- Chronic nonmalignant pain can be treated successfully, with the patient and neurologist working together to improve the patient's quality of life.
- Education and documentation will help to prevent any diversion of medication—a safeguard that is critical to the patient, neurologist, patient's family, and regulatory agencies.

KEY WORDS

Addiction—a neuropsychologic disease with genetic, psychosocial, and environmental components that is reflected in aberrant behavior, including drug cravings, compulsive drug use, impaired control of drug use, and continuous use, despite injury to self and others.

Chronic nonmalignant pain—persistent pain and suffering that lasts months to years without a relation to cancer.

Pseudoaddiction—inadequate dosing of the patient that elicits behavior that appears to be "drug-seeking" but clears with appropriate dosing of pain medication. The quality of life of the patient improves without evidence of addiction.

Tolerance—the expected physiologic response to a medication such as an opiate. It can be seen within months, with the patient requiring increased doses of the medication to obtain the same symptomatic relief. No evidence of change in disease status or addiction is observed.

NOTE

The case described in this chapter was previously published by Peter Lars Jacobson, MD, in *CONTINUUM: Lifelong Learning in Neurology*.[1] The discussion has been modified and updated. We wish to thank the AAN for permission to reuse the case.

REFERENCES

1. Jacobson PL. Ethical Perspectives in Neurology. *CONTINUUM: Lifelong Learning in Neurology* 2006; 12(6):285–9.
2. Jacobson PL, Mann JD. Evolving role of the neurologist in the diagnosis and treatment of noncancer pain. Mayo Clinic Proc 2003; 78:80–4.
3. Portenoy RK. Opioid therapy for chronic nonmalignant pain: A review of the critical issues. J Pain Symptom Manage 1996; 11:203–17.
4. The use of opioids for the treatment of chronic pain. A consensus statement from the American Academy of Pain Medicine and the American Pain Society. Clin J Pain 1997; 13:6–8.
5. McLeod DB, Swanson R. A new approach to chronic pain in the ED. Am J Emerg Med 1996; 14:323–6.
6. Federation of State Medical Boards of the United States, Inc. Model policy for the use of controlled substances for the treatment of pain, May 2004. Available at www.fsmb.org/pdf/2004_grpol_Controlled_Substances.pdf. Accessed March 21, 2012.
7. Jacobson PL, Mann JD. The valid informed consent–treatment contract in chronic non-cancer pain: Its role in reducing barriers to effective pain management. Comp Ther 2004; 30(2):101–4.
8. American Academy of Neurology Ethics, Law and Humanities Committee. Ethical consideration for neurologists in the management of chronic pain. Neurology 2001; 57:2166–7. [*PECN* document S available at www.aan.com/view/PECN]
9. Bernat, 52, Ch. 3.
10. Bernat, 51–6, Ch. 3.
11. Bernat, 24–7, Ch. 2.
12. Cassel EJ. The nature of suffering and the goals of medicine. N Engl J Med 1982; 306:639–45.

SUGGESTION FOR FURTHER READING

Pain & Policy Study Group. Available at www.painpolicy.wisc.edu/. Accessed March 21, 2012.

29 THE CLINICAL INVESTIGATOR AND INVOLVEMENT IN CLINICAL RESEARCH

Amalia M. Issa, PhD, MPH

LEARNING OBJECTIVES

Upon completion of this chapter, participants will be able to:

1. Define blinding, randomization, and placebo-controlled trials.
2. Explain the concept of equipoise.
3. Describe and identify experimental bias.
4. Identify the key ethical issues associated with involvement in clinical trials.

LEARNING RESOURCES

Key chapters in Bernat's third edition—19

Key relevant AAN documents available at www.aan.com/view/PECN

A   D

CLINICAL VIGNETTE

The dean of admissions at a medical school has been diagnosed with amyotrophic lateral sclerosis (ALS) and is eligible to participate in a randomized, placebo-controlled phase III clinical trial of a novel ALS drug being conducted at his institution by a neurologist who also is his treating physician. The dean requests a special meeting with the neurologist, who is the principal investigator (PI), and indicates that he wants "professional courtesy" extended so that he is guaranteed assignment to the active drug as opposed to placebo. In this trial, a pharmacist working with the PI is responsible for these assignments.

The pharmaceutical company sponsoring this drug trial has had difficulty recruiting and enrolling ALS patients. In addition to compensating investigators the standard fee of $4,000 per subject, which covers the time and effort of the PI to perform research-related activities for the study, the company is offering investigators an extra incentive of $500 per subject for enrolling at least 15 subjects in the first 3 months.

QUESTIONS FOR GROUP DISCUSSION

GETTING STARTED

1. Is the dean's request consistent with traditional notions of professional courtesy? Why or why not?

ASSESSMENT

2. What does "blinding" mean in a clinical trial, and why is it important?
3. What is randomization? What is its purpose?
4. What are placebo-controlled trials, and what are some of their salient ethical aspects?
5. What is a conflict of interest? What are the relevant conflicts of interest in this case?

MORAL DIAGNOSIS

6. Identify the ethical issues in this case. Discuss the ethical principles that can be used to address them.
7. What is informed consent and how is it relevant to this case?
8. What established guidelines exist for addressing the ethical problems in this case?

GOAL SETTING, DECISION MAKING, AND IMPLEMENTATION

9. What are ethically acceptable options to resolve the problems in this case?
10. How do you justify the options that you have selected?
11. What process or procedures would you recommend to achieve a satisfactory resolution to this case?

COMMENTARY ON DISCUSSION QUESTIONS

GETTING STARTED

1. Is the dean's request consistent with traditional notions of professional courtesy? Why or why not?

"Professional courtesy" originally described the practice of providing medical care to other physicians and their immediate families.[1] However, the term is sometimes construed more broadly, as extending privileges to other members of the same profession that would not be extended routinely to non-physicians. Many healthcare professionals encounter situations in which either they or their colleagues are the recipients of professional courtesy, such as not waiting to be examined, being seen after regular office hours, or calling in a prescription on behalf of a colleague who is not a patient. The dean's request for assignment to the active drug in the context of a clinical research protocol, which is subject to stricter ethical and regulatory oversight than is clinical practice, thus cannot be construed as a request for professional courtesy. More importantly, because of the power differential between the dean and the neurologist, the neurologist could feel coerced into breaking the protocol to honor the dean's request.

ASSESSMENT

2. What does "blinding" mean in a clinical trial, and why is it important?

Clinical trials are experiments that involve humans as research participants. Considered the "gold standard" of evidence for the approval and marketing of new therapeutics, randomized controlled clinical trials involve the assignment of a group of patients to either an experimental group or the control group. Subjects can then be prospectively observed to compare treatment effects. The characteristics of the phases of clinical trials are outlined in Box 29-1.

To yield information that is clinically useful, it is important that clinical trials are designed to take into consideration several factors, including blinding, which is the process of masking the study arm to which the research participants are assigned in order to minimize the effect of

---

BOX 29-1

Characteristics of the Phases of Clinical Trials

PHASE	KEY CHARACTERISTICS
1	Primary purpose is to provide pharmacokinetic/pharmacodynamic information Focused on safety Useful in identifying minimal and maximal dosages
2	Primary purpose is to assess clinical efficacy measures and establish a dose range Collection of additional safety data
3	Typically involves a large randomized controlled trial Usually a comparison of a new therapeutic intervention (drug) with standard treatment (or placebo in certain cases) Usually a blinded study Typically the final phase prior to regulatory approval and marketing
4	Post-marketing study involving a large population Primary purpose is to identify adverse events, morbidity, and mortality May sometimes identify new indications for the drug being tested

experimenter bias and participant expectation about the effects of the treatment. In a blinded trial, a member of the research team who is not directly involved in assessing the research participants may know the assignment of each research participant to active drug or placebo, but the other investigators and the research participants do not know the assignment. In this case, the pharmacist is unblinded because he knows which subjects have been assigned to which intervention; however, the pharmacist does not interact with subjects. The potential for a placebo effect is minimized when subjects do not know if they are receiving the experimental treatment, standard treatment, or a control. If researchers know to which treatment arm participants are assigned, they may, knowingly or not, interpret the participants' treatment response differently based on this knowledge, which could bias the study outcome.

In a double-blind study, neither the investigators nor the subjects know whether the subjects are in the experimental or control arm. Blinding is usually used in conjunction with randomization to avoid bias in the conduct of the trial and the interpretation of the data.

3. What is randomization? What is its purpose?

Bernat, 476, Ch. 19

Randomization is a method used to assign clinical trial participants to a study arm based on chance.[2] The purpose is to create comparable intervention groups, minimizing differences in baseline characteristics by equally distributing participants among the different arms of the trial. Trial participants are randomly assigned (by predetermined statistical methods) to be in either the intervention arm or control arm of the trial. Randomization mitigates systematic bias of non–treatment-related factors, allowing researchers to draw more reliable conclusions on drug effects and arrive at better-informed ethical judgments concerning these drugs. Randomization is not necessary for a trial to be ethically sound, as many ethically valid research protocols do not incorporate randomization. However, randomized controlled trials are often considered the "gold standard" in terms of evidentiary standards.

4. What are placebo-controlled trials, and what are some of their salient ethical aspects?

A placebo is an agent that is not active and has no expected treatment effect. It is usually made to look, taste, and feel as close to the active drug as possible. The ethics of placebo controls in research are in dispute. The Declaration of Helsinki by the World Medical Association regarding Ethical Principles for Medical Research Involving Human Subjects advises researchers to "test against the best current prophylactic, diagnostic, and therapeutic methods" and to conduct placebo-controlled trials only in situations or studies in which no proven treatment exists. The rationale is that a true placebo (i.e., one that is an inactive agent) is

Bernat,
478–80,
Ch. 19

equivalent to no treatment, and because most research is conducted on participants with a specific medical condition or symptom, it is unethical to withhold treatment for the sake of research. Bernat points out that many advocate strict adherence to the "no placebo" principle for clinical research studies in the United States.[3] Proponents of placebo controls in clinical trials, including FDA scientists, argue that they are justified based on scientific necessity.[4,5]

5. **What is a conflict of interest? What are the relevant conflicts of interest in this case?**

The Association of American Medical Colleges defines conflicts of interest as "situations in which financial or other personal considerations may compromise, or have the appearance of compromising, an investigator's judgment in conducting or reporting research."[6,7] Conflicts of interest are a special concern in human-subjects research because researchers are responsible for protecting the rights and welfare of research participants. As an example, a conflict of interest can occur when an investigator is both the treating physician and the PI for the same trial participants.[8]

Bernat,
481–4,
Ch. 19

According to the AAN Code of Professional Conduct, Section 8.2:

> The neurologist who is paid for treating patients in a clinical research project should inform the patient of any compensation the neurologist receives for the patient's participation. The compensation for patient treatment should be reasonable in amount. The neurologist should not bill the patient or the insurer for services already compensated by the study sponsor.[9]

Given that the elements of scientific integrity, research-subject safety, and objectivity of the investigator are paramount in clinical research, any conflicts of interest that might unduly influence researchers' conduct are of particular concern. The case presented involves several conflicts of interest. The sponsor of this clinical trial is offering money as an incentive to the clinical investigators to enroll patients within a specific time frame. Although the incentive presumably has been deemed "appropriate" by the Institutional Review Board (IRB) prior to approval of the protocol, the incentive nonetheless presents a conflict of interest to the investigators, as it is possible that the monetary incentive could influence the researchers to enroll participants who do not meet the entry criteria for the study.

The neurologist has a conflict of interest or, more appropriately, a role conflict by being both the researcher and the treating physician for the dean. The primary obligation of treating physicians is to improve the health and well-being of *individual patients under their care*, whereas the primary role and interest of clinical researchers is to advance scientific knowledge for the benefit of *groups of future patients*, while minimizing potential burdens for research participants within the context of the research protocol.[10] Strong arguments maintain that this conflict is irreconcilable and that clinical investigators who face this conflict should help the patient find another treating physician so that the investigator can serve only a single role as a researcher.[11,12] Achieving an appropriate and adequate balance between the interests of individual patients and those of future patients is challenging. One approach involves creating a "firewall" to mitigate the conflict, whereby a member of the research team *other* than the clinical investigator, explains the research protocol and obtains informed consent.

MORAL DIAGNOSIS

6. **Identify the ethical issues in this case. Discuss the ethical principles that can be used to address them.**

Several ethical issues must be considered in evaluating a clinical research study; among them are the conflict-of-interest concerns discussed above, relative risks and benefits to the research participants, availability of effective treatment (beyond placebo), method of randomization, and equipoise. Researchers are obliged to conduct trials in a scientifically and ethically sound manner to minimize the risk to human research participants.[2] An IRB is a group that has been formally designated to approve, monitor, and review research involving humans. IRBs have critical scientific, ethical, and regulatory oversight functions and are empowered to approve, require modifications in (to secure approval), or disapprove research under Title 45 CFR (Code of Federal Regulations) Part 46.[13] Although these are not issues for the case as presented, key issues considered by an IRB prior to approval of a study are:

Bernat,
476,
Ch. 19

a. Whether the trial is designed in such a way as to be able to answer the primary research question.
b. Whether effective treatment already exists for the disease under consideration.
c. The severity of the disease for which the intervention trial is being conducted.
d. The probability and magnitude of possible benefits to society and to the research participants.
e. The probability and magnitude of any possible risks or harms to the research participants.
f. The balance of risks and benefits to the research participants and to others (particularly the target group, in this case, ALS patients).

Equipoise is among the most important justifications for undertaking a comparative efficacy drug study. In research, equipoise describes a state of uncertainty about whether the efficacy of the experimental intervention being tested in the trial is unknown or uncertain as compared with the control arm.[14] Equipoise does not exist if either study arm is already known to be superior. "A trial is ethical if there is genuine uncertainty within the expert medical community—not necessarily on the part of the individual investigator—about the preferred treatment."[14]

Another ethical issue involves the *therapeutic misconception*,[15] in which the research participant believes that enrolling in a clinical trial will provide direct therapeutic benefit, despite being informed that it may not.[16,17] As many as 70% of subjects in clinical research studies may hold a therapeutic misconception.[18] Minimizing this problem demands a rigorous informed-consent process in which researchers clearly distinguish between clinical research and clinical therapy. The dean's request to be assigned to the treatment arm probably stems from the therapeutic misconception.

7. What is informed consent and how is it relevant to this case?

In general, patients who participate in research must provide informed consent to enroll in the study. Informed consent involves informing potential research participants of the purpose of the study in terms that they can understand, how the research study is to be conducted, the risks and benefits of the trial, and the alternatives that exist to participating in the research study. Prospective research participants are also informed that they have a right to withdraw from the trial at any time without consequences to their relationship with their healthcare providers or to their receipt of medical care. Further, participants are informed that they will be randomly assigned to an arm of the trial (e.g., active treatment, placebo, or experimental treatment versus standard therapy). The principles of informed consent are an integral component of all clinical research with human participants, and informed consent in research is held to a higher standard than informed consent in clinical practice. All potential research participants receive identical IRB-approved consent documents that detail all critical aspects of their participation in the research.

8. What established guidelines exist for addressing the ethical problems in this case?

Numerous guidelines for the conduct of clinical research exist. In the United States, basic principles of research ethics are described within the Belmont Report.[19] The current US Code of Federal Regulations, particularly Title 45 CFR Part 46, is based in large part on the Belmont report, and all clinical researchers must be familiar with it.[13,19] Well-known international guidelines and regulations include the Nuremberg Code, the Declaration of Helsinki, the International Conference on Harmonization Guideline for Good Clinical Practice, the Council for International Organizations of Medical Sciences International Ethical Guidelines, and the Canadian Tri-Council Policy Statement. Additional resources include the journal *IRB: Ethics & Human Research* and the *Oxford Textbook of Clinical Research Ethics*.

GOAL SETTING, DECISION MAKING, AND IMPLEMENTATION

9. What are ethically acceptable options to resolve the problems in this case?

Bernat, 9–11, Ch. 1

Bernat, 477, Ch. 19

Strong scientific and ethical reasons exist for the neurologist not to honor the dean's request to assign him specifically to the treatment arm of the research protocol. Others might argue that his request should be allowed to preserve the principle of autonomy.[20] According to Bernat, "enrollment in a RCT [randomized controlled trial] may diminish a patient's autonomy. True autonomy can be exercised only when the patient has the freedom to choose into which arm of the protocol to enroll."[21] However, it would be erroneous to infer that autonomy is not honored by preventing the participant from selecting the research arm. The potential research participant is free to choose whether to participate in the research protocol *as it is designed and approved by the IRB*, and researchers can uphold the participant's autonomy by respecting that choice while simultaneously upholding the ethical obligation to conduct research rigorously. The most ethically acceptable option is to inform the dean that he must be treated like every other research subject. He must meet eligibility criteria, provide informed consent, demonstrate that he understands the purpose of the research study, and its risks and benefits, and agrees to random assignment into the intervention or the placebo control.

10. How do you justify the options that you have selected?

The dean should be treated like any other ALS patient who participates in this clinical trial and be accorded no special privilege, which respects the ethical principle of justice. Scientifically and ethically sound clinical research must strictly adhere to the randomization process to place research participants in different arms of a trial with equal chance, and to ensure that the trial remains blinded (or masked) from the beginning of the trial until the study is completed.

11. What process or procedures would you recommend to achieve a satisfactory resolution to this case?

To resolve the dilemmas in this case, the site PI should have a frank discussion with the dean to explain the above points. To resolve the potential for coercion by the dean, as well as the physician–researcher role conflict for the neurologist, the possibility of enrolling the dean in the same protocol at another institution should be considered. If eligible, once assigned to a research arm, he can then continue the protocol in the same arm at his institution in the appropriately blinded manner. It may also help for the neurologist to discuss concerns with the chair of the IRB, especially if the dean persists in his request to be assigned to the active treatment arm. Should threats of coercion become overt, the neurologist may have little choice but to discuss the dean's conduct with the medical school committee responsible for hearing and reviewing allegations of professional misconduct.

KEY POINTS

- Understanding the phases and ethical issues inherent in clinical trials at each phase of a study is critical.
- Conflicts of interest are a special concern in human-subjects research because researchers are responsible for protecting the rights and welfare of human participants.
- The principles of informed consent are an integral component of all clinical research with human research participants.

KEY WORDS

Conflict of interest—a set of conditions in which professional judgment concerning a primary interest (such as a patient's welfare or the validity of research) tends to be unduly influenced by a secondary interest (such as financial gain).

Equipoise—a state of uncertainty about whether the efficacy of the experimental intervention being tested in the trial is unknown or uncertain as compared with the control arm.

Placebo—an agent that is not active and has no expected treatment effect.

Randomization—a method used to assign participants of clinical trials to a study arm based on chance. The purpose is to create comparable intervention groups, minimizing differences in baseline characteristics by equally distributing participants among the different arms of the trial.

REFERENCES

1. Jones JG. Medical professional courtesy: A crumbling freemasonry? BMJ Careers Aug 25, 2007;72. Available at http://careers.bmj.com/careers/advice/view-article .html?id=2556. Accessed April 10, 2012.
2. Bernat, 476, Ch. 19.
3. Bernat, 478–80, Ch. 19.
4. Temple R, Ellenberg SS. Placebo-controlled trials and active-control trials in the evaluation of new treatments. Part 1. Ethical and scientific issues. Ann Intern Med 2000; 133(6):455–63.
5. Holton T. FDA uneasy about placebo revision. Nat Med 2001; 7:7.
6. DeAngelis CD, Fontanarosa PB, Flanagin A. Reporting financial conflicts of interest and relationships between investigators and research sponsors. JAMA 2001; 286(1):89–91.
7. Association of American Medical Colleges. In the interest of patients: Recommendations for physician financial relationships and clinical decision making: Report of the task force on financial conflicts of interest in clinical care. Washington, DC: AAMC, 2010. Available at www.aamc.org/download/157030/data/coi_in_clinical_care.pdf. Accessed March 16, 2012.

8. Bernat, 481–4, Ch. 19.
9. American Academy of Neurology. Code of Professional Conduct, Section 8.2, Disclosure of Potential Conflicts. [*PECN* appendix document A. Also available at www.aan.com/view/PECN]
10. Williams MA, Haywood C. Critical care research on patients with advance directives or DNR status: Ethical challenges for clinician investigators. Crit Care Med 2003; 31(Suppl.):S167–71.
11. Miller FG, Brody H. A critique of clinical equipoise. Therapeutic misconception in the ethics of clinical trials. Hastings Cent Rep 2003; 33(3):19–28.
12. Miller FG, Rosenstein DL. The therapeutic orientation to clinical trials. N Engl J Med 2003; 348:1383–6.
13. Department of Health and Human Services. "Protection of Human Subjects." Title 45 Code of Federal Regulations, Pt. 46, 2005.
14. Freedman B. Equipoise and the ethics of clinical research. N Engl J Med 1987; 317(3):141–5.
15. Appelbaum PS, Roth LH, Lidz C. The therapeutic misconception: Informed consent in psychiatric research. Int J Law Psychiatry 1982; 5(3–4):319–29.
16. Appelbaum PS, Roth LH, Lidz C, et al. False hopes and best data: Consent to research and the therapeutic misconception. Hastings Cent Rep 1987; 17(2):20–4.
17. Henderson G, Churchill LR, Davis AM, et al. Clinical trials and medical care: Defining the therapeutic misconception. PLoS Medicine 2007; 4:1735–8.
18. Appelbaum, Paul S. Clarifying the ethics of clinical research: A path toward avoiding the therapeutic misconception. Am J Bioethics 2002; 2(2):22–3.
19. The National Commission for the Protection of Human Subjects of Biomedical and Behavioral Research. The Belmont Report: Ethical Principles and Guidelines for the Protection of Human Subjects of Research. US Department of Health, Education and Welfare, DHEW Publication No. (OS) 78-0012, 1979.
20. Bernat, 9–11, Ch. 1.
21. Bernat, 477, Ch. 19.

SUGGESTIONS FOR FURTHER READING

Canadian Institutes of Health Research, Natural Sciences and Engineering Research Council of Canada, and Social Sciences and Humanities Research Council of Canada, Tri-Council Policy Statement: Ethical Conduct for Research Involving Humans, December 2010. Available at www.pre.ethics.gc.ca/pdf/eng/tcps2/TCPS_2_FINAL_Web.pdf. Accessed March 21, 2012.

Emanuel EJ, Wendler D, Grady C. What makes clinical research ethical? JAMA 2000; 283(20):2701–11.

International Ethical Guidelines for Biomedical Research Involving Human Subjects, CIOMS, 2002. Available at www.cioms.ch/publications/guidelines/guidelines_nov_2002_blurb.htm. Accessed March 21, 2012.

Levy MA, Arnold RM, Fine MJ, et al. Professional courtesy — current practices and attitudes. N Engl J Med 1993; 329(22):1627–31.

Nuremberg Code. Reprinted from Trials of War Criminals before the Nuremberg Military Tribunals under Control Council Law No. 10, Vol. 2, pp. 181–2. Washington, DC: US Government Printing Office, 1949. Available at www.hhs.gov/ohrp/archive/nurcode.html. Accessed March 21, 2012.

Steinbrook R. Rethinking professional courtesy. N Engl J Med 1993; 329(22):1652–3.

World Medical Association's Declaration of Helsinki on Ethical Principles for Medical Research Involving Human Subjects. J Postgrad Med 2002; 48(3):206–8.

ACRONYMS

ACRONYM	DEFINITION
AAMC	Association of American Medical Colleges
AAN	American Academy of Neurology
AAP	American Academy of Pediatrics
ABIM	American Board of Internal Medicine
ACCME	Accreditation Council for Continuing Medical Education
ACP–ASIM	American College of Physicians–American Society of Internal Medicine
AD	advance directive
AD	Alzheimer disease
ADHD	attention deficit hyperactivity disorder
AdvaMed	Advanced Medical Technology Association
AHRQ	Agency for Healthcare Research and Quality
AIDS	acquired immune deficiency syndrome
ALS	amyotrophic lateral sclerosis
AMA	American Medical Association
AMSA	American Medical Student Association
ANH	artificial nutrition and hydration
CBC	complete blood (cell) count
CDR	clinical dementia rating
CIOMS	Council for International Organization of Medical Sciences
CME	Continuing Medical Education
CNS	central nervous system
CPR	cardiopulmonary resuscitation
CSF	cerebrospinal fluid
CT	computed tomography
DCD	organ donation after cardiac death
DEA	Drug Enforcement Administration
DMC	decision-making capacity
DMV	Department of Motor Vehicles
DNR	do not resuscitate
DPOA	durable power of attorney (for healthcare decisions)
ED	emergency department
EEG	electroencephalogram
EFIM	European Federation of Internal Medicine
ELHC	Ethics, Law and Humanities Committee of the AAN
EMG	electromyography
EMU	epilepsy monitoring unit
FDA	US Food and Drug Administration
FTD	frontotemporal dementia
GBS	Guillain–Barré syndrome
HCP	healthcare provider
HCT	healthcare team
HD	Huntington disease
HIPAA	Health Insurance Portability and Accountability Act
HIV	human immunodeficiency virus

(continued)

340

ACRONYM	**DEFINITION**
ICU	intensive care unit
INR	international normalized ratio
IQ	intelligence quotient
IRB	Institutional Review Board
IV	intravenous
IVC	intraventricular catheter
LCME	Liaison Committee on Medical Education
LP	lumbar puncture
LST	life-sustaining treatment
MCS	minimally conscious state
MMSE	Mini-Mental State Examination
MRA	magnetic resonance angiography
MRI	magnetic resonance imaging
MS	multiple sclerosis
NCS	nerve conduction study
NIH	National Institutes of Health
NSAID	nonsteroidal anti-inflammatory drug
OPO	organ procurement organization
OPTN/UNOS	Organ Procurement and Transplantation Network/ United Network for Organ Sharing
OR	operating room
PAS	physician-assisted suicide
PEG	percutaneous endoscopic gastrostomy
PhRMA	Pharmaceutical Research and Manufacturers of America
PT	prothrombin time
PVS	persistent vegetative state
REB	Research Ethics Board
SICU	surgical intensive care unit
SMA	spinal muscular atrophy
TCD	transcranial Doppler
tPA	tissue plasminogen activator
UDDA	Uniform Determination of Death Act
UMHS	University of Michigan Health System
VS	vegetative state

A AAN Code of Professional Conduct

B AAN Disciplinary Action Policy

C Upholding professionalism: The disciplinary process of the AAN
Neurology 2010; 75:2198–203

D AAN policy on conflicts of interest

E AAN policy on pharmaceutical and device industry support
Neurology 2012; 78:750–4

F Principles governing academy relationships with external sources of support

G AAN policy on consent issues for the administration of IV tPA

H Certain aspects of the care and management of profoundly and irreversibly paralyzed patients with retained consciousness and cognition
Neurology 1993; 43:222–3

I Ethical issues in the management of the demented patient
Neurology 1996; 46:1180–3

J Evaluation and management of driving risk in dementia: Report of the Quality Standards Subcommittee of the AAN
Neurology 2010; 74:1316–24

K AAN position statement on physician reporting of medical conditions that may affect driving competence
Neurology 2007; 68:1174–7

L Responding to requests from adult patients for neuroenhancements
Neurology 2009; 73:1406–12

M Position statement on laws and regulations concerning life-sustaining treatment, including artificial nutrition and hydration, for patients lacking decision-making capacity
Neurology 2007; 68:1097–100

N Certain aspects of the care and management of the persistent vegetative state patient
Neurology 1989; 39:125–6

O Palliative care in neurology
Neurology 1996; 46:870–2

P Assisted suicide, euthanasia, and the neurologist
Neurology 1998; 50:596–8

Q Evidence-based guideline update: Determining brain death in adults
Neurology 2010; 74:1911–8

R Practice parameter: genetic testing alert
Neurology 1996; 47:1343–4

S Ethical considerations for neurologists in the management of chronic pain
Neurology 2001; 57:2166–7

All documents are accessible at www.aan.com/view/PECN

AMERICAN ACADEMY OF NEUROLOGY CODE OF PROFESSIONAL CONDUCT

Appendix A

DECEMBER 2009

PREFACE

The American Academy of Neurology developed the Code of Professional Conduct to formalize the standards of professional behavior for neurologist members of the Academy. The primary goal of the Code is to promote the highest quality of neurologic care. The Code is framed to outline the set of professional standards that neurologists must observe in their clinical and scientific activities.

The Code embodies traditional medical ethical standards dating from the time of Hippocrates as well as more contemporary standards. It includes general principles of medical ethics and provides their application to the specific demands of neurologic practice. The Code is delineated to be generally consistent with the American Medical Association Code of Medical Ethics and the American Medical Association Current Opinions of the Council on Ethical and Judicial Affairs.

The Code is written in relatively broad language. It is designed to be a dynamic instrument that can grow and change in response to future developments in the practice and science of neurology. While ethical principles do not change with time, developments in science, technology, and clinical practice may lead to a change in application of these ethical principles.

The Code outlines the standards of professional conduct for Academy members. Violations of these standards may serve as the basis for disciplinary action as provided in the Bylaws of the Academy.

If any provision of this code conflicts with state or federal law, the state or federal laws will govern.

1.0 THE NEUROLOGIST–PATIENT RELATIONSHIP

1.1 The Practice of Neurology

The profession of neurology exists primarily to study, diagnose, and treat disorders of the nervous system. The neurologist–patient relationship forms the foundation for neurologic care.

1.2 Fiduciary and Contractual Basis

The neurologist has fiduciary and contractual duties to patients. As a fiduciary, the neurologist has an ethical duty to consider the interests of the patient first. As a party to an implied contract, the neurologist has a duty to practice competently and to respect patients' autonomy, confidentiality, and welfare.

1.3 Beginning and Ending the Relationship

The neurologist is free to decide whether or not to undertake medical care of a particular person. The neurologist must not decline a patient on the basis of race, religion, nationality, sexual orientation, or gender. Once the relationship has begun, the neurologist must provide care until care is complete, the patient ends the relationship, or the neurologist returns the patient to the care of the referring physician. If the neurologist justifiably desires to end the relationship, and if continued neurologic care is appropriate, he/she should assist in arranging care by another neurologist.

1.4 Informed Consent

The neurologist must obtain the patient's consent for tests or treatment. The neurologist should disclose information that the average person would need to know to make an appropriate medical decision. This information should include benefits, risks, costs, and alternatives to the proposed treatment. If the patient lacks medical decision-making capacity, the neurologist must obtain informed consent from an appropriate proxy.

1.5 Communication

The neurologist has a duty to communicate effectively with the patient. The neurologist should convey relevant information in terms the patient can understand and allow adequate opportunity for the patient to raise questions and discuss matters related to treatment.

1.6 Emergency Care

In an emergency situation, the neurologist should render services to the patient to the best of his/her ability. While obtaining informed consent is desirable before beginning treatment, the neurologist should not delay urgently needed treatment because of concerns about informed consent.

1.7 Medical Risk to the Physician

A neurologist should not refuse to care for a patient solely because of the real or perceived medical risk to the neurologist. The neurologist should take appropriate precautions to minimize his/her medical risk.

1.8 Medical Decision Making

The patient has the ultimate right to accept or reject the neurologist's recommendation about medical treatment. The neurologist should respect decisions made by patients with decision-making capacity and by the lawful proxy of patients who lack decision-making capacity. If the neurologist cannot honor the patient's or proxy's decision, the neurologist should seek to arrange transfer of the patient's care to another physician.

2.0 GENERAL PRINCIPLES OF NEUROLOGIC CARE

2.1 Professional Competence

The neurologist must practice only within the scope of his/her training, experience, and competence. The neurologist should provide care that represents the prevailing standards of neurologic practice. To this end, neurologists should participate in a regular program of continuing education.

2.2 Consultation

The neurologist should obtain consultations when indicated. The neurologist should refer patients only to competent practitioners and should assure that adequate information is conveyed to the consultant. Any differences of opinion between the neurologist and consultant or between the neurologist and the referring physician should be resolved in the best interest of the patient.

2.3 Confidentiality

The neurologist must maintain patient privacy and confidentiality. Details of the patient's life or illness must not be publicized.

2.4 Patient Records

The neurologist should prepare records that include relevant history, neurologic findings, assessment, and plan of evaluation and treatment. Patients are entitled to information within their medical records.

2.5 Professional Fees

The neurologist is entitled to reasonable compensation for medical services to or on behalf of patients. The neurologist should receive compensation only for services actually rendered or supervised. The neurologist must not receive a fee for making a referral ("fee-splitting") or receive a commission from anyone for an item or service he/she has ordered for a patient ("kickback"). The agreed upon division of practice income among members of an organized medical group is acceptable.

2.6 Appropriate Services

The neurologist should order and perform only those services that are medically indicated.

3.0 SPECIAL CATEGORIES OF NEUROLOGIC CARE

3.1 The Dying Patient

The neurologist should strive to relieve the suffering of dying patients. The neurologist should respect the expressed wishes of dying patients about life-prolonging therapy, including lawful advance directives.

3.2 The Profoundly Paralyzed Patient

The neurologist should attempt to enhance the independence and communication of profoundly paralyzed patients. Patients with advanced degrees of paralysis who retain decision-making capacity should be encouraged and assisted to participate in decisions about their medical care including decisions about withdrawing life-support.

3.3 The Demented Patient

The neurologist should define a course of treatment that respects the wishes expressed by the patient before dementia has impaired decision-making capacity. If such wishes are not ascertainable, the neurologist should be guided about appropriate treatment by the patient's lawful proxy.

3.4 The Patient in a Persistent Vegetative State

The neurologist managing the patient in a persistent vegetative state should follow the provisions of lawful advance directives for medical care and, in their absence, the healthcare decisions of a lawfully authorized proxy.

3.5 The Brain-Dead Patient

The neurologist should determine brain death using accepted tests and techniques. The neurologist should be mindful that some patients may have religious or other strongly held objections to the concept of brain death. Compassionate management in these situations is desirable.

4.0 PERSONAL CONDUCT

4.1 Respect for the Patient

The neurologist must treat patients with respect, honesty, and conscientiousness. The neurologist must not abuse or exploit the patient psychologically, sexually, physically, or financially.

4.2 Respect for Agencies and the Law

The neurologist should observe applicable laws. Because agencies may impact on patients' welfare, the neurologist should cooperate and comply with reasonable requests from insurance, compensation, reimbursement, and government agencies within the constraints of patient privacy and confidentiality.

4.3 Maintenance of the Neurologist's Personal Health

The neurologist should strive to maintain physical and emotional health. The neurologist should refrain from practices that may impair capacities to provide adequate patient care.

5.0 CONFLICTS OF INTEREST

5.1 The Patient's Interest is Paramount

Whenever a conflict of interest arises, the neurologist must attempt to resolve it in the best interest of the patient. If the conflict cannot be eliminated, the neurologist should withdraw from the care of the patient.

5.2 Avoidance and Disclosure of Potential Conflicts

The neurologist must avoid practices and financial arrangements that would, solely because of personal gain, influence decisions in the care of patients. Financial interests of the neurologist that might conflict with appropriate medical care should be disclosed to the patient.

5.3 Dispensing Medication

The neurologist may dispense medication, assistive devices, and related patient-care items as long as this practice provides a convenience or an accommodation to the patient without taking financial advantage of the patient. The patient should be given a choice to accept the dispensed medication or device or to have a prescription filled outside the neurologist's office.

5.4 Healthcare Institutional Conflicts

The neurologist generally should support his patient's medical interests when they are compromised by policies of a healthcare institution or agency. Physicians employed by healthcare institutions should represent the patient's medical interests and serve as their medical advocate to the institutional administration.

5.5 Conflicting Ethical Duties

While a neurologist ordinarily must respect a patient's confidentiality, there are circumstances in which a breach of confidentiality may be justified. When the neurologist is aware that an identifiable third party is endangered by a patient, the neurologist must take reasonable steps to warn the third party. When the neurologist is aware that members of the general public are endangered by a patient, the neurologist must take reasonable steps to advise responsible public officials or agencies of that danger.

6.0 RELATIONSHIPS WITH OTHER PROFESSIONALS

6.1 Cooperation with Healthcare Professionals

The neurologist should cooperate and communicate with other healthcare professionals, including other physicians, nurses, and therapists, in order to provide the best care possible to patients.

6.2 Peer Review

The neurologist should participate in peer review activities in order to promote the best care possible of patients.

6.3 Criticism of a Colleague

The neurologist should not unjustifiably criticize a colleague's judgment, training, knowledge, or skills. Neurologists should not knowingly ignore a colleague's incompetence or professional misconduct, thus jeopardizing the safety of the colleague's present and future patients.

6.4 Legal Expert Testimony

The neurologist called upon to provide expert medical testimony should testify only about those subjects for which the neurologist is qualified as an expert by training and experience. Before giving testimony the neurologist should carefully review the relevant records and facts of the case and the prevailing standards of practice. In providing testimony, the neurologist should provide scientifically correct and clinically accurate opinions. Compensation for testimony should be reasonable and commensurate with time and effort spent, and must not be contingent upon outcome.

6.5 Healthcare Organizations

The neurologist may enter into contractual agreements with managed healthcare organizations, prepaid practice plans, or hospitals. The neurologist should retain control of medical decisions without undue interference. The patient's welfare must remain paramount.

6.6 The Impaired Physician

The neurologist should strive to protect the public from an impaired physician and to assist the identification and rehabilitation of an impaired colleague.

7.0 RELATIONSHIPS WITH THE PUBLIC AND COMMUNITY

7.1 Public Representation

The neurologist should not represent himself/herself to the public in an untruthful, misleading, or deceptive manner. A patient's medical condition must not be discussed publicly without the patient's consent.

7.2 Duties to Community and Society

Neurologists should work toward improving the health of all members of society. This may include participation in educational programs, research, public health activities, and the provision of care to patients who are unable to pay for medical services. The neurologist should be aware of the limitation of society's healthcare resources and should not squander those finite resources by ordering unnecessary tests and ineffective treatments.

7.3 Disclosure of Potential Conflicts

Neurologists who make written or oral public statements concerning a product of a company from which they receive compensation or support, or in which they hold a significant equity position, have a duty to disclose their financial relationship with the company in that public statement.

7.4 Prohibition against Participating in Legally Authorized Executions

A neurologist should not be a participant in a legally authorized execution.

8.0 CLINICAL RESEARCH AND SCHOLARLY WORKS

8.1 Institutional Review

The neurologist who participates in clinical research must ascertain that the research has been approved by an Institutional Review Board (IRB) or other comparable body and must observe the requirements of the approved protocol.

8.2 Disclosure of Potential Conflicts

The neurologist who is paid for treating patients in a clinical research project should inform the patient of any compensation the neurologist receives for the patient's participation. The compensation for patient treatment should be reasonable in amount. The neurologist should not bill the patient or the insurer for services already compensated by the study sponsor.

8.3 Individual Patient Experimentation

The neurologist who begins a patient on an experimental therapy that has not been approved as a valid clinical study by an IRB should obtain informed consent from the patient.

8.4 Reporting Research Results

The neurologist should publish research results truthfully, completely, and without distortion. In reporting research results to the news media, the neurologist should make statements that are clear, understandable, and supportable by the facts. Neurologists should not publicize results of research until after the data have been subjected to appropriate peer review.

8.5 Misrepresentation of authorship (ghostwriting)

The neurologist should not claim authorship of any scholarly work submitted for publication if an undisclosed author wrote that work in whole or in part.

The neurologist who authors a scholarly work, in whole or in part, must disclose this fact when the work is submitted for publication. Scholarly work includes, but is not limited to, work that claims research findings or carries recommendations for diagnosis, treatment, or prevention of medical conditions.

HISTORY

Portions of this Code were modified from the following codes of professional ethics and professional conduct: 1. American Academy of Orthopaedic Surgeons: Guide to the Ethical Practice of Orthopaedic Surgery, 1990. 2. American Association of Neurological Surgeons: American Association of Neurological Surgeons Code of Ethics. 3. American Academy of Ophthalmology: Code of Ethics of the American Academy of Ophthalmology, Inc., 1991. 4. American College of Physicians: American College o Physicians Ethics Manual. Part I: history; the patient; other physicians; Annals of Internal Medicine; 1989; 111:245–252. 5. American College of Physicians: American College of Physicians Ethics Manual. Part II: the physician and society; research; life-sustaining treatment; other issues. Annals of Internal Medicine; 1989; 111:327–335. 6. American College of Surgeons: American College of Surgeons Statements on Principles, 1989. 7. American Psychiatric Association: The Principles of Medical Ethics with Annotations Especially Applicable to Psychiatry, 1989. 8. American Medical Association: Code of Medical Ethics and Current Opinions of the American Medical Association Council on Ethical and Judicial Affairs, 1992. Approved Practice Committee and AAN Board of Directors February 1993. Section 7.4, was added in 2008 when the AANPA Board of Directors also endorsed E-2.06 (Capital Punishment) in the AMA Code of Ethics. Amendments approved by the Ethics, Law and Humanities Committee on January 12, 2008, the AANPA Executive Committee on February 21, 2008, and the AANPA Board of Directors on March 7, 2008 (AANPA Policy 2008-06). Section 8.5 was approved by the Ethics, Law and Humanities Committee in October 2009 and by the AANPA Executive Committee on December 17, 2009 (AANPA Policy 2009-14).

The AAN General Counsel edited the Code to reflect the governance changes adopted by the Membership in April 2010 and the Board of Directors on December 2, 2010 (effective December 6, 2010).

MGS:20101221

INDEX